The Little Black Book of

Gastroenterology

Series Editor: Daniel K. Onion

SECOND EDITION

David W. Hay, MD
Adjunct Assistant Professor of Community
  and Family Medicine
Dartmouth Medical School
MaineGeneral Medical Center
Waterville, Maine

JONES AND BARTLETT PUBLISHERS
Sudbury, Massachusetts
BOSTON   TORONTO   LONDON   SINGAPORE

World Headquarters

Jones and Bartlett Publishers	Jones and Bartlett Publishers Canada	Jones and Bartlett Publishers International
40 Tall Pine Drive	6339 Ormindale Way	Barb House, Barb Mews
Sudbury, MA 01776	Mississauga, ON L5V 1J2	London W6 7PA
978-443-5000	CANADA	UK
info@jbpub.com		
www.jbpub.com		

Jones and Bartlett's books and products are available through most bookstores and online booksellers. To contact Jones and Bartlett Publishers directly, call 800-832-0034, fax 978-443-8000, or visit our website www.jbpub.com.

Substantial discounts on bulk quantities of Jones and Bartlett's publications are available to corporations, professional associations, and other qualified organizations. For details and specific discount information, contact the special sales department at Jones and Bartlett via the above contact information or send an email to specialsales@jbpub.com.

Library of Congress Cataloging-in-Publication Data
Hay, David W.
    The little black book of gastroenterology / David W. Hay. — 2nd ed.
        p. ; cm.
    Rev. ed. of: Blackwell's primary care essentials. Gastrointestinal and liver disease / by David W. Hay.   c2002.
    Includes bibliographical references and index.
    ISBN 0-7637-3457-8
1. Gastrointestinal system—Diseases—Handbooks, manuals, etc.
    [DNLM: 1. Gastrointestinal Diseases—Handbooks.   2. Evidence-Based Medicine—Handbooks.   3. Gastroenterology—Handbooks.   WI 39 H412L 2006]   I. Hay, David W. Blackwell's primary care essentials. Gastrointestinal and liver disease.   II. Title.
    RC802.H37 2006
    616.3′3—dc22

                                                                    2005017210

Production Credits

Executive Publisher: Christopher Davis	Composition: ATLIS Graphics
Production Director: Amy Rose	Cover Design: Anne Spencer
Associate Editor: Kathy Richardson	Cover Images: © Photos.com
Production Assistant: Alison Meier	Printing and Binding: Malloy, Inc.
Associate Marketing Manager: Laura Kavigian	Cover Printing: Malloy, Inc.
Manufacturing Buyer: Therese Connell	

Printed in the United States of America
09   08   07   06   05   10 9 8 7 6 5 4 3 2 1

Dedication

The first edition was dedicated:
To my parents, William Hay (1927–1998) and Elizabeth
Bethune Hay, who gave me every opportunity and taught me the
value of kindness
To my children, Gillian and Colin, who make me proud and bring
me joy

The second edition is dedicated:
To Nancy I. Belanger with love and gratitude

Contents

Chapter 3 Stomach and Duodenum 105

Chapter 4 Inflammatory, Functional, and Other Intestinal Disorders 153

Chapter 5 Neoplastic Intestinal Disorders 219

Preface

This short text is intended to be a practical resource for clinicians treating adults and adolescents. I have written the text from my viewpoint as a clinical gastroenterologist with a love of teaching. I expect that this text will also be of value to medical students and residents on gastroenterology or medicine rotations. It should not be difficult to read the entire volume over the course of a typical clerkship. Gastroenterology fellows will find it helpful as a quick reference and as a valuable resource for reviewing prior to board certification examinations. Gastrointestinal nurses and assistants will find concise discussions relevant to their daily work. There are more than 2000 references cited so that the reader can quickly find the most relevant clinical evidence on a topic.

The first section deals with the approach to common clinical problems such as abdominal pain, gastrointestinal bleeding, and jaundice. In these sections, a practical diagnostic approach is suggested. The individual diseases are discussed in the remainder of the text. There are many cross-references to take the reader from a complaint (e.g., abdominal pain) to a specific diagnosis (e.g., biliary colic).

For each chapter, I have listed one or two review articles. These were usually the papers that I found most helpful in understanding the topic. *The Little Black Book of Gastroenterology* uses the concise format outlined below:

Review Articles: Lists valuable review articles
Cause: Agent, if known
Epidemiology
Pathophysiology
Symptoms
Signs

Course of Disease
Complications
Differential Diagnosis: The differential diagnosis of diseases with similar presentations
Laboratory Tests: The available tests and their interpretation
X-ray: Imaging studies
Endoscopy: Endoscopic findings
Treatment

The last chapter is a brief list of "pearls" of clinical gastroenterology. Each pearl is cross-referenced to the appropriate chapter so that the reader can understand the evidence on which the pearl is based.

I would like to thank and acknowledge the work of those who helped me complete this project. The task would have been impossible without the expertise and tireless good cheer of librarian Cora Damon. I would like to thank Nancy Belanger for her extensive assistance in the preparation of the manuscript and tables. The text was vastly improved by the revisions suggested by Diane Brandt, Michael Saletta, Stephen Frost, and Michael Griffin. I am grateful to Dan Onion for offering me the opportunity to write the text and for his many practical suggestions. The first edition was published by Blackwell Science. The editorial expertise of Julia Casson, Irene Herlihy, and Erin Whitehead at Blackwell Science, Inc., is acknowledged with thanks.

I am grateful to Chris Davis for his editorial guidance in the creation of a second edition of this text and for his support of the series. I would like to thank Alison Meier and the editorial staff at Jones and Bartlett for their meticulous work. Many others, including Steve Diaz and the employees of Mid Maine Gastroenterology, are thanked for their assistance, encouragement, and advice.

David W. Hay

Medical Abbreviations

<	less than
<<	much less than
>	more than
>>	more more than
μ	micron
5′ NT	5′ nucleotidase
5-HIAA	5-hydroxyindoleacetic acid
5-HT	5-hydroxytryptophan
6MP	6-mercaptopurine
ab	antibody
ac	before meals
ACBE	air contrast barium enema
ACE	angiotensin converting enzyme
ACG	American College of Gastroenterology
ACS	American Cancer Society
ACTH	adrenocorticotropic hormone
ADH	antidiuretic hormone
AFB	acid-fast bacillus
AFP	alpha fetoprotein
ag	antigen
AGA	American Gastroenterological Association
AHCPR	U.S. Agency for Healthcare Policy and Research
AIH	autoimmune hepatitis
AIP	acute intermittent porphyria
aka	also known as
ALA	5-aminolevulinate
ALD	alcoholic liver disease
alk phos	alkaline phosphatase
ALT	SGPT; alanine aminotransferase
AMA	antimitochondrial antibodies
ANA	antinuclear antibody
ANCA	antineutrophil cytoplasmic autoantibodies
AP	acute pancreatitis
APC	adenomatous polyposis coli
ARDS	adult respiratory distress syndrome
ASA	aspirin
ASGE	American Society for Gastrointestinal Endoscopy
ASMA	anti-smooth muscle ab
AST	SGOT; aspartate aminotransferase
ATPase	adenosine triphosphatase
AVM	arteriovenous malformation
Ba	barium
BE	barium enema

BICAP	bipolar electrocautery	CREST	calcinosis, Raynaud's, esophageal reflux, sclerodactyly, telangiectasias
bid	twice a day		
BM	bowel movement		
BP	blood pressure		
BUN	blood urea nitrogen	crs	course
bx	biopsy	CT	computerized tomography
		Cu	copper
C&S	culture and sensitivity	CVP	central venous pressure
C. diff	*Clostridium difficile*	CXR	chest x-ray
CA 19-9	Carbohydrate antigen 19-9		
Ca	cancer or calcium, depending on context	DES	diffuse esophageal spasm
		DIC	disseminated intravascular coagulation
CAD	coronary artery disease		
cAMP	cyclic AMP	diff dx	differential diagnosis
CBC	complete blood count	DJD	degenerative joint disease
cc	cubic centimeter		
CCK	cholecystokinin	DNA	deoxyribonucleic acid
CEA	carcinoembryonic antigen	DS	double strength
Cfu	colony forming units	DU	duodenal ulcer
CHF	congestive heart failure	DVT	deep venous thrombosis
Cl	chloride	dx	diagnosis or diagnostic
CMP	comprehensive metabolic profile[1]		
		EBV	Epstein-Barr virus
cmplc	complications	eg	for example
CMV	cytomegalovirus	EGD	esophagogastro- duodenoscopy
CNS	central nervous system		
COPD	chronic obstructive pulmonary disease	EKG	electrocardiogram
		ELISA	enzyme-linked immunosorbent assay
COX	cyclooxygenase		
CPK	creatinine phosphokinase	EMG	electromyography
Cr	creatinine	epidem	epidemiology
CRC	colorectal cancer	ERCP	endoscopic retrograde cholangio- pancreatography
		EUS	endoscopic ultrasound
		EVL	endoscopic variceal ligation

[1]A **CMP,** or comprehensive metabolic profile, consists of glucose, electrolytes, albumin, total protein, Ca^{++}, BUN, Cr, bilirubin, alk phos, and trans- aminases.

F	female or Fahrenheit	Hg	mercury
f/u	follow-up	Hgb	hemoglobin
FAP	familial adenomatous polyposis	HIDA	hepatobiliary iminodiacetic acid
FB	foreign body	HIV	human immunodeficiency virus
FDA	(U.S.) Food and Drug Administration	HLA	human leukocyte antigens
Fe	iron	HMG-CoA	hydroxymethyl-glutaryl-coenzyme A
FH	family history		
flex sig	flexible sigmoidoscopy	HNPCC	hereditary nonpolyposis colon cancer
FOBT	fecal occult blood test		
		Hp	*Helicobacter pylori*
GAVE	gastric antral vascular ectasia	hr	hour/s
		HRS	hepatorenal syndrome
GE	gastroesophageal	hs	at bedtime
GERD	gastroesophageal reflux disease	HSV	herpes simplex virus
		HTN	hypertension
GGTP	gamma-glutamyl transpeptidase	HUS	hemolytic uremic syndrome
gi	gastrointestinal	hx	history
GIST	gastrointestinal stromal tumor		
		IBD	inflammatory bowel disease
gm	gram		
GU	gastric ulcer	IBS	irritable bowel syndrome
		IDDM	insulin-dependent diabetes mellitus
H&E	hematoxylin and eosin		
H&P	history and physical	ie	that is
h/o	history of	IEU	idiopathic esophageal ulcer
H2RA	histamine-2 receptor antagonist		
		Ig	immunoglobulin
HBIG	hepatitis B immune globulin	im	intramuscular
		INR	international normalized ratio
HCC	hepatocellular carcinoma		
HCO₃	bicarbonate	ITP	idiopathic thrombocytopenic purpura
hct	hematocrit		
HCV	hepatitis C virus		
hep	hepatitis	IU	international units

iv	intravenous	Na	sodium
IVC	inferior vena cava	NaOH	sodium hydroxide
IVP	intravenous pyelogram	NASH	nonalcoholic steatohepatitis
K	potassium	neg	negative
kg	kilogram	NG	nasogastric
KUB	abdominal x-ray (kidneys, ureters, bladder)	NGT	nasogastric tube
		NH3	ammonia
		NNT	number needed to treat
L	liter	no.	number
LDH	lactate dehydrogenase	npo	nothing by mouth
LES	lower esophageal sphincter	NS	normal saline
LFTs	liver function tests (bilirubin, AST/ALT, alk phos, albumin)	NSAID	nonsteroidal antiinflammatory drug
		NUD	nonulcer dyspepsia
LLQ	left lower quadrant	O&P	ova and parasites
LUQ	left upper quadrant	O_2	oxygen
lytes	electrolytes	OCG	oral cholecystogram
M	male	OH	hydroxyl
MAI	mycobacterium avium intracellulare	osm	osmoles
		OTC	over the counter
MALT	mucosa associated lymphoid tissue	P	pulse
		patho-phys	pathophysiology
MCV	mean corpuscular volume		
meds	medications	PBC	primary biliary cirrhosis
mEq	milliequivalent	PBG	porphobilinogen
mets	metastases	pc	after meals
Mg	magnesium	PCR	polymerase chain reaction
mg	milligram	PE	physical examination
MI	myocardial infarction	PEG	percutaneous endoscopic gastrostomy
min	minute		
mOsm	milliosmole	PET	positron emission tomography
MRCP	magnetic resonance cholangio-pancreatography		
		PG	prostaglandin
MRI	magnetic resonance imaging	PHG	portal hypertensive gastropathy

PMN	polymorphonuclear leukocytes	s/p	status post
po	by mouth	SBFT	small bowel follow through
PO4	phosphate	SBP	spontaneous bacterial peritonitis
PPI	proton pump inhibitor		
pr	by rectum	sc	subcutaneous
prn	as needed	ScleroRx	sclerotherapy
PSC	primary sclerosing cholangitis	sens	sensitivity
		si	signs
PT	prothrombin time	SLE	systemic lupus erythematosis
pt(s)	patient(s)		
PTHC	percutaneous transhepatic cholangiography	specif	specificity
		SPEP	serum protein electrophoresis
PTT	partial thromboplastin time	staph	staphylococcus
PUD	peptic ulcer disease	STD	sexually transmitted disease
q	every	Supps	suppositories
qam	every morning	SVC	superior vena cava
qd	daily	sx	symptom/s
qid	4 times a day		
qod	every other day	tab	tablet
qpm	every evening	TG	triglycerides
		TIBC	total iron-binding capacity
r/o	rule out	tid	3 times a day
RAST	radioallergosorbent test	TIPS	transjugular intrahepatic portosystemic shunt
rbc	red blood cell		
RCT	randomized controlled trial	tiw	three times a week
		Tm/S	trimethoprim/ sulfamethoxazole
RIA	radioimmunoassay		
RIBA	radioimmunoblot assay	TNM	tumor, nodes, metastases
RLQ	right lower quadrant	TPN	total parenteral nutrition
RNA	ribonucleic acid	TSH	thyroid-stimulating hormone
ROS	review of systems		
RR	relative risk		
RUQ	right upper quadrant	U	units
rx	treatment	U.S.	United States

UA	urinalysis	vs	versus
UC	ulcerative colitis		
UDCA	ursodeoxycholic acid	wbc	white blood cells or white
UGI	upper gastrointestinal		blood count
UGIS	upper gi series	WNL	within normal limits
US	ultrasound		
UTI	urinary tract infection	ZE	Zollinger-Ellison syndrome
		Zn	zinc
VIP	vasoactive intestinal peptide		

Journal Abbreviations

Most of the journal abbreviations are in the format used by the National Library of Medicine. Several frequently used journals have been more concisely abbreviated. These include:

Am Fam Phys	American Family Physician
Am J Med	American Journal of Medicine
Am J Surg	American Journal of Surgery
Arch IM	Archives of Internal Medicine
BMJ	British Medical Journal
Clin Perspect Gastro	Clinical Perspectives in Gastroenterology
Curr Gastroenterol Rep	Current Gastroenterology Reports
Curr Opin Gastro	Current Opinion in Gastroenterology
Dig Dis Sci	Digestive Diseases and Sciences
Dis Mo	Disease-a-Month
GE	Gastroenterology
Hepatogastro	Hepatogastroenterology
Jama	Journal of the American Medical Association
Nejm	New England Journal of Medicine

Notice

The authors, editor, and publisher have made every effort to provide accurate information. However, they are not responsible for errors, omissions, or for any outcomes related to the use of the contents of this book and take no responsibility for the use of the products described. Drugs and medical devices are discussed that may have limited availability controlled by the Food and Drug Administration (FDA) for use only in research study or clinical trial. The drug information presented has been derived from reference sources, recently published data, and pharmaceutical tests. Research, clinical practice, and government regulations often change the accepted standard in this field. When consideration is being given to use of any drug in the clinical setting, the health care provider or reader is responsible for determining FDA status of the drug, reading the package insert, and prescribing information for the most up-to-date recommendations on dose, precautions, and contraindications and determining the appropriate usage for the product. This is especially important in the case of drugs that are new or seldom used.

Chapter 1

Approaching Common Clinical Problems

1.1 Abdominal Pain

Sx: The hx is the cornerstone of the efficient dx of abdominal pain. There are many different ways to obtain a hx and everyone develops an individual style. It is best to begin by letting the pt describe the pain without any leading questions. Ask the pt to "Tell me the whole story about your pain beginning with the first time in your life you had a pain anything like this." Many pts will give a neat, chronological story and others will wander. It is worthwhile to give the pt some time to present the story in his or her own way, but it often becomes necessary to direct the pt to establish the following points:

- *Timing:* When did the pain first begin? How often does it occur? When an episode occurs how long does it last? Is the pt entirely well between episodes, or is the pain always present to some degree? Is the pain present 24 hours a day, 7 days a week? A pain present for years is unlikely to be malignant. Upper abdominal pain that occurs in discrete attacks is more likely to be biliary. Pain that is constant is often functional (eg, IBS in the setting of sexual abuse) or is readily diagnosed with imaging studies, hx, and physical exam (eg, malignancy, musculoskeletal pain, intraabdominal inflammation or infection).
- *Character:* Ask the pt to describe the pain. If the pt finds the pain indescribable, offer a multiple choice list, such as, "Is the

pain sharp, dull, aching, burning, or stabbing?" Asking the pt to characterize the pain is helpful in evaluating pts who have multiple pain complaints, since each of the pains can be referred to separately.

- *Radiation:* Ask the pt if the pain radiates anywhere. Upper abdominal pain radiating to the back suggests biliary colic, PUD, or an esophageal source. Acute perforation of a viscus can cause shoulder pain. Pain radiating to the groin or testicle suggests a urinary tract source. Pain radiating to the leg or thigh suggests a nonabdominal cause. Pain radiating to the neck or arm suggests a cardiac cause.

- *Relieving or exacerbating factors:* Ask the pt, "Is there anything that makes the pain predictably worse, such as eating, bms, stressful situations, or any kind of position or activity?" Identify factors that predictably bring relief, such as OTC remedies. These points help to establish if the pain is of gi origin and if it is more likely related to the bowel or to the upper gi tract.

- *Associated sx:* A complete ROS is necessary. Depending on the nature of the sx it is important to establish whether or not there has been weight loss, fever, anorexia, nausea, melena, or hematochezia.

- *Medications:* Many abdominal sx are related to medications, including OTC preparations. The duration of use should be determined.

- *Past medical and family history:* These histories help to establish risk factors for specific disorders and the safety and appropriateness of invasive tests.

Si: A complete physical exam is done, including assessment of vitals, skin, lymph nodes, the neck, heart, lungs, joints, and where indicated, a neurologic evaluation. The abdomen is usually the most informative part of the exam in creating a differential diagnosis.

- *General abdominal exam:* Bowel sounds are evaluated. Very active bowel sounds suggest the possibility of infection or early obstruction. Bowel sounds may be absent with intra-abdominal catastrophe or ileus. The abdomen is assessed for tenderness to percussion. Percussion tenderness suggests peritoneal irritation. Palpation is done to look for masses or tenderness. If a pt seems to react with surprising drama, the exam can be continued while the pt is distracted with questions. If the abdomen is tender, the pt is asked to lift the head and shoulders a few inches off the table to see if the tenderness on palpation changes. Pain that worsens with this maneuver is often from the abdominal wall. Pain that is unchanged or that improves with tensing the abdominal muscles is often from an intraabdominal cause. The costal margins should be carefully examined with firm palpation to look for evidence of the painful rib syndrome (p 356). The aorta should be palpated for tenderness or enlargement.

- *Inflammation and peritonitis:* Percussion tenderness, rebound tenderness, or pain with shaking of the pelvis suggests peritoneal irritation. In diffuse peritonitis, the abdomen may become rigid. A positive **psoas sign** (pain on extension of the thigh with the pt lying laterally on the opposite hip) may occur with retroperitoneal inflammation. A positive **obturator sign** (pain on internal rotation of the flexed thigh) may indicate an inflammatory process in the pelvis. A **Murphy's sign** (the abrupt cessation of inspiration when examiner is palpating the RUQ because of worsening of the pain) strongly suggests cholecystitis.

- *Liver and spleen:* Hepatomegaly can be assessed by percussion and palpation. Percussion of the upper border should be firm and that of the lower border lighter. The normal liver span is 12-15 cm in the midclavicular line. The normal liver is usually palpable with deep inspiration. It is often easier to palpate the liver edge by using both hands with palms lying on the rib cage and the fingers hooked over the edge of the costal margin. A similar technique is helpful for the spleen. The spleen is usually not palpable, and percussion in the LUQ may reveal its lower margin.

- *Stigmata of liver disease:* see p 42.
- *Rectal and pelvic exams* are often needed depending on the differential being considered.

Approach to Dyspepsia: Chronic or recurrent pain centered in the upper abdomen is usually referred to as dyspepsia. Many pts with dyspepsia have GERD, and this can be suspected based on clues such as retrosternal burning pain, gross regurgitation, or dysphagia to solids. Some GERD pts will have sx exclusively in the epigastrium, and this group may be difficult to identify without additional tests such as EGD, a therapeutic trial of a PPI, or pH probe (p 53). About 15-25% of pts with dyspeptic sx have peptic ulcer disease (p 114) (GE 1998;114:579). About 60% of pts with dyspepsia never have an organic cause found and are said to have nonulcer dyspepsia (p 128). The remainder of the differential is listed in Table 1.1. The painful rib syndrome (p 356) should be easily identified on physical exam but is often overlooked.

Pts should have a CBC, CMP, amylase, and lipase. The AGA has published guidelines for evaluating dyspepsia (GE 1998;114:579). In pts >45 years of age who have new onset dyspepsia, EGD is appropriate to rule out gastric cancer. Pts with alarm sx of weight loss, recurrent vomiting, dysphagia, bleeding, or anemia should also undergo EGD. Pts under 45 years of age with no alarm features should be tested for *Helicobacter pylori* (Hp) (p 106) with serology or breath testing. If positive, they are treated and undergo EGD only if sx fail to improve or sx recur within 8 weeks. If a young pt is Hp negative, an empiric 4-8 week course of a PPI or H2RA is appropriate. EGD is done only if the pt fails to improve or if sx rapidly recur after stopping rx. There is little point to obtaining a UGI barium study since it is not sensitive enough to be a reliable negative test and a UGI series showing GU or a possible cancer requires EGD.

Table 1.1   Causes of Dyspepsia

Condition	Discussed on Page
Gastroesophageal reflux disease	53
Peptic ulcer disease	114
Nonulcer dyspepsia	128
Pancreatitis	311
Biliary colic	335
Gastroparesis	130
Pancreatic cancer	327
Lactose intolerance	172
Air swallowing	14
Giardia	274
Gastric Cancer	137
Other intra-abdominal neoplasms	—
Crohn's disease	177
Irritable bowel syndrome	153
Sphincter of Oddi dysfunction	352
Celiac disease	200
Chronic mesenteric ischemia	305
Porphyria	409
Lead poisoning	—
Painful rib syndrome	356
Other parasites	283
Angina	—
Somatization disorder	—

If no cause of sx is identified at EGD, clinical judgment is used to determine how vigorously to pursue the rest of the differential diagnosis. CT scan and ultrasound of the abdomen, gastric emptying scan, 24-hour pH probe, SBFT, testing for *Giardia* and other parasites, or dietary trials may be selectively indicated.

Approach to Attacks of Upper Abdominal Pain: If pain comes in discrete attacks, in between which the pt feels well, then biliary colic (p 335) should be strongly considered. CBC, CMP, amylase, and lipase are generally indicated and an RUQ ultrasound should be obtained. If the ultrasound is negative, the differential may need to be broadened to include the causes of dyspepsia (Table 1.1). If further evaluation shows no convincing cause of pain, the possibility of a false-negative ultrasound needs to be considered. About 80% of pts with a good story for biliary colic, a negative ultrasound, and no other evident cause of dyspepsia will get relief with cholecystectomy. Some physicians use gallbladder emptying tests to select pts for cholecystectomy (Am J Surg 1997;63:769). A radionuclide scan (p 340) with an ejection fraction of <35% (in response to CCK stimulation) is considered abnormal. However, there is no high-quality evidence (ie, an RCT) showing that radionuclide scanning improves outcome for this challenging group of pts (Am J Gastro 2003;98:2605).

Approach to Acute Abdominal Pain: If hx suggests that the pain is entirely new (not an exacerbation of a chronic problem) and that the pain is of very recent onset (typically hours), the differential considerations are different (Table 1.2). Appendicitis typically presents with midabdominal pain that later moves to the RLQ but can be variable. Biliary colic, cholecystitis, pancreatitis, and cholangitis usually present with acute upper abdominal pain. Bowel obstruction usually presents as severe, crampy pain and distension usually in a pt with a prior hx of abdominal surgery. In acute mesenteric ischemia, the pain is severe and out of proportion to the initial physical exam findings. In ischemic colitis there is usually intense, crampy lower abdominal pain with bloody diarrhea. In dissecting abdominal aortic aneurysm, there may be a pulsatile mass and hypotension, but these findings are not universal. In diverticulitis the pain is usually (but not always) in the LLQ and associated with fever. The pain of renal colic is often in the flank and may radiate to the groin in a pt with a benign belly. Other considerations include perforated ulcer disease, ectopic pregnancy, ruptured ovarian cyst, ovarian abscess or torsion, drug seeking, epiploic appendagitis, and acute presentations of Crohn's disease.

Table 1.2   Causes of Acute Abdominal Pain

Category	Condition	Discussed on Page
Gastrointestinal		
	Appendicitis	174
	Perforated ulcer disease	114
	Bowel obstruction	206
	Acute mesenteric ischemia	303
	Ischemic colitis	306
	Infectious gastroenteritis	259
	Diverticulitis	165
	Perforated bowel	—
	Acute presentations of Crohn's disease	177
	Epiploic appendagitis	217
Pancreatic and Biliary		
	Biliary colic	335
	Cholecystitis	335
	Cholangitis	345
	Pancreatitis	311
Urologic	Renal colic	—
	Pyelonephritis	—
	UTI	—
Gynecologic	Ectopic pregnancy	—
	Pelvic inflammatory disease	—
	Ruptured ovarian cyst	—
	Ovarian abscess	—
	Ovarian torsion	—
Retroperitoneal		
	Retroperitoneal hemorrhage	—
	Dissecting aortic aneurysm	305
	Psoas abscess	
Thoracic	Myocardial infarction	—
	Lower lobe pneumonia	—
Other	Drug seeking	—
	Narcotic withdrawal	—
	Diabetic ketoacidosis	—

A CBC, CMP, amylase, lipase, pregnancy test, and UA are generally indicated. A flat and upright view of the abdomen may demonstrate obstruction. In some cases an upright film centered on the diaphragm is done to look for free air. Depending on the severity of the sx, studies such as a CT scan may be warranted.

These considerations are reviewed separately for each disease entity.

Approach to Chronic Lower Abdominal Pain: Pain centered in the lower abdomen often has a colonic source. Crampy pain, diarrhea, relief of pain with passage of bms, change in bms, and rectal bleeding are features that suggest a colonic source of sx. Chronic pain from the colon is most often due to irritable bowel syndrome (p 153) or constipation (p 17). Rectal bleeding, weight loss, or a change in bowel habits (bm frequency, caliber) may suggest colorectal cancer (p 219). Diverticulitis usually presents with acute pain, but in some pts onset of sx can be more gradual (p 165). If diarrhea is prominent, infectious colitis is a possibility, though most pts with infectious colitis present with acute sx. Chronic bloody diarrhea and weight loss suggest ulcerative colitis (p 190) or Crohn's colitis (p 177).

If pain seems unrelated to bms, gynecologic and urinary tract causes should be considered. Musculoskeletal causes of pain are usually evident by hx and exam.

If the hx suggests a high probability of cancer or inflammatory bowel disease, colonoscopy is warranted. The approaches to suspected irritable bowel (p 153) and constipation (p 17) are discussed in separate sections.

Approach to Chronic Diffuse Pain: Pts with chronic diffuse pain that occurs 24 hours a day, 7 days a week are challenging. They fall broadly into two groups. The first group includes pts with illnesses such as intra-abdominal malignancy or inflammation who undergo imaging studies or have findings on exam that are diagnostic. The second, more difficult group includes pts with chronic abdominal pain, typically with multiple pain complaints, many prior physician visits, and many diagnostic tests that have been unrevealing. A careful hx and physical is done to categorize the complaints. It is essential to obtain records of *all* prior evaluations prior to any new studies. Many of these pts will turn out to have functional or psychiatric diagnoses. It is vital not to overlook the connection between this pattern of complaints, medical evaluations, and hx of physical or sexual abuse (p 162). It is important for the pt to see that the physician has considered each complaint carefully. Do not appear dismissive or trivialize the pt's difficulties.

1.2   Dysphagia and Odynophagia

GE 1999;117:229

Sx and Si: **Dysphagia** is the sensation that a swallowed food bolus sticks in the chest. Ask the pt, "If I gave you a bite of steak, bread, or apple to eat and told you that you had to wolf it down, would it stick in your chest?" Pts may perceive the sticking at the sternal notch even though the bolus is at the GE junction. Sometimes the sticking is relieved by swallowing liquid or by lifting the arms over the head or with other body position changes. Amazingly, some pts do not identify the bolus as stuck, but instead will complain of pain and excessive salivation. Pts often do not report these episodes unless specifically asked. Some pts have dysphagia to liquids as well as solids. They may experience nasal regurgitation. Many of these pts have motor disorders of the esophagus. Another group has problems with the initial nonesophageal phases of swallowing, called **oropharyngeal dysphagia.** Sx are usually above the sternal notch, sometimes with aspiration, coughing, or drooling. The physical exam is usually not helpful in the evaluation of swallowing except for revealing neurologic disease in some pts with oropharyngeal dysphagia.

Odynophagia, or painful swallowing, is less common than dysphagia. Acute odynophagia suggests the possibility of infections (candida, herpes, CMV) or pill esophagitis. There may be evidence of oral thrush or herpes infection of the oropharynx in some pts.

Diff Dx: The causes of **dysphagia** are listed in Table 1.3. Strictures due to GERD and benign esophageal rings (Schatzki rings) are the most frequent causes. In dysphagia due to GERD without a stricture, the sx are usually brief and not associated with prolonged food impaction. Esophageal cancer is often associated with weight loss. Extrinsic compression of the esophagus is usually due to malignancy. A Zenker's diverticulum can be associated with a mass in the neck or coughing food debris hours after it was eaten. In congenital esophageal stenosis, the pt may describe a lifetime of being a slow eater.

Dysphagia to liquids raises the possibility of achalasia, diffuse esophageal spasm, and related spastic disorders. The evaluation of oropharyngeal dysphagia usually results in a diagnosis of a neuromuscular or other disorder not related to the gi tract and is not

Table 1.3   Causes of Dysphagia and Odynophagia

Dysphagia	Found on Page	Odynophagia	Found on Page
Esophageal strictures and rings	72	Pill esophagitis	—
GERD without stricture	53	Herpetic esophagitis	99
Esophageal cancer	80	Candida esophagitis	98
Extrinsic compression	—	CMV esophagitis	101
Benign esophageal tumors	103	Idiopathic esophageal	102
Zenker's diverticulum	95	ulcer	
Other esophageal diverticula	96		
Eosinophilic esophagitis	75		
Congenital esophageal stenosis	76		
Achalasia	87		
Diffuse esophageal spasm	93		
Other spastic disorders	93		
Oropharyngeal causes	—		

further discussed in this text (see GE 1999;116:455 for a comprehensive review).

Pill esophagitis is a frequent cause of **odynophagia.** Doxycycline, alendronate, quinidine, ASA, other NSAIDs, and potassium tabs are the most frequent offenders (J Clin Gastroenterol 1999; 28:298). Esophagitis due to candida, herpes, or CMV often presents with painful swallowing. Idiopathic esophageal ulcer is seen in HIV infection. The other listed causes of dysphagia should also be considered in pts with painful swallowing.

Approach to Dx and Rx: Most pts with intermittent solid food dysphagia are best served with EGD for diagnosis and possible rx with esophageal dilatation. Pts with severe sx, and those with a story suggestive of a Zenker's diverticulum, other proximal lesions or achalasia should have a barium swallow. Some pts with severe sx have long and complex strictures and a barium swallow helps the endoscopist decide on how to proceed with dilatation. A Zenker's diverticulum presents a perforation risk during endoscopy, since it can be difficult to pass the scope beyond the diverticulum. If EGD is not readily available, a barium swallow with a 13-mm barium tablet is a good test to detect stricture and rule out a mass. However, barium swallow is not therapeutic and is insensitive for esophagitis. Pts with sx suggesting a motor disorder may be candidates for esophageal manometry testing after a structural abnormality has been excluded.

Pts who are awaiting evaluation need to be cautioned to cut food in small pieces and to chew carefully to avoid food impaction. If sx of GERD are present it is reasonable to begin a PPI while awaiting diagnostic testing.

1.3 Nausea and Vomiting

GE 2001;120:263

Diff Dx: Nausea is a nonspecific sx with an enormous differential diagnosis. Acute nausea and vomiting without substantial abdominal pain are most often related to infectious gastroenteritis, food poisoning, drugs, systemic infection, metabolic abnormalities, migraine, increased intracranial pressure, labyrinthitis, or any cause of acute pain. Many other acute illnesses can cause vomiting with pain (eg, obstruction) but usually there are obvious clues. In most cases the cause of acute nausea and vomiting can be readily determined.

Chronic nausea can be a more difficult problem. Vomiting increases the probability that a structural cause will be found. Some of the many causes of nausea and vomiting are listed in Table 1.4. Morning sickness of pregnancy must not be overlooked. Numerous drugs cause nausea. These include cancer chemotherapy, analgesics, hormonal preparations, antibiotics, antivirals, and cardiovascular drugs. Structural diseases of the stomach, such as gastric outlet obstruction due to malignancy or ulcer disease, are usually associated with pain or weight loss. Gastroparesis is often considered as a cause of chronic nausea, but the pathogenesis is unclear and gastroparesis should not be accepted as the cause without excluding other etiologies. GERD is associated with nausea and pts may interpret gross regurgitation as vomiting. Labyrinthine disorders are usually associated with clues on exam or hx, such as vertigo or nystagmus. A syndrome of cyclical vomiting that may be a migraine equivalent occurs in children (Dig Dis Sci 1999;44:23S). While many other diseases can present with nausea and vomiting (bowel obstruction, pancreatitis, cholecystitis, hepatitis, adrenal insufficiency, renal failure, electrolyte disorders, narcotic withdrawal), they rarely do without offering some other substantial clinical or laboratory clue to diagnosis.

Approach to Dx and Rx: The most efficient approach is usually evident after a careful hx, physical exam, and selective use of laboratory tests (CBC, CMP, pregnancy test, amylase, lipase). In most cases the cause can be identified and treated. If a dx is not evident

Table 1.4 Causes of Nausea and Vomiting

Category	Disorder	Found on Page
Gastrointestinal		
	Infectious gastroenteritis	259
	Food poisoning	285
	Gastric outlet obstruction	12
	Gastroparesis	130
	Gastroesophageal reflux disease	53
	Nonulcer dyspepsia	128
	Bowel obstruction	206
	Intraabdominal inflammation	—
	Intraabdominal malignancy	—
	Eosinophilic gastroenteritis	215
	Gastric volvulus	135
	Pseudo-obstruction	210, 212
Medications	Cancer chemotherapy	—
	NSAIDs	—
	Antibiotics	—
	Digoxin	—
	Many others	—
Central Nervous System		
	Eating disorders	—
	Rumination syndrome	97
	Migraine	—
	Increased intracranial pressure	—
	Psychiatric disorders	—
Endocrine and Metabolic		
	Fluid and electrolyte disorders	—
	Acute intermittent porphyria	405
	Hyperthyroidism	—
	Addison's disease	—
	Renal failure	—
Postoperative	Postoperative	—
Other	Systemic infection	—
	Morning sickness	—

after initial evaluation, empiric rx with an antiemetic or prokinetic such as metoclopramide may be appropriate for some pts.

Very few trials have compared **antiemetic** regimens and several classes of agents are available (Am Fam Phys 2004;69:1169).
Anticholinergics (scopolamine), and antihistamines (meclizine,
diphenhydramine, hydroxyzine) are popular for motion sickness
and labyrinthine disorders. Phenothiazines (eg, prochlorperazine
5-10 mg po tid to qid or 25 mg supps pr bid or 2.5-10.0 mg iv
q 3-4 h to a maximum of 40 mg daily) are effective in many
causes of nausea and vomiting. Other phenothiazines include
prometh-azine, triethylperazine, chlorpromazine, and per-
phenazine. Serotonin antagonists (eg, ondansetron and others)
are effective, expensive, and widely used in chemotherapy pts.
The choice of prokinetics is limited and metoclopramide
(5-10 mg po qid) is most frequently used.

For many pts empiric rx is not appropriate and further evaluation is needed. The selective use of EGD, gastric emptying scan,
abdominal CT scan, plain films of the abdomen, MRI of the
brain, SBFT, and psychiatric evaluation may be appropriate. The
nature, duration, and severity of complaints guide the extent of
the evaluation.

1.4   Belching

Postgrad Med 1997;101:263

Diff Dx: Belching (eructation) is the involuntary expulsion of air from
the esophagus and stomach. Regurgitation of swallowed air from
the stomach is a normal physiological event. Some pts swallow
air into the esophagus/hypopharynx and immediately expel it in a
belch. Several organic disorders can be associated with belching,
including GERD (p 53), gastroparesis (p 130), gastric outlet
obstruction due to malignancy (p 137) or PUD (p 114), and
achalasia (p 87). Aerophagia (air swallowing) is an unconscious
habit or is related to anxiety, chewing gum, tobacco, postnasal

drip, COPD, asthma, or ill-fitting dentures. Aerophagia can also be a response to pain in the stomach or esophagus.

Approach to Dx and Rx: If the hx or physical suggests an organic etiology, further testing is needed. A trial of a PPI may be considered for the question of GERD (p 61). If an organic etiology seems unlikely, air swallowing is discussed with the pt. It is most effective if the physician masters air swallowing and is able to match the pt belch for belch during the interview.

Those with suspected aerophagia should be counseled to minimize swallowed air by avoiding chewing gum, hard candy, smoking, and carbonated beverages. Pts should be educated that their sx are not caused by production of gas by the stomach. A pencil held clenched between the teeth is said to decrease air swallowing but the value of this technique has been questioned (Am J Gastroenterol 1998;93:2276).

1.5 Bloating

Clin Perspect Gastro 2000;July:209; Postgrad Med 1997;101:263

Diff Dx: Bloating can be a sx associated with many organic diseases including GERD, gastroparesis, PUD, pancreatic disease, malabsorption, intestinal infection, constipation, diverticular disease, drug side effects, and intra-abdominal malignancy. While this is a daunting list, it is rare that bloating would be the sole sx in these disorders. Bloating as a single sx (or associated with generalized discomfort) is usually not related to the excess production of gas (Gut 1991;32:662), but is probably a manifestation of IBS (p 153). Dietary management to minimize gas production may benefit these pts because they have abnormal sensitivity to volumes of gas that pts without IBS do not find distressing.

Approach to Dx and Rx: The H&P is used to determine if there are clues that may take the clinician in a direction other than irritable bowel. Dietary hx as detailed for the flatulent pt (see 1.6) is appropriate. In the absence of other clues the approach is that outlined for IBS (p 153). Measures to decrease flatus (see 1.6) can be tried.

1.6 Flatulence

Clin Perspect Gastro 2000;July:209; Postgrad Med 1997;101:263

Diff Dx: Normal subjects produce up to 2500 mL of flatus a day and pass it up to 20 times daily. Rectal gas is a combination of swallowed air (rich in nitrogen) and gas produced from colonic bacterial metabolism that produces hydrogen, methane, and malodorous sulfur gases (Gut 1998;43:100). Some pts will complain of frequent passage of flatus because of poor sphincter tone. A small number of pts will have excess gas from serious malabsorptive diseases (p 30) such as celiac disease, small bowel bacterial overgrowth, and pancreatic insufficiency. The remainder have an anatomically normal gut and have excessive flatus either from air swallowing or from gas produced by bacterial fermentation of carbohydrates.

Excessive colonic production of gas may be of a variety of dietary sources. **Lactose** intolerance is a frequent cause (p 172). **Fructose** (found in high concentration in figs, dates, prunes, pears, apples, grapes, some vegetables, and in soft drinks sweetened with high fructose corn syrup) can cause flatulence because it is less efficiently absorbed than other sugars (Am J Gastro 2004;99:2046). **Sorbitol** (found in sugarless gum, many hard candies, food sweetened for diabetics, and in apples, pears, prunes, and peaches) is minimally absorbed and causes distressing sx due to bacterial fermentation (Gut 1988;29:44). Legumes (such as beans, broccoli, cabbage, and cauliflower) have complex carbohydrates that cannot be fully digested because humans lack α-galactosidase. Starches and dietary fiber also provide substrates for intestinal gas production.

Approach to Dx and Rx: The H&P is used to look for clues to serious underlying disease and to assess rectal tone. Dietary hx is obtained for lactose, fructose, sorbitol, legumes, and fiber. The pt is watched for evidence of air swallowing. If there are clues to serious disease, further evaluation is indicated (see Malabsorption, p 30). Those with poor sphincter tone are educated as to the nature of the problem, and incontinence is treated (p 294). Flatus passed more than 20 times daily is abnormal. Colonic fermentation should be suspected if the flatus is especially malodorous, nocturnal, or meal related. The pt can be evaluated for lactose intolerance (p 172) and can be given diets low in offending carbohydrates. Those with odorless flatus, belching, and bloating may be suspected of air swallowing, but dietary trials are still worthwhile. Collection of rectal gas to distinguish air swallowing (flatus high in nitrogen) from colonic fermentation (high in methane and hydrogen) has been reported but is impractical for widespread use (Am J Gastroenterol 1998;93:2276).

Oral activated charcoal is of no benefit (Am J Gastroenterol 1999;94:208), but a charcoal lined pillow (Toot-trapper) is effective at reducing noxious odor (Gut 1998;43:100). Beano, a commercially available α-galactosidase preparation, is effective in reducing flatulence associated with legumes.

1.7 Constipation

GE 2000;119:1766; Cleve Clin J Med 1999;66:41

Sx: Constipation is a term used by pts to describe a wide variety of complaints related to defecation. To the physician, constipation is usually defined as a bm frequency of less than 3 per week. More complex definitions have been proposed but are not of practical significance except for scientific study (Gut 1999; 45[suppl 2]:II43). Pts may use the term constipation to mean excessive straining, painful defecation, hard stools, abdominal pain, or the failure to have a daily bm. The quality and time course of each complaint should be noted. The use of mechanical means (vaginal or perineal pressure, a finger in the rectum, enemas) to evacuate stool suggests pelvic floor dysfunction. Dietary hx is crucial since in many cases dietary fiber is inadequate. Ask the pt to describe a typical breakfast, lunch, and dinner. Determine servings of cereal, whole-grain bread, rice, pasta, vegetables, and fruit as a rough method of determining dietary fiber. Many pts will eat only 1 or 2 servings daily of high-fiber foods and the most likely cause of their sx becomes evident quickly.

Si: Rectal exam is done to look for evidence of masses, fissures, strictures, painful spasm of the sphincter, or impaction. The pt is asked to strain in simulated defecation while the examiner watches for prolapse or paradoxical contraction of the anal sphincter. Paradoxical contraction of the sphincter when simulating defecation suggests pelvic floor dysfunction. Rectocele is detected by vaginal examination. Neurologic exam may be appropriate.

Diff Dx: (Am J Gastroenterol 1999;94:567) The common causes of constipation are listed in Table 1.5. There are two **primary** mechanisms for constipation. In **slow transit constipation,** feces is moved slowly from cecum to rectum because of decreased contractions. Alternatively, uncoordinated contractions of the left colon may act as a functional barrier. In **pelvic floor dysfunction** feces is stored in the rectum for an excessive period because of lack of coordinated mechanisms for rectal emptying. There are numerous secondary causes of constipation. Inadequate dietary fiber, inadequate fluid, and ignoring the urge for a bm are frequent causes. Constipation can be secondary to structural lesions, drugs, IBS, neurologic diseases, or metabolic causes.

Approach to Dx: The H&P are used to evaluate the probability of a secondary cause of constipation. In general, obstructing colon cancer should be ruled out in new onset constipation in a pt over

Table 1.5 Causes of Constipation

Cause	Example
Slow transit constipation	—
Pelvic floor dysfunction	—
Dietary	Inadequate fiber, inadequate fluids
Behavioral	Ignoring urge for bm
	Psychiatric illness
Structural	Colon cancer
	Colonic stricture
	Volvulus
	Anal fissure with spasm
	Rectal prolapse
	Rectocele
Systemic	Hypercalcemia
	Hypothyroidism
	Hypokalemia
	Diabetes
	Addison's disease
	Scleroderma
Neurologic	Parkinson's disease
	Multiple sclerosis
	Spinal cord injury
	Autonomic neuropathy
	Hirschsprung's disease
Drugs	Multiple causes including:
	Iron
	Narcotics
	Cholestyramine
	Calcium channel blockers
	Anticholinergics
Functional	IBS

40 years and in selected younger pts. Colonoscopy has the advantage in older pts of allowing highly effective CRC screening (by detection and removal of polyps incidental to the pts sx) but flex sig and BE are adequate if the only purpose is to rule out obstruction. BE alone is not adequate because of poor visualization of

the rectum and limited views of overlapping loops of sigmoid colon. A TSH, electrolytes, and serum Ca^{2+} should be obtained routinely and other labs may be selectively needed.

If no secondary cause of constipation is found, empiric rx with a 25-gm fiber diet, six 8-oz glasses of water daily, moderate exercise, and planned time for bms (15 minutes twice daily) is appropriate. If pts do not respond to these measures, a **colonic transit study** should be done. Pts are given a gelatin capsule containing 24 radio-opaque rings (commercially available in the U.S. as Sitzmarks [Konsyl Pharmaceuticals, New Jersey]) and 5 days later a KUB is done (Gut 1969;10:842). If there are 5 or fewer markers remaining, transit is normal. There are numerous variations of this test in which markers are ingested on multiple days to allow colonic transit times to be calculated for right and left colon. This may yield additional diagnostic information (GE 1987;92:40). If transit time is normal, "constipation" may be IBS (p 153) or the problem may be of psychogenic origin. Slow transit constipation is diagnosed when more than 5 markers are scattered through the colon. Pelvic floor dysfunction is suspected when markers bunch up in the rectosigmoid. Other clues to pelvic floor dysfunction include excessive straining, paradoxical tightening of the sphincter with attempts to simulate defecation on physical exam, and manual attempts using pressure or a finger to evacuate stool. Some pts have features of both disorders.

Some specialized centers perform **anorectal manometry, balloon expulsion tests,** and **barium defecography** to evaluate pelvic floor dysfunction, rectocele, and Hirschsprung's disease. These techniques are not widely available and their role in selecting rx is not well established (GE 1999;116:735).

Rx:

- *General measures:* Pts are instructed to slowly increase fiber to a goal of 25 gm daily. They may feel bloated or gassy at the outset, but generally this improves. A list of common high-fiber foods is provided and pts are encouraged to read food labels. A diary of fiber intake and bms can be helpful in reaching the target. In pts who cannot reach target with diet, fiber supplements can be given. Popular choices include psyllium (eg, Metamucil 1 tsp po up to tid provides 3 gm fiber/dose), methylcellulose (eg, Citrucel 1 tbsp po up to tid which provides 2 gm of fiber/dose) and polycarbophil (eg, FiberCon 500-mg tabs, up to 6 gm daily). Pts should be instructed to drink at least six 8-oz glasses of water. Daily, moderate exercise and planned time for bms (15 minutes twice daily) should be encouraged.

Osmotic laxatives: Osmotic laxatives are used in pts who fail to improve with general measures. These agents cause fluid to be retained in the gut lumen. Milk of Magnesia 1-2 tbsp po qd-bid is inexpensive, but the taste is a problem and renal failure is a contraindication. Sorbitol (usually 1-2 tbsp po bid) and lactulose (1-3 tbsp po up to tid) are effective but cause flatulence, cramps, and are very sweet tasting. Sorbitol is cheaper than lactulose. Polyethylene glycol (6-32 oz daily) is highly effective but expensive. It is available in a palatable, single-dose form (17 gm powder in 8 oz liquid daily to start).

Stimulant laxatives: The agents promote motility and colonic secretion. There is suggestive evidence that these agents may damage the enteric nervous system (Dis Colon Rectum 1973;16:455). For that reason, these agents are the last choice for chronic use. Common choices are senna (eg, Senokot 2 tabs qd to 4 tabs bid), and bisacodyl (eg, Dulcolax 5 mg po qd). Misoprostol 300 mcg po qid is another alternative in refractory pts (Dig Dis Sci 1994;39:929).

- *Biofeedback:* This modality can be used to train pts to relax their pelvic floor during defecation. Programs are not readily available and are labor intensive. However, they are safe and often effective (Dig Dis Sci 1993;38:1953). Biofeedback should be used prior to surgery in pelvic floor dysfunction.

- *Surgery:* Carefully selected pts with chronic, disabling sx of slow transit constipation that is refractory to medical rx and who have no evidence of pseudo-obstruction (p 212) can be treated with ileorectal anastomosis with good results (Ann Surg 1991;214:403). Pts with evidence of pelvic floor dysfunction usually get relief with surgery, though straining is still common postoperatively (Gut 1988;29:969).

1.8 Acute Diarrhea

Dis Mo 1999;45:268; Am J Gastroenterol 1997;92:1962

Sx and Si: This discussion focuses on the approach to acute diarrhea in adults from developed nations. Acute diarrhea refers to the abrupt onset of passage of frequent, poorly formed stools. It is an illness that generally lasts <2 weeks but may last up to a month. Only pts with more severe illness require medical evaluation. Clues to severe illness include profuse watery stool with dehydration, dysentery (the passage of many small volume stools with blood and often pus), temp >101° F, illness >48 hours, more than 6 stools/day, severe pain, and illness in an immunocompromised or elderly host.

The epidemiologic and medical hx guides the evaluation. It is important to determine: (1) the duration and severity of sx, (2) a history of recent antibiotic use, (3) the travel history, (4) current medicines, especially OTC preparations and new medicines, (5) whether a male pt has sex with men, (6) whether the illness is part of an outbreak, (7) the pt's water source, (8) recent ingestion of suspicious food or undercooked meat, and (9) if the pt is immunocompromised.

On exam the pt's volume status should be assessed (postural vital signs, mucous membranes). Abdominal findings should be noted and impaction ruled out by rectal exam at which time FOBT can be done.

Diff Dx: Acute diarrhea is most often infectious. Infections and other common causes of acute diarrhea are listed in Table 1.6. Food poisoning is usually of short duration and is often associated with vomiting. Ischemic colitis is often associated with pain and bloody diarrhea. Many drugs cause diarrhea. In recipients of anal intercourse with sx of proctitis (small frequent stools, sense of painful rectal spasm, and incomplete emptying), gonorrhea,

Table 1.6   Causes of of Acute Diarrhea

Disorder	Agent	Found on Page
Food poisonings	Many	285
Viral infections	Many	281
Bacterial infections	*Salmonella*	266
	Campylobacter	264
	Shigella	268
	E. coli O157:H7	269
	Yersinia	272
	Aeromonas	273
	Plesiomonas	273
	Other *E. coli*	273
Protozoan infections	*Amebiasis*	275
	Giardia	274
	Cyclospora	279
	Cryptosporidium	277
	Isospora	280
Sexually transmitted disease		—
Drugs		—
Partial bowel obstruction		206
Fecal impaction		297
Ischemic colitis		306
Bacterial overgrowth		283

herpes, *Chlamydia,* and syphilis are considerations. Diarrhea in HIV infected pts is discussed on p 282.

Approach to Dx: Pts with mild illness do not need additional evaluation. In those with high fever, blood in the stool, illness as part of an outbreak, or other suggestions of an invasive pathogen, it is reasonable to culture the stool and treat presumptively with a quinolone for a bacterial pathogen. Some prefer to skip the culture in these circumstances, but a positive culture may guide rx if the pt fails to do well or relapses. Most laboratories now culture routinely for *E. coli* O157:H7 in submitted stool samples, but it is important to check your lab. This pathogen should be sought in bloody diarrhea (especially if fever is absent or low grade), after eating undercooked hamburger, in outbreaks, or when there is evidence of HUS (p 269). Some authors use stool wbc or stool lactoferrin to select pts for stool culture or empiric rx, but the poor performance characteristics of these tests (Ped Infect Dis J 1996;15:486) makes this common practice questionable. If the epidemiology suggests *Giardia* or the illness has lasted more than 1-2 weeks, testing the stool for *Giardia* antigen is appropriate. Testing the stool for *C. difficile* is needed if there is recent antibiotic use or the pt is hospitalized, and empiric rx pending the result should be considered if the pt is ill. In the pt who has diarrhea for more than 1-2 weeks, testing the stool for *Cryptosporidia, Cyclospora,* and *Isospora* may be worthwhile. Stool for O&P is very low yield in acute diarrhea. Testing may be appropriate in travelers returned from endemic areas.

Approach to Rx:
- *Fluid and diet:* Sport drinks, diluted fruit juice, broths, and soups augmented with saltine crackers are usually adequate to meet salt and fluid needs. In substantially volume depleted pts, oral rehydration solutions can be used but iv fluids are commonly used for rapid, effective relief. As the illness subsides, noodles, rice, potatoes, boiled vegetables, bananas, and yogurt

can be tried. Caffeine is avoided and milk products are commonly withheld, though acute lactase deficiency is not common.

- *Empiric rx for invasive infection:* It is reasonable to consider empiric rx of pts with features suggesting invasive diarrhea (temp >101°F, dysentery, FOBT positive, positive for wbc, or lactoferrin if done) because rx shortens the duration of illness by about a day (Clin Infect Dis 1996;22:1019; Arch IM 1990;150:541). Ciprofloxacin 500 mg po bid or norfloxacin 400 mg po bid for 3-5 days are common choices. If *E. coli* O157:H7 is suspected, antibiotics are avoided (see p 269).

- *Antimotility rx:* Loperamide 4 mg followed by 2 mg after each loose stool to a maximum of 16 mg per 24 hours is given in most cases for symptomatic relief. It had been a concern that pts with invasive pathogens may worsen with antimotility agents (Jama 1973;226:1525), but this is uncommon. Loperamide should be avoided in pts with dysentery or *E. coli* O157:H7 for fear of inducing HUS (p 269) (J Pediatr 1990;116:589).

- *Traveler's diarrhea* (Nejm 1993;328:1821): Travelers to high-risk areas should take dietary precautions and only eat steaming hot food, carbonated beverages (skip the ice), dry foods (bread), acidic foods (citrus), and high-sugar foods (jellies and syrups). Since most episodes are due to bacterial pathogens, the traveler should bring a quinolone and loperamide. Treatment is begun promptly if diarrhea occurs. Chemoprophylaxis is not routinely recommended for healthy travelers unless a short duration diarrheal illness would be intolerable. Many pts going on a hard earned international vacation would prefer to avoid diarrhea and request prophylaxis. Medically ill pts and those taking a PPI (which reduces stomach acid content and predisposes to infection) should receive prophylaxis. Bismuth subsalicylate 2 tabs po qid is 65% effective (Jama 1987;257:1347). A single dose of a quinolone daily (eg, ciprofloxacin 500 mg po qd) is >90% effective.

1.9 Chronic Diarrhea

GE 1999;116:1464; Nejm 1995;332:725

Sx and Si: Chronic diarrhea is usually defined as diarrhea lasting >4 weeks and characterized by 4 or more loose stools daily. Stool weight is typically in excess of 250 gm/day. The diff dx is long and can be narrowed substantially by the hx and exam. The hx is used to broadly categorize the sx. The clinician should assess if the sx suggest an illness that is (1) functional, (2) structural (eg, IBD), (3) colonic, (4) malabsorptive/small bowel, (5) infectious, (6) related to important psychiatric or psychosocial factors, or (7) present in an immunocompromised or HIV-infected host.

Stool frequency and character are determined. Periods of constipation alternating with diarrhea suggest a functional illness such as IBS or a low-fiber diet. Blood in the stool, weight loss, and nocturnal diarrhea argue against a functional cause. Extraintestinal manifestations of IBD (joint sx, perianal disease, skin, or eye sx [p 179]) can be helpful clues. Frequent small-volume stools, crampy lower abdominal pain, and a sense of incomplete evacuation suggest a distal colonic process. Diarrhea with crampy mid-abdominal pain, large-volume stools, bloating, and borborygmi (bowel sounds audible at a distance) suggest a small bowel or malabsorptive cause. Stools that are oily, greasy, and difficult to flush may contain fat, suggesting malabsorption. Abrupt onset of sx with large-volume diarrhea and fever may suggest an infectious cause. Inquiries must be made about stress, depression, and sexual abuse (p 162).

Dietary hx is crucial. Determine the consumption of lactose (milk, frozen yogurt, ice cream, other dairy products), sorbitol (breath mints, sugarless gum, apples, pears, prunes, peaches, diabetic foods), fructose (figs, dates, prunes, pears, apples, grapes, and soft drinks sweetened with high fructose corn syrup), and dietary fiber.

The physical exam identifies localized tenderness, masses, and evidence of systemic disease. The rectal exam is crucial in the evaluation of sphincter tone and impaction. A complaint of "chronic diarrhea" is often undiagnosed incontinence.

Diff Dx: The causes of chronic diarrhea are listed in Table 1.7. Dietary causes include excessive caffeine, lactose (p 172), sorbitol (p 16), and fructose (p 16). Causes of malabsorption are discussed on p 30. Fecal incontinence (p 294) or fecal impaction (p 297) are missed without a proper rectal exam. Bile salt malabsorption may occur as a result of defects in the ileal bile salt transporter (J Clin Invest 1997;99:1807) or due to ileal resection. Bile salts that are malabsorbed cause diarrhea in pts with an intact colon by stimulating colonic fluid secretion.

Approach to Dx: Based on the sx and si, the disease is characterized and the approach varies:

- *Sx and si suggest functional causes:* If the sx sound diet related or are those of longstanding IBS, consider a CBC, CMP, and FOBT. Dietary trials (exclude milk products, caffeine, sorbitol; consider fiber if diarrhea alternates with constipation) and a follow-up office visit are often adequate. If sx persist additional evaluation and rx as detailed in the IBS section are appropriate (p 153). Laxative screening may be needed.
- *Sx and si suggest IBD:* If the sx suggest IBD, colonoscopy and SBFT are usually needed to make a dx and assess the extent and severity of illness. The approach is outlined in the sections on Crohn's (p 177) and ulcerative colitis (p 190).
- *Sx and si suggest colonic causes:* Colonic sx are those of crampy lower abdominal pain, an uncomfortable sensation of rectal spasm (tenesmus), and frequent small-volume stools. Infection

Table 1.7   Causes of Chronic Diarrhea

Common Causes	Found on Page
Irritable bowel syndrome	153
Fecal incontinence	294
Fecal impaction	297
Chronic infection	See Table 1.6
Inflammatory bowel disease	177, 190
Drugs	—
Dietary	—
Malabsorption	30
Colon cancer	219
Collagenous colitis	198
Microscopic colitis	199
Surreptitious laxative use	—
Diabetic neuropathy	—
Postgastrectomy diarrhea	120
Radiation enteritis	213
Bile salt malabsorption	27
Hyperthyroidism	—
Hormone secreting tumors	332, 145
HIV infection	282
Scleroderma	—
Amyloid	—
Carcinoid	254
Mastocytosis	—

vs IBD vs IBS are the main considerations. Consider CBC, CMP, TSH, stool c&s, and stool for C. *diff*. If these are negative, a colonoscopy with biopsies (for IBD or microscopic colitis [p 198]) may be needed. If the sx are those of proctitis (small-volume stools with urgency and blood but without systemic illness), a flex sig may be adequate.

- *Sx and si suggest malabsorption or disease of the upper gut:* See p 30 regarding the evaluation of malabsorption.
- *Sx and si suggest an infectious cause:* Extensive stool testing may be worthwhile if the onset was very abrupt with a large volume of stool, fever, and systemic sx. Consider stool tests for C&S,

C. diff, Giardia antigen, test stool for Cryptosporidium, Cyclospora, and determination of stool O&P on three samples. The yield of the O&P studies is very low. If amebiasis is a consideration, the antigen test may be superior (p 275). The technique for detection of Cryptosporidium and C. diff will depend on the local lab. Antigen tests or special stains may be used. An empiric trial of metronidazole for Giardia is often reasonable. If a dx is not made, colonoscopy or SBFT may be needed to rule out abrupt onset IBD.

- *Immunocompromised host:* Consider HIV testing and testing for unusual causes of infection (p 30).
- *Additional studies are warranted if sx persist after focused evaluation.* If the sx sound functional but are refractory, consider a stool laxative screen and reexplore the abuse history. A TSH should be obtained. It may be necessary to do a low-yield colonoscopy and SBFT to rule out IBD. A trial of cholestyramine (4 gm po tid) for possible bile salt malabsorption should be tried. Loperamide, antidepressants, and antispasmodics may need to be considered. If the sx warrant further evaluation, the considerations for testing include:
  - *72-hour stool collection:* This study is done on a 100-gm fat diet (p 30) at which time a laxative screen and total weight and fat are recorded. If stool weight and fat are normal then the yield for organic disease with more extensive testing is very low. If diarrhea is large volume then evaluation for hormone secreting tumors and reevaluation of possible malabsorption or small bowel disease (with SBFT or bx) may be warranted.
  - *Test stool for electrolytes and osmoles:* This is done to calculate the stool osmolar gap, which equals $(290 - 2x([Na^+] + [K^+])$ in mOsm/kg. The value of 290 mOsm/kg in this equation is the normal expected osmolality of stool. If diarrhea is due to an osmotically active particle (such as Mg^{++} antacids, lactulose, sorbitol) the gap is usually >125 mOsm/kg. In a

pure, secretory diarrhea, nearly all the osmotic particles are related to Na^+ and K^+, and the gap is <50 mOsm/kg. If the measured osmolality is less than 290 mOsm/kg, water may have been added to the stool.

- *Laxative screen:* Commercially available tests are available to screen stool liquid for bisacodyl and urine for anthraquinones. Phenolphthalein (now off the U.S. market) is detected by a pink color when NaOH is added to the stool supernatant. Room searches (after asking the pt) are a consideration.
- *Tests for small bowel bacterial overgrowth:* see p 283.
- *Tests for hormone secreting tumors:* See Islet Cell tumors (p 332), Gastrinoma (p 145), and Carcinoid (p 254). A urine for pheochromocytoma testing (metanephrines and VMA) is a consideration.
- *Small bowel bx:* This may uncover unusual diseases such as Whipple's or celiac disease missed by other means (see Malabsorption and Maldigestion, next chapter).
- *Evaluation for mesenteric ischemia:*See p 305.
- *Consider HIV* even in the absence of risk factors or clues.

General Rx: While completing an evaluation, minimizing caffeine, milk products, and using loperamide (2-4 mg up to qid) is reasonable to give some sx relief.

1.10 Malabsorption and Maldigestion

Compr Ther 1997;23:672

Pathophys: Malabsorption is often a term used very loosely by clinicians to include maldigestion and malabsorption. Normal **digestion** involves the hydrolysis of proteins, fats, and carbohydrates by pancreatic enzymes in the gut lumen. Digestion creates amino acids, fatty acids, monoglycerides, and monosaccharides. Fatty acids and monoglycerides are held in solution in the aqueous environment by bile salts secreted from the liver into bile. The products of digestion are moved into the epithelial cells by active transport in the process called **absorption.** Fatty acids and monoglycerides are reassembled into triglycerides and transported via the **lymphatics** to the systemic circulation. Interference with the process at any of these three levels can result in clinical evidence of malabsorption/maldigestion.

Sx and Si: Pts with malabsorption typically present with weight loss and diarrhea. The stool is of high fat content so it might look greasy, oily, or be difficult to flush. There may be bloating, excessive flatus, and borborygmi. In very advanced cases there may be a syndrome associated with specific nutrient deficiencies such as anemia associated with folate or B_{12} deficiency, bleeding with vitamin K deficiency, or metabolic bone disease from vitamin D deficiency. However, it is now uncommon for pts to present with these advanced findings.

Diff Dx: The causes of **maldigestion** include: (1) pancreatic insufficiency due to chronic pancreatitis (p 322) or pancreatic cancer (p 327), (2) poor mixing due to gastric or weight reduction surgery (causing unregulated release of stomach contents, bypassing the duodenum or parts of jejunum), or (3) ZE syndrome (p 145), in which low duodenal pH inactivates enzymes. **Malabsorption** is most often due to celiac disease (p 145) because of loss of absorptive surface. In bacterial overgrowth (p 283), malabsorption is the result of mucosal damage and bile salt deconjugation by bacteria. Some infections, notably *Giardia* (p 274), can cause a malabsorptive picture by mucosal inflammation. In short bowel syndrome (p 204), malabsorption comes from inadequate surface area. Crohn's disease can cause malabsorption, but there are usually ample clues to its presence. Rare but important causes include Whipple's disease (p 286), eosinophilic gastroenteritis (p 215), radiation enteritis (p 213), and small bowel lymphoma. Abetalipoproteinemia (Jama 1993;270:865) and lymphangiectasia (Am J Gastroenterol 1993;88:887) cause malabsorption by preventing fat from being transported from the enterocyte via the lymphatics to the systemic circulation.

Approach to Dx: If a pt has sx or si suggestive of malabsorption but with no clues to a more specific etiology (such as celiac disease), a CBC and CMP are appropriate. If anemia is present, levels of folate, B_{12}, and iron should be determined. A 72-hour fecal fat study should be done. The sample is collected after 3 days of a 100-gm fat diet that is continued throughout the collection. More than 7 gm/day is abnormal, but mild increases of up to 14 gm are very common in any cause of diarrhea. In steatorrhea (fat malabsorption), there is typically >14 gm of fat/24 hr in the stool (GE 1999;116:1464). If steatorrhea is not present, then the dx might not be malabsorption. If the pt is reluctant to do a 72-hour collection, a qualitative fecal fat on a single sample can be a helpful positive but is not a reliable negative.

If the fecal fat is elevated, the etiology must be determined. A trial of pancreatic enzymes (p 326) is a practical way to evaluate for pancreatic insufficiency. If enzyme replacement results in improvement, then the cause of pancreatic insufficiency is determined with imaging tests and hx. If enzyme replacement is not helpful, then a small bowel bx and/or tests for bacterial overgrowth (p 283) are appropriate. Small bowel bx will detect the rare conditions listed in the differential. Some experts would use serologic tests for celiac disease (p 200) prior to considering bx. If a small bowel bx is normal, then an SBFT to look for other structural abnormalities can be helpful. Tests for pancreatic insufficiency that are more sensitive than a trial of pancreatic enzymes may need to be considered (p 322).,

1.11 Gastrointestinal Bleeding

Med Clin N Am 2000;84:1183; Am J Gastroenterol 1998;93:1202

Sx and Si: The H&P are used to assess the acuity and severity of bleeding and to determine if bleeding is from an upper or lower source. It is important to determine if the pt has risk factors for bleeding such as NSAID use, anticoagulant use, or liver disease. Blood loss can present as: (1) hematemesis (bloody vomitus, either red and fresh or coffee grounds), (2) melena (stool that looks black and shiny like tar and is sticky, malodorous and difficult to flush), (3) hematochezia (maroon stool or bright red bleeding with or without stool), or (4) sx related to the effects of blood loss such as syncope, MI, dyspnea, or weakness. Upper tract bleeding is easily diagnosed if there is hematemesis. Melena also suggests upper bleeding but can be seen in slow, lower bleeds. Melena can be confused with the dull black stool of iron, bismuth subsalicylate, beets, and greens. Hematochezia can be from a lower bleed or from a brisk upper bleed.

Vital signs are taken. If pulse and blood pressure are normal, it may be useful to obtain postural vital signs. The pt is asked to sit up and dangle the legs for a few minutes and pulse and blood pressure are repeated. In rough terms, a rise in pulse of >10 points generally indicates that the pt is at least one liter volume depleted. The greater the pulse rise the more specific (and less sensitive) the test, and some authors use a pulse rise of 30 points to signify volume depletion (Jama 1999;281:1022). A postural drop in systolic blood pressure >20 mm Hg (which should generally go along with a pulse rise) may indicate volume depletion of a couple of liters. However, postural vital signs are neither sensitive nor specific and need to be one piece of data in context. Up to 10% of euvolemic pts have postural hypotension, especially if they have chronic hypertension. It is unnecessary to check posturals in the bleeding pt with resting tachycardia or hypotension since they are clearly volume depleted. Postural vitals can be misleading in pts on beta blockers, those with intrinsic heart disease, and those with autonomic dysfunction (Jama 1999;281:1022). Other important findings on exam include stigmata of chronic liver disease (p 42), abdominal findings, the appearance of the stool, and evidence of systemic illness.

Diff Dx: The causes of gi bleeding are listed in Table 1.8. Upper gi bleeding is bleeding that arises proximal to the ligament of Treitz. Aortoduodenal fistula is a very rare cause of bleeding not discussed elsewhere in the text (Am J Surg 1980;46:121). The small bowel is an uncommon cause of acute bleeding. Most acute lower bleeding is from colonic diverticula.

Approach to Acute Bleeding: Laboratory assessment includes CBC, platelet count, CMP, and PT/PTT to look for coagulopathy. An EKG is reasonable in pts over 50 years or for those with cardiac risk factors. In the acute setting, a type and crossmatch should be done for 2-6 units depending on the fitness of the pt, the initial

Table 1.8   Causes of Gastrointestinal Bleeding

Cause	Found on Page
Upper gi Bleeding	
Peptic ulcer disease	114, 126
Erosive gastritis	105
Esophageal/gastric varices	429
Esophagitis	53
Mallory-Weiss tear	93
Gastric cancer	137
Portal hypertensive gastropathy	430
Gastric antral vascular ectasias	149
Angiodysplasia	308
Dieulafoy's lesions	150
Gastric lymphoma	140
Other gastric malignancies	—
Benign gastric tumors	—
Aortoduodenal fistula	34

Table 1.8   continued

	Cause	Found on Page
Small Bowel Bleeding		
	Angiodysplasia	308
	Tumors	—
	Ulcers	—
	Meckel's diverticulum	216
	Other diverticula	—
	Crohn's disease	177
	Intussusception	300
	Parasites	283
Colonic gi Bleeding		
	Colonic diverticula	165
	Angiodysplasia	308
	Ischemic colitis	306
	Inflammatory bowel disease	177, 190
	Colon cancer	219
	Colonic ulcers due to NSAIDs	—
	Stercoral ulcers	297
	Infectious colitis	23
	Radiation colitis	213
	Hemorrhoids	289
	Anal fissure	292
	Postpolypectomy bleeding	—
	Solitary rectal ulcer	298
	Colonic varices	429
	Vasculitis	—
	Endometriosis	216

hemoglobin, and the estimated magnitude of the bleed. The blood bank should be instructed to crossmatch a unit each time one is transfused in the critically ill pt. This ensures that blood stays available if the bleeding is massive. The hgb may markedly underestimate blood loss in an acute bleed. At equilibrium, every 1 gm below normal represents about 1 unit (500 mL of whole

blood) of blood lost (Ann IM 1994;121:278). An elevation
of the ratio of BUN/Cr >36:1 is a strong clue that the bleeding
is from the upper tract if the pt is not on diuretics and does
not have renal failure (Am J Gastroenterol 1997;92:1777).
An isolated elevation in the PT should suggest the possibility of
liver disease and varices. This finding may prompt the use of
octreotide (p 429) in the massively bleeding pt who is awaiting
EGD. Some clinicians use NGT aspirate to identify upper bleeds.
However, an aspirate can be negative from an actively bleeding
DU or from other lesions not actively bleeding at the time of the
passage of the tube. The clinical and lab data are used to determine if the bleeding is more likely to be upper or lower and if it is
acute or chronic.

- *Acute upper bleeding:* If bleeding is thought to be upper tract in
  origin, the pt is stabilized and undergoes EGD. Not only is
  EGD generally diagnostic, but it is also therapeutic for
  bleeding ulcer disease (p 126) and varices (p 429). The endoscopic findings can also be used to predict the likelihood of
  ongoing bleeding and can be used in determining the safety of
  prompt discharge in acute upper bleeding. If the pt with suspected upper bleeding has a normal endoscopy, then colonic or
  small bowel sources need to be considered. The most likely
  causes of upper bleeding missed at initial EGD are Dieulafoy's
  ulcer (p 150) and angiodysplasia (p 308). There is no role for
  barium studies in acute bleeding.
- *Acute lower bleeding:* In large volume hematochezia, the evaluation depends on the severity of the bleed and whether or not
  colonoscopy is possible. In pts with large volume hematochezia
  and hemodynamic instability, bleeding from the upper tract
  needs to be considered. In this very select group it is reasonable
  to do EGD after volume resuscitation. Some clinicians forgo
  EGD if an NG aspirate shows copious amounts of bile. If
  ongoing active bleeding prevents colonoscopy, a tagged rbc
  scan is appropriate. The pt's red cells are labeled with

technetium-99 and reinjected. If bleeding occurs at rates of >0.1 mL/minute, extravasation into the bowel lumen can be identified (AJR Am J Roentgenol 1987;148:869). The scan is highly accurate if positive within 2 hours and an upper tract source has been excluded by EGD (Am J Gastroenterol 1994;89:345). The scan is more likely to be misleading if long scanning times are required (J Nucl Med 1992;33:202). If the site is localized by a high-quality scan and bleeding does not stop, a surgical resection is performed. Blind colectomy should be avoided because of the high morbidity (Dis Colon Rectum 1982;25:441). Angiography can be diagnostic and therapeutic but is associated with a high incidence of complications, requires more vigorous bleeding than a rbc scan requires for visualization (≥0.5 mL/min), and surgery is still frequently required (GE 2000;118:978). The use of angiography varies widely among institutions and its role is undefined. If bleeding stops, the pt should undergo colonoscopy to look for a treatable cause of the bleeding and possibly for endoscopic rx (p 166). If colonoscopy is negative, evaluation of the small bowel may be needed.

Approach to Obscure Bleeding: (Gastro Endosc 2003;58:650) When the source of continued bleeding (either recurrent visible bleeding or occult bleeding) is not evident from an initial EGD/colonoscopy, it is reasonable to consider repeating these exams. The yield of repeat endoscopy may be as high as 35% (Brit J Surg 1983;70:489). The quality of the initial exam and the experience of the endoscopist should be considered in the decision. If the bleeding is acute and the pt is young, a Meckel's diverticulum is a possibility and nuclear scanning is considered (p 216). An SBFT may show Crohn's disease, diverticular disease, or tumors. If an SBFT is normal, the small bowel can be evaluated with push enteroscopy. In this exam, the scope can be passed up to 100 cm beyond the ligament of Treitz with use of an overube.

Enteroscopy has a yield of 38-75% in obscure bleeding. The development of wireless capsule endoscopy has revolutionized imaging of the small intestine. It is superior to push enteroscopy in the detection of bleeding lesions. Limitations include the inability to precisely locate the lesion or to provide therapy of bleeding lesions. The chief risk is failure of the capsule to pass through narrow areas of intestine, thereby requiring surgical removal. Intraoperative endoscopy may be needed in some cases of small bowel bleeding (Am J Surg 1992;163:94). Enteroclysis (in which aqueous methylcellulose containing contrast is administered by nasoenteric tube) has a yield of only 10% (GE 1989;97:58)). If obscure bleeding occurs in recurrent discrete episodes, a technetium-99 labeled rbc scan at the onset of bleeding may be of use.

Approach to Visible Small-Volume Rectal Bleeding: (Jama 1997;277:44) This is a common complaint in primary care practice. About 3% of the population report having blood in the toilet and 12-15% report blood on tissue within the prior 6 months. The optimal strategy for evaluation has not been established. The major uncertainty is whether to examine all or part of the colon. In an older age primary care population, blood mixed with stool and short duration of bleeding are associated with serious disease. In older pts, the clinical hx does not identify a subgroup well served by a limited exam such as sigmoidoscopy. A practical approach is to offer colonoscopy to any pt over age 50 who has not had CRC screening. For younger pts with a long-standing complaint, a sigmoidoscopy can be a less expensive alternative to a low-yield colonoscopy (Am J Gastroenterol 2000;95:1184). Flex sig will detect proctitis, distal polyps (such as in FAP, p 246), and the unusual distal cancer. If sigmoidoscopy is chosen, the pt should be informed of the limitations of the test. The need for further study if bleeding persists must be emphasized, since a small proportion of young pts have a neoplastic cause of bleeding. The advantages of choosing colonoscopy as the initial test in a young pt are that it usually provides an immediately reassuring negative test and that young pts generally tolerate sedated colonoscopy much better than unsedated sigmoidoscopy.

Approach to FOBT Positive Stool: (Nejm 1999;341:38) Pts with a positive FOBT obtained in screening should have colonoscopy because it is more accurate than barium enema and flexible sigmoidoscopy. The yield in the screening setting is about 3% for CRC and 30% for adenomatous polyps (Nejm 1993;328:1365). Pts with normal colonoscopies and localizing upper tract sx, weight loss, or anemia may benefit from EGD. The yield of EGD is 25-40% in asymptomatic pts. EGD may result in changes in management such as the discontinuation of NSAIDs or the addition of acid blocking rx (Nejm 1998;339:153). However, EGD adds substantially to the costs of screening for colon cancer with FOBT. The AGA position statement recommends EGD for pts with positive FOBT and negative colonoscopy (GE 2000; 118:197). The position statement concedes that the clinical and economic impact requires further study. The cost of EGD would add substantially to the cost of colon cancer screening with FOBT if all pts with normal colonoscopies have EGD. It seems reasonable to educate the asymptomatic pt who has no need for NSAIDs regarding the purpose of EGD. Many will opt not to proceed with a test that generally does not change the quality of their lives. Neither NSAIDs nor warfarin can be accepted as a cause of positive FOBT because the yield of full investigation is similar to that seen in pts not on those agents (Am J Med 1996; 100:598).

Approach to Iron Deficiency Anemia: In women in their reproductive years, iron deficiency is usually related to menses and pregnancy losses. In males and postmenopausal women, gi tract blood loss is the most common cause. The cause of iron deficiency is found in the upper tract in 40%, in the small bowel in 3%, in the colon in

22%, and not found in 34% of pts (Nejm 1999;341:38). The initial endoscopic evaluation can be directed to the site of sx (Nejm 1993;329:1691), but the other end should be examined if the initial exam is normal. Celiac disease can present as iron deficiency in the absence of other sx. The use of random bx of the duodenum at EGD to detect celiac disease is controversial. The yield was 3% in one large series (Gut 1993;34:1102). The practice was not advocated in an AGA position paper because of the low yield (GE 2000;118:197). Nevertheless, the practice seems reasonable in populations with a high prevalence of celiac disease, such as northern Europeans.

The optimal evaluation of iron deficiency in **premenopausal women** has not been determined. A retrospective study from a referral center suggested that 12% of such pts had important gi lesions, including gastric cancer (3%) (Am J Med 1998;105:281). Referral bias limits the value of these observations. Since iron deficiency is most commonly related to menses, these women usually can be managed with iron and regulation of menses. However, endoscopic evaluation should be considered in women over age 40 years, in those with abdominal sx, in those with substantial anemia (hgb <10 gm/dL), FOBT positive stool, or in whom the anemia seems out of proportion to the perceived menstrual losses (Lancet 1998;352:1953).

Approach to Rx: The specific cause of bleeding is identified and treated. Some general guidelines include:

- *Initial resuscitation in acute bleeding:* Volume resuscitation is performed by rapid infusion of NS through large bore (18 gauge or greater) peripheral ivs. Fluids can be wide open until pulse and blood pressure are acceptable. Postural vital signs after each liter may be helpful. At least two reliable IVs should be maintained until the acute illness is resolved.
- *Transfusion:* The appropriate threshold for transfusion of red blood cells has not been established in clinical studies. The goal is to transfuse only as much blood as is needed to mini-

mize the risk of end organ damage (eg, MI). Transfusion is almost never indicated if hgb >10.0 gm/dL and is almost always indicated if hgb is <6 gm/dL (Arch Pathol Lab Med 1998;122:130). It is common clinical practice to keep the hgb of a young healthy pt with acute bleeding >7.0 and to aim for a hgb >9.0 in pts with known coronary disease and those thought to be at risk for ischemia. Chronic blood loss is often well tolerated and transfusion is needed at lower levels of hgb than with acute blood loss. Symptoms, age, and the expected course of bleeding also affect the decision. The threshold to transfuse will be lower in a pt who has bleeding that is likely to continue.

Fresh frozen plasma should also be given to pts with active bleeding and an INR >1.5 (Jama 1994;271:777). Fresh frozen plasma is also indicated after replacement of more than one blood volume (about 10 units in a 70-kg adult) if continued bleeding and a coagulopathy are present (Jama 1994;271:777). The usual starting dose is 2 units (unless coagulopathy is severe), and the effect is measured by repeating the INR within an hour of transfusion. Additional units are given if the INR does not fall below 1.5. The half-life of factor VII is only 5-6 h (longer for most other factors) and repeat dosing may be needed. The INR is followed serially if the pt is actively bleeding. In some cases (warfarin use, malabsorption, poor diet, recent antibiotics) an elevated INR is due to vitamin K deficiency. Vitamin K 10 mg sc qdx3 should be given, though a full response will usually take 1-3 days. Platelet transfusion is appropriate in major acute bleeding if platelet count is <50,000/mm^3. A dose of 6 units will raise platelet counts by 50,000/mm^3 (Jama 1994;271:777).

- *Hospital length of stay:* In Ugi hemorrhage there is an excellent clinical tool for determining the appropriate length of stay (Am J Med 1996;100:313). A risk score based on endoscopic findings, timing of bleeding, hemodynamics, and comorbidities is generated. The risk score can be used to predict the safety of discharge from the hospital. There is no similar guideline for lower gi bleeding.

1.12 Evaluating Suspected Liver Disease

Sx: (Sherlock S and Dooley J. Diseases of the liver and biliary system. 10th ed. Boston: Blackwell Science, 1997:5-6.) Several aspects of the hx and exam should be emphasized in the pt with suspected liver disease. Abdominal pain and fever may be a clue to biliary obstruction from stones or mass. Risk factors for viral hepatitis should be identified (blood transfusion, sexual practices, iv drug abuse, travel). Pruritus may suggest a chronic cholestatic disease. Nonspecific sx of liver disease include fatigue, arthralgias, decreased libido, impotence, and ovulatory failure. Alcohol consumption should be carefully evaluated, and a complete list of current and past prescription medicines, OTC remedies, and herbal remedies should be obtained. Herbal hepatotoxicity is of growing importance (Jama 1995;273:502). Occupational hx and the family hx of liver disease should be obtained.

Si: On exam the liver span is determined by **percussion** and is usually 12-15 cm. The liver margin is **palpated** by standing facing the supine pt's feet and hooking the fingers over the right upper quadrant. A liver palpable with deep inspiration is a normal finding. Rarely, a friction **rub** may be heard or felt due to tumor, recent biopsy, or inflammation. The liver may be **pulsatile** from tricuspid insufficiency. The **venous hum** of portal HTN (heard between umbilicus and xiphoid) and the arterial murmur of hepatocellular carcinoma are rare. Jaundice may first be evident as scleral icterus. **Vascular spiders** are red lesions that are seen on the upper trunk, neck, face, and hands. They have a central arteriole and smaller radiating branches that look like a spider's legs and can be made to blanch with central pressure. They usually indicate cirrhosis but can be seen in pregnancy, viral hepatitis, or rarely in normal pts. **Palmar erythema** may be noted. **Dilated veins** over the abdominal wall may indicate portal HTN. Testes may be atrophic in cirrhosis. Gynecomastia is rare.

Massive **ascites** due to portal HTN is easily detected, but the exam can be misleading. The flanks bulge due to fluid and there is stony dullness to percussion. The line on the flank where there is a change from dullness to tympany should be determined. By rolling the pt obliquely and repeating percussion, the line of dullness shifts as the fluid moves to a dependent position. This finding of **shifting dullness** confirms ascites, but false positives (with bowel contents and movement of the mesentery) and false negatives occur. A **fluid wave** is identified in the supine pt by tapping briskly on one side of the abdomen while a receiving hand waits on the other end for the fluid wave. There is a perceptible delay between tapping and receiving the wave. Fat can cause a similar finding so an assistant must press down on the abdominal wall to prevent confusion.

Asterixis (a flapping tremor caused by momentary loss of muscle tone) is associated with hepatic encephalopathy. It is best brought out by having the pt hold the wrist dorsiflexed with arms outstretched. **Fetor hepaticus** is a sour fecal smell in the breath due to exhaled mercaptans that should have been cleared by the liver.

Diff Dx: Pts come to an evaluation for suspected liver disease in several ways. The largest group have asymptomatic elevations of LFTs. Others will present with jaundice, evidence of cirrhosis on physical exam, an abnormal imaging test, or fulminant hepatic failure. The liver diseases that need to be considered are listed in Table 1.9.

Approach to Asymptomatic, Persistently Abnormal Transaminases:
(Nejm 2000;342:1266) If there is no obvious cause (such as alcohol or recent hepatotoxic drugs), studies should be obtained (see Table 1.10). These routinely include tests for hepatitis B

Table 1.9 Causes of Liver Disease

Disease	Discussed on Page
Alcoholic liver disease	421
Drug hepatotoxicity	425
Hepatitis A	359
Hepatitis B	362
Hepatitis C	370
Other viral agents	377
Fatty liver	383
Nonalcoholic steatohepatitis	383
Autoimmune hepatitis	395
Hemochromatosis	399
Wilson's disease	405
Primary biliary cirrhosis	386
Primary sclerosing cholangitis	391
Alpha-1 antitrypsin deficiency	408
Ischemic hepatitis	453
Budd-Chiari syndrome	451
Hepatocellular carcinoma	413
Other hepatic neoplasms	418
Disorders of pregnancy	457
Occupational hepatotoxins	—
Herbal and other ingested hepatotoxins	—
Biliary obstruction	47
Hepatic masses	418

(HBsAg, and Anti-HBc), hepatitis C (serum antibody), hemochromatosis (Fe/TIBC, ferritin), Wilson's (ceruloplasmin if pt <40 yrs old), autoimmune hepatitis (ANA, ASMA, SPEP), and alpha-1 antitrypsin deficiency (optional and low yield). The liver should be imaged with ultrasound to look for structural abnormalities (eg, tumor, echogenicity suggesting hepatocellular disease, the irregular contour of cirrhosis) and bile duct dilatation due to obstruction. A PT and albumin evaluate synthetic function and can be a clue to serious chronic disease. Thrombocytopenia may suggest cirrhosis. If no cause is found with this testing,

Table 1.10 Evaluation of Persistently Elevated Transaminases

Disease	Test
ROUTINELY OBTAIN THE FOLLOWING:	
Hep B	Hep B surface antigen
	Hep B IgM core ab
Hep C	Hep C ab[1]
Autoimmune hepatitis	Antinuclear ab
	Antismooth muscle ab
	IgG level
Hemochromatosis	Fe/TIBC and ferritin
Wilson's disease	Ceruloplasmin (if pt <40)
Mass/Obstruction/Cirrhosis	Ultrasound or CT scan
Evaluate ? of cirrhosis	Prothrombin time, platelets
	Albumin
CONSIDER THE FOLLOWING:	
Alpha-1 antitrypsin deficiency	Alpha-1 antitrypsin level
Primary biliary cirrhosis	Antimitochondrial ab
Primary sclerosing cholangitis	MRCP/ERCP
Prolonged hep A	Hep A IgM ab
Missed dx of hep C	Hep C by PCR
Older onset Wilson's	Ceruloplasmin
Celiac disease	Tissue transglutaminase
	Antigliadin ab
	IgA level
Muscle disease	CPK, aldolase
Sarcoid	ACE level, chest x-ray
Disorders of pregnancy	HCG level

the most likely diagnosis is nonalcoholic fatty liver disease
(p 383). Rarely, hepatitis C is missed by antibody testing. A
hep C viral RNA determination by PCR is reasonable, especially
if risk factors are present. Other lower-yield considerations are an
ACE level and CXR for sarcoid, and an AMA for PBC even if
alk phos is normal. Consideration should be given to nonhepatic
causes of abnormal transaminases, such as celiac disease (see

p 200 for dx testing [Lancet 1998;352:26]) and primary diseases of muscle (check CPK and aldolase). Muscle disease is more likely to be the çause if AST>>ALT.

If abnormalities persist for greater than 6 months, the traditional approach has been liver bx. However, in the current era of extensive and accurate serum testing, bx does not appear to effect management. In a study of 1124 adults referred for abnormal LFTs, 81 had negative serum testing (all the studies listed previously) and underwent bx. There were 8 normal biopsies, and all the remaining biopsies showed evidence of fatty liver or of NASH (with varying degrees of fibrosis) (Am J Gastroenterol 1999;94:3010). In light of this study, it is difficult to justify the morbidity of bx unless effective therapies for NASH make the distinction between NASH and milder forms of fatty liver disease more important.

Approach to Abnormal Alkaline Phosphatase: (Mayo Clin Proc 1996;71:1089) Alk phos is secreted by bile duct epithelial cells. Synthesis increases when bile ducts are obstructed. However, increases can come from bone disease (Paget's, malignancy, fractures), in pregnancy from the placenta (causing levels twice normal), in growing children, and in adolescents (up to 3 times normal). Alk phos also increases with age, and the yield of chasing a value <20% above the upper limit of normal is very low.

The first step in evaluation is to confirm that it is of liver origin by obtaining a GGTP or a 5-nucleotidase (5'NT). If GGTP or 5'NT is normal, then the alk phos elevation is not of hepatic origin. A bone scan may be helpful to evaluate elevated alk phos of bony origin. If alk phos and GGTP or 5'NT are elevated, then diagnostic possibilities include: (1) bile duct obstruction (from stones, strictures, or neoplasia), (2) infiltrative liver disease (sarcoid, lymphoma, tbc, fungal infections), (3) intrahepatic obstruction from tumor, and (4) cholestatic liver disease (drugs, PBC, PSC, occasionally hepatitis A). Hyperthyroidism, renal cell cancer, and CHF can also increase alk phos. Ultrasound and AMA should be obtained. If there is obstruction, then ERCP is generally indicated to identify and remove stones or to diagnose and stent obstructing tumors. If alk phos levels are <50% above normal and the initial studies are normal, then observation is appropriate (Nejm 2000;342:1266). If alk phos is >50% elevated and initial studies are normal, then MRCP (or selectively ERCP) is done to look for PSC or other evidence of obstruction. If MRCP is normal, then a liver bx to look for evidence of PBC with a negative antimitochondrial antibody is usually indicated.

Approach to Jaundice: Jaundice can arise from mechanical obstruction, intrinsic liver disease, or overproduction of bilirubin from hemolysis. **Hemolysis** is suspected when (1) the bilirubin is <6.0 mg/dL, (2) the indirect (unconjugated) fraction is >50% of the total (usually 80%), (3) the remainder of the LFTs are normal, (4) splenomegaly is present (a variable finding), and (5) there is anemia with a reticulocytosis. **Mechanical obstruction** presents acutely in the form of common duct stones. These pts usually have sudden pain sometimes radiating to the back, and may have fever if there is associated cholangitis (infected bile). In the first few days of illness the transaminases may be as high as 300-1000, sometimes raising the question of viral hepatitis. As obstruction persists, the alk phos climbs and the transaminases fall. Obstruction from malignancy often presents as painless jaundice. Jaundice from **intrinsic liver disease** can present in a **hepatocellular** pattern (transaminases >5-10 times normal, alk phos <3 times normal) or a **cholestatic** pattern (transaminases <5 times normal, alk phos >3-5 times normal). Hepatocellular patterns are seen with viral hepatitis, some drug hepatitis (especially acetaminophen), autoimmune hepatitis, ischemic hepatitis, Wilson's disease, mononucleosis, and environmental toxins. Cholestatic patterns are seen with alcoholic hepatitis (in which transaminases are usually <300 mg/dL and AST>ALT), PBC, PSC, some drug hepatitis, and, on occasion, hep A.

The initial evaluation of jaundice includes a CBC, CMP, PT, and ultrasound. If there is no evidence of hemolysis and the hx and ultrasound do not suggest obstruction or a mass, then the studies detailed above for abnormal transaminases (plus hep A IgM antibody) are obtained. If the pattern is cholestatic, an AMA is also obtained. If obstruction is seen, it is generally evaluated with ERCP. If the presentation is acute and ascites is seen on the ultrasound, Budd-Chiari should be considered. Ascites should be evaluated (p 436). If the story suggests obstruction and the ultrasound shows normal ducts, it is important to consider that bile duct dilatation may be minimal early in the course of obstruction from stones. If there is underlying cirrhosis, the bile ducts may not dilate at all despite obstruction.

Evaluation of Cirrhosis: The evaluation of an adult pt with stigmata of cirrhosis or with an imaging test suggesting cirrhosis is similar to that of asymptomatic elevated transaminases (p 43). Testing for hep A is not necessary since that illness is never chronic. Alcohol, hep B, and hep C are the most common causes. Studies should be obtained for hepatitis B (HBsAg, and Anti-HBc), hepatitis C (serum antibody and PCR study if the ab is negative and the cause is not found), hemochromatosis (Fe/TIBC, ferritin), Wilson's (ceruloplasmin if pt <40 yrs), autoimmune hepatitis (ANA, ASMA, SPEP), and alpha-1 antitrypsin deficiency. An AMA should be obtained if there is substantial elevation of alk phos or other features of PBC (p 386). The liver should be imaged to rule out mass or obstruction. Long-standing obstruction can cause cirrhosis. MRCP or ERCP may be appropriate to evaluate the question of PSC (p 391) if the alk phos is very high or the pt has IBD. Evaluation for hepatic vein thrombosis (Budd-Chiari syndrome) is very selectively indicated (p 451). Endoscopy is indicated in established cirrhosis to look for varices that may benefit from medical rx to prevent bleeding (p 429). Liver bx confirms the presence of cirrhosis and may give clues to the etiology. However, in most cases the etiology is evident from the hx and lab studies and liver bx is not needed. In about 5-10% of cases the etiology is not determined (so-called "cryptogenic cirrhosis").

Approach to Isolated Elevated Bilirubin: The most common cause of an isolated elevated bilirubin is **Gilbert's syndrome.** Hyperbilirubinemia in Gilbert's syndrome is caused by an inherited deficiency in enzymes for bilirubin glucuronidation. The diagnosis is made by the presence of an unconjugated hyperbilirubinemia (>60% indirect/unconjugated fraction), no evidence of hemolysis, and otherwise normal LFTs. It effects >2% of the population and is found incidentally on biochemical testing. Life expectancy is normal and there is no clinical illness (Scand J Gastroenterol 1989;24:617). Rare causes of isolated hyperbilirubinemia include Crigler-Najjar syndrome, Dubin-Johnson, and Rotor syndrome (Sherlock S and Dooley J. Diseases of the liver and biliary system. 10th ed. Boston: Blackwell Science, 1997: 210-213).

Approach to Fulminant Hepatic Failure (FHF): (Lancet 1997;349:1081) This condition is defined by the abrupt onset of massive hepatic necrosis. It usually occurs in pts without underlying liver disease, but can be seen in Wilson's disease, hep D infection in hep B carriers, and autoimmune hepatitis. The most common causes are acetaminophen overdose, viral hepatitis, acute fatty liver of pregnancy, Reye's syndrome, *Amanita phalloides* mushroom poisoning, hyperthermia, vascular occlusion, and rarely other drugs or other viruses (Am J Gastroenterol 1993;88:1000). The course is complicated by cerebral edema in 80%. Cerebral edema is the most common cause of death in these pts. Other complications include renal failure, bacterial infection, hypoglycemia, hemorrhage, and circulatory collapse. Management is complex and pts should be treated in referral centers with a liver transplant program. The outlook is grim, with 60-80% mortality.

Approach to Elevated Prothrombin Time (PT): The question of liver disease is often raised by the finding of an elevated PT. The differential is largely between vitamin K deficiency and hepatic disease. The pt should be given vitamin K 10 mg sc qdx3 and the PT repeated. If the PT normalizes with vitamin K within a few days (typically improvement is seen in 24 hours), the cause was vitamin K deficiency. Otherwise intrinsic liver disease is likely.

Approach to Cholangitis: Pts with cholangitis present with the combination of fever, upper abdominal pain, and jaundice. In elderly, demented, or immunosuppressed pts, pain and fever may not be obvious. The most common cause of cholangitis is bacterial infection secondary to bile duct obstruction from stones (p 345). Ascariasis is a common cause of cholangitis in Asia (p 283). When cholangitis is suspected, ultrasound is obtained to rule out hepatic abscess and to look for evidence of obstruction. ERCP is usually needed for dx and rx.

Table 1.11   Child-Pugh Classification of Severity of Liver Disease

Clincal Feature	Points Scored		
	1 Point	2 Points	3 Points
Encephalopathy	None	Grades 1 and 2	Grades 3 and 4
Ascites	Absent	Slight	Moderate
Bilirubin (mg/dL)	1–2	2–3	>3
Albumin (gm/dL)	>3.5	2.8–3.5	<2.8
Prothrombin time (sec prolonged)			
	1–3	4–6	>6

Grade A: 5–6 points
Grade B: 7–9 points
Grade C: 10–15 points

Approach to Hepatic Mass: See p 418.

Child-Pugh Classification: (Hepatology 1987;7:660) This classification is commonly used to grade severity of cirrhosis. It is used to varying degrees in clinical studies and in assessing surgical risk. The system is presented in Table 1.11 (Brit J Surg 1973;60:646). To use the system, encephalopathy must be graded. Encephalopathy is called Grade 3 if there is somnolence to semistupor, confusion, and gross disorientation. It is called Grade 4 if coma is present. In Grades 1-2, mental status changes are less severe (Aliment Pharmacol Ther 1996;10:681).

Chapter 2
Esophagus

2.1 Gastroesophageal Reflux Disease

Am Fam Phys 1999;59:1161; Jama 1996;276:983; Arch IM
1995;155:2165; Am J Gastro 1999;94:1434

Cause: Episodes of gastroesophageal reflux occur normally in asymptomatic individuals. However, excessive duration and frequency of
reflux events lead to a symptomatic illness referred to as gastroesophageal reflux disease (GERD).

Epidem: Lack of a gold standard for GERD makes epidemiologic
studies difficult to perform, and data are limited (Digestion
1992;51:24). In the general population, reflux symptoms occur
monthly in 15-44%, weekly in 10-14%, and daily in 4-7%.
Reflux sx occur with equal frequency in males and females,
though Barrett's is more frequent in males. The prevalence of
endoscopic esophagitis is about 1.1%. The incidence of GERD
rises steadily after the age of 40. The mortality is low at 0.10 per
100,000 per year (excluding adenocarcinoma from Barrett's)
(World J Surg 1992;16:288).

Pathophys:
- Transient relaxation of the lower esophageal sphincter (LES) is
  an important cause of reflux events both in normals (J Clin
  Invest 1980;65:256) and in pts with esophagitis (Nejm
  1982;307:1547). Newer evidence suggests that the frequency of
  these transient relaxations is not higher in GERD pts than
  normal but that when relaxations occur they are more likely to

be associated with reflux of acid in GERD pts (Am J Gastro 2001;96:2569). Transient relaxation is not the mechanism of GERD in hiatus hernia (GE 2000;119:1439).

- Some episodes of reflux are due to abrupt increases in intra-abdominal pressure that overcomes LES pressure (Nejm 1982;307:1547). This is probably a greater factor in pts with more severe grades of esophagitis than in those with mild disease (Gut 1995;36:505).
- Hiatal hernia has been convincingly implicated as a contributor to reflux. The right diaphragmatic crus, which encircles the LES, augments LES pressure, particularly with sudden increases in abdominal pressure that occur with coughing and inspiration. Hiatal hernia interferes with this increased LES pressure, and the larger the hernia, the smaller the benefit of the crus in preventing reflux (Ann IM 1992;117:977).
- About 30% of pts with heartburn severe enough to require self-medication with antacids have sensitivity to esophageal acid infusion or balloon distension despite normal endoscopies and pH probes. A lower threshold for esophageal pain may play a role in this subgroup of pts (Am J Gastroenterol 1999;94:628).
- Delayed gastric emptying is an important mechanism for GERD in a small subgroup of pts (GE 1981;80:285).
- In progressive systemic sclerosis (scleroderma), impaired esophageal acid clearance due to poor motility in the distal esophagus and a hypotensive esophagus are the primary defects (Dig Dis Sci 1992;37:833).
- Emotional stress (caused by stressful tasks like playing video games and doing math problems!) increases the subjective severity of reflux symptoms but not the actual number or duration of reflux events. The data suggest that pts who are anxious or subjected to stress may perceive minimal esophageal reflux as major symptomatic events.
- Reflux in smokers is most often due to the combination of a decreased resting LES pressure and the abrupt increases in

intra-abdominal pressure associated with coughing and deep inspiration (Gut 1990;31:4).

- *H. pylori* infection limited to the antrum might worsen reflux by increasing acidity but more commonly (especially in the developing world), *H. pylori* gastritis infects the antrum and body of the stomach and the resultant gastritis reduces acid production and reduces the incidence of GERD (Am J Gastro 2004;99:1222). There is strong inverse relationship between *H. pylori* infection and severe forms of GERD such as Barrett's esophagus (Am J Gastro 2004;99:1213).

Sx: Frequencies of sx are difficult to establish because of the lack of a clear gold standard defining GERD and the lack of population-based studies. Important sx include:

- *Heartburn* (a retrosternal burning sensation) is the most common sx for which pts will use many synonyms, including indigestion and sour stomach.
- *Gross regurgitation* of gastric contents, particularly after bending or with recumbency. Pts will often incorrectly report this as vomiting. It is distinguished from vomiting by the lack of the intense nausea that generally precedes vomiting, by the lack of force, and seemingly spontaneous nature of the sx. Minor episodes might only leave a bitter, hot taste in the mouth, especially upon awakening.
- *Dysphagia*, the sensation that food sticks in the chest (see p 9). Dysphagia is one of the most helpful clues to a dx of GERD if pts have primarily high epigastric pain or nausea.
- *Odynophagia*, painful swallowing, is less common than dysphagia and suggests the possibility of infections (candida, herpes) or pill esophagitis, especially if sx are of sudden onset.
- *Belching*, a frequent cause of reflux events in normal pts.
- *Nausea* is not rare, and intractable nausea can be the primary presenting complaint (Ann Intern Med 1997;126:704).

- *Chest pain*, with or without other typical reflux sx, that may be difficult to distinguish from cardiac chest pain by history alone (p 90).
- *Hoarseness*, repetitive throat clearing, sensation of fullness in the back of the throat (globus sensation), and chronic cough are associated with GERD (Gastrointest Endosc 1995;43:225; Clin Gastroenterol Hepatol 2003;1:333).
- *Asthma* is frequently found in association with GERD with up to half of pts in asthma clinics having symptomatic GERD and up to 80% of asthma pts having abnormal pH probes (Chest 1998;114:275).
- *Water brash*, the abrupt, episodic salivation of large volumes filling the mouth is an uncommon sx.

Si: Usually none.

Crs: GERD is a chronic illness and chronic rx is needed except in mild disease. Erosive esophagitis has a relapse rate of 50-80% in 6-12 months without maintenance (Arch IM 1996;156:477).

Cmplc: Esophageal stricture (see p 72) and Barrett's esophagus (see p 67).

Diff Dx: The dx is usually made on the basis of the H&P. With a wide variety of presenting sx, the diff dx for GERD can be quite broad. For typical sx (heartburn, regurgitation, dysphagia), consider PUD, especially with secondary reflux due to gastric outlet obstruction, esophageal infection (expect some odynophagia/dysphagia), gastroparesis, non ulcer dyspepsia, massive hiatal hernia, esophageal cancer, achalasia (fermenting food debris in esophagus), angina, and biliary tract disease (p 4).

Lab:
- *Technique for pH probe:* (Am J Med 1997;103:130S; GE 1996;110:1982). In ambulatory pH probe studies, a pH probe is passed through the nostril and positioned 5 cm above the manometrically determined LES. The pH is recorded every 6-8 seconds. The accurate placement of the probe is crucial.

The extra step of determining the location of the LES with manometry is necessary, because determining the LES location by fluoroscopy, endoscopy, or by seeing the step-up in pH that occurs when the catheter is pulled back from stomach to esophagus is not reliable (GE 1996;110:1982). Pts usually find the probe tolerable, though not pleasant. It is attached to a recorder worn by the pt. The pt indicates the occurrence of events such as meals, sleeping, or symptoms (heartburn, chest pain, cough) by pushing an event marker on the device and by means of a diary. Pts who pull the probe out after an hour because they cannot stand it are also providing their physicians with valuable information about their tolerance of discomfort. A wireless system using a pH telemetry device placed endo-scopically (Bravo pH System) is an alternative to an indwelling catheter (Am J Gastro 2003;98:740). Reflux episodes are defined as drops in pH to below a value of 4.0. Commercial probes provide information on percent total time $pH<4$, percent upright time $pH<4$, percent recumbent time $pH<4$, total number of episodes, and number of episodes longer than 5 minutes. The most important of these is percent time $pH<4$, which discriminates between abnormal and physi-ologic reflux. Most of the clinical application of pH probe is in the correlating of symptoms with reflux episodes.

- *Indications for pH probe:* Only a tiny proportion of pts with reflux need pH probe as part of their evaluation. AGA guide-lines (GE 1996;110:1981) suggest that pH probe is indicated for (1) proving abnormal reflux prior to sending a patient with a negative endoscopy to antireflux surgery, (2) evaluating recurrent reflux symptoms in pts who have had antireflux surgery, (3) evaluating symptoms that persist despite a month of a PPI, (4) evaluating noncardiac chest pain or throat symp-toms that do not resolve with a PPI trial, and (5) evaluating whether or not reflux episodes are associated with adult onset nonallergic asthma.

- *Intraluminal Impedance Monitoring:* This technique measures electrical impedance between pairs of electrodes attached to a plastic catheter in the esophageal lumen. During reflux of liquid, impedance falls rapidly and during reflux of gas, it rises rapidly. Thus impedance monitoring can provide information about reflux unrelated to acidity and may be of value in evaluating pts with sx unrelieved by PPIs or with atypical sx. Its clinical application has yet to be clearly defined (GE 2001;120:1862)

- *Omeprazole test:* The response of symptoms to a 14-day trial of omeprazole 40 mg daily in pts with symptoms suggestive of GERD has a positive predictive value of 68% and a negative predictive value of 63% when compared to pH probe as a gold standard (Am J Gastroenterol 1997;92:1997). The fact that this number is not higher reflects problems using pH probe as a gold standard. As a practical matter, if it sounds like GERD and gets better with omeprazole, it is probably GERD.

- *Indications for EGD:* Pts with typical GERD symptoms who respond to a course of rx usually do not benefit from endoscopy (Gastrointest Endosc 1999;49:834). EGD is clearly indicated in pts with **dysphagia** so that strictures can be found and dilated. EGD is needed in pts who show evidence of gastrointestinal blood loss, iron deficiency, or symptoms suggestive of malignancy, such as weight loss. Many physicians offer EGD to pts with sx of several years' duration, because they are at a higher risk of developing Barrett's esophagus. The benefit of this widely used approach is unproven (see Barrett's esophagus, p 67). Endoscopy is also appropriate for pts whose symptoms do not respond to a course of rx. Endoscopy in this group may demonstrate esophagitis, stricture, Barrett's, or there may be an alternative explanation of symptoms, such as PUD, gastric outlet obstruction, gastroparesis with retained food, malignancy, candida, or herpetic esophagitis.

- *Grading of esophagitis:* Several grading systems for esophagitis exist and serve as important tools for clinical studies. Grades are commonly used in endoscopy reports. The Savary-Miller system (Gastrointest Endosc Clin N Am 1994;4:677) and the Los Angeles classification (Gut 1999;45:172) are two common grading systems.
- *Endoscopic bx* should be performed in pts with endoscopic esophagitis if they are immunosuppressed (Nejm 1994;331:656). Biopsy is less likely to be helpful if there is visible erosive change in a normal host. Pts with grossly normal esophageal mucosa may benefit from biopsy. If biopsy shows convincing histologic evidence of reflux, the pt may be spared a pH probe for definitive diagnosis. Intraesophageal eosinophils are perhaps the most useful diagnostic findings in reflux, though basal zone thickness and height of papillae are also helpful if specimens are properly oriented (Gastroenterol Clin North Am 1990;19:631).

X-ray: UGI series may show evidence of free reflux, a patulous gastroesophageal junction, esophageal fold thickening due to esophagitis, esophageal ulcer, or stricture. However, UGI series is not a sensitive test for GERD, and the mere occurrence of reflux during an exam is not specific. Therefore, UGI series is rarely useful for diagnosis in pts with GERD.

Rx:

- *Patient teaching:* There is no simple therapeutic recipe appropriate for all pts with GERD. The most common error is failing to appreciate the severity and chronicity of a pt's complaints and offering him inadequate rx. Rx begins by teaching pts the basic pathophys of GERD so that they understand why their sx are likely to be chronic without appropriate rx. Most physicians suggest diet and lifestyle modifications despite the lack of critical evidence that such measures change outcomes (Am J Gastroenterol 2000;95:2692). Pts should be advised to

(1) avoid large meals, (2) avoid eating within 3 hours of bed-time, (3) stop smoking, and (4) if tolerable, elevate the head of the bed by 6 inches. Diet can be modified to minimize high fat foods, chocolate, caffeine, citrus, alcohol, and tomato products (Mayo Clin Proc 2001;76:1002). Coffee produces reflux greater than that of tea containing equal caffeine concentrations. Decaffeination reduces the reflux caused by coffee, probably by removing substances in coffee other than just the caffeine (Aliment Pharmacol Ther 1994;8:283). The milder the GERD sx, the more likely that these modifications will make an impact on the need for drug therapy.

- *Drug rx:* There are two approaches to drug rx. In some cases it is best to start with a PPI for rapid sx relief and to switch to an H2RA after sx are completely relieved. Alternatively, one can begin with H2RA and intensify rx if sx are not relieved. Severity of sx and cost of rx are major factors.
- *Histamine-2 blockers:* There are four available H2RAs in the U.S. (see Table 2.1). For pts with mild to moderate symptoms, H2RAs are often effective for sx control. Because they do not suppress acid production completely, the H2RAs are less effec-tive for healing esophagitis, especially if the esophagitis is high grade (Jama 1996;276:983). **Ranitidine** and **famotidine** are currently the most sensible choices. They are available generi-cally, thus reducing cost, and do not have the many drug inter-actions seen with cimetidine. For pts without prescription insurance, it is sometimes cheaper to shop for the OTC H2RA

Table 2.1   H2 Receptor Antagonists

Drug	Rx Dosage	OTC Dosage
Cimetidine	400 mg po bid	200 mg po bid
Ranitidine	150 mg po bid	75 mg po bid
Famotidine	20 mg po bid	10 mg po bid
Nizatidine	150 mg po bid	75 mg po bid

blockers and double up on the dose, because competitive market forces have driven the cost down. H2RAs are usually given twice a day, before breakfast and before supper. They can be supplemented with antacids as needed.

- *Proton pump inhibitors:* There are 5 PPIs available in the U.S. (see Table 2.2). PPIs should be offered to pts who require the most rapid relief, to those with advanced degrees of esophagitis, and to those with strictures. Little differentiates the drugs clinically, and cost (often a function of the patient's insurance) is frequently the deciding factor in choosing an agent. The availability of OTC omeprazole (Prilosec OTC 20 mg) has made PPIs much more affordable to the uninsured.

The differences between PPIs may be most evident in pts with the most severe disease. Esomeprazole, the S-isomer of omeprazole, when used in a dose of 40 mg, is more effective than 20 mg omeprazole in healing esophagitis and controlling sx (Am J Gastro 2001;96:656). Esomeprazole (40 mg) is slightly more effective than 30 mg of lansoprazole in healing erosive disease with differences greatest in severe disease (Am J Gastro 2002;97:575).

Correct dosing instructions are crucial. The PPIs are pro-drugs that require an acidic environment for binding (GE 2000;118:S9). This occurs when the parietal cell is activated by the stimulation of meals. PPIs are most effective after an overnight fast when levels of the proton pump on canalicular

Table 2.2 Proton Pump Inhibitors

Drug	Sizes	Usual Total Daily Dose
Omeprazole	10, 20, 40 mg	20-40 mg
Lansoprazole	15, 30 mg	30-60 mg
Rabeprazole	20 mg	20-40 mg
Pantoprazole	40 mg	40-80 mg
Esomeprazole	20, 40 mg	20-80 mg

membranes are highest. Therefore, single doses should be taken 30 min to 1 hour ac breakfast. The drugs should not be given concomitantly with H2RAs or prostaglandins that will reduce PPI binding. Steady state occurs in a few days and bid dosing may be useful in the first few days. If a second dose is needed, it should be given 30 min to 1 hour ac supper. The PPIs can be expected to heal esophagitis in 80% or more of pts (versus about 50% with H2RAs) and free pts of heartburn in a similar proportion (GE 1997;112:1798). If one PPI fails, it is worthwhile trying another, because individual response varies.

- *Promotility agents*: Promotility agents are appealing in theory because they more directly address the pathophysiology of reflux. Delayed gastric emptying, inadequate LES pressure, and esophageal acid clearance are all potentially reversible with the ideal agent. As first line rx, cisapride (Propulsid) was shown to be as effective as H2RAs for mild disease (Arch IM 1995;155:2165) and it was used in maintenance rx (Nejm 1995;333:1106). However, cisapride was withdrawn from the U.S. market because it caused life-threatening arrhythmias related to drug interactions and because of the drug's effect in prolonging the QT interval. Metoclopramide (Reglan) should only be tried as a last resort in selected pts because of its limited effectiveness and the possibility of serious irreversible movement disorders (mostly tardive dyskinesia) (Arch IM 1989;149:2486).

- *Sucralfate*: This agent binds to ulcer bases and binds to pepsin and bile salts. It has efficacy similar to H2RAs in some trials (Am J Med 1991;91:2A). Its most frequent use may be in pregnant pts where its minimal absorption is perceived as a possible benefit.

- *Maintenance therapy*: GERD is a chronic disorder that usually requires chronic therapy. Maintenance rx is sensible to (1) control symptoms of relapsing disease or (2) to prevent complications of erosive esophagitis. For pts with symptomatic disease but minimal endoscopic esophagitis, intermittent rx with either omeprazole or ranitidine works well for about half of pts (BMJ 1999;318:502). Rapid recurrence of symptoms or slow response to retreatment should lead to continuous maintenance rx with the lowest dose of an antisecretory agent that controls symptoms.

The first step in tapering rx is to reduce PPI use to once daily. Most pts requiring multiple dose PPIs can be tapered to single dose rx with good relief (Am J Gastro 2003;98:1940). If daily PPI rx is well tolerated for a month or two, the patient can switch to ranitidine 150-300 mg bid or famotidine 20-40 mg bid. This can be tapered further if symptoms remain well controlled. If sx recur with the taper, therapy with the previously effective agent at the previously effective dose is resumed.

For pts with endoscopic esophagitis, a very strong argument can be made for maintenance rx to prevent symptomatic relapses and complications (Arch IM 1995;155:1465). It is intuitive, though not well proven, that preventing the relapse of erosive esophagitis might prevent progression to the more severe complications of stricture and Barrett's esophagus. For erosive disease, the PPIs are clearly superior to H2RAs, and if one chooses to control esophagitis rather than sx, then chronic PPI rx is rational (Arch IM 1999;159:649; Ann Intern Med 1996;124:859; GE 1994;107:1305).

- *Long-term PPI safety:* Initially, omeprazole was released in the U.S. with a warning on its package insert cautioning against prolonged use. Animal models raised the concern that long-term rx may cause carcinoid tumors of the stomach. Widespread human use has not borne this out. There is an increased risk of atrophic gastritis (and therefore theoretically gastric cancer) in pts infected with *H. pylori* and maintained on omeprazole, though dysplasia associated with atrophy is rare (GE 2000;118:661). This has prompted many clinicians to eradicate the organism if a long-term PPI is used. B_{12} malabsorption may occur (Ann IM 1994;120:211), though it is usually not a clinically evident problem and can usually be prevented with an oral B_{12} supplement. Because of decreased gastric acidity, pts may be more susceptible to small intestinal bacterial overgrowth (Gut 1996;39:54) or acute infectious gastroenteritis.

• *Refractory GERD symptoms:* Some pts will not respond to conventional once-a-day dosing of PPIs with the relief of symptoms. In this case the dx should be carefully reconsidered. Malignancy, esophageal infection, gastroparesis, achalasia, and heart disease must be excluded. The most common reason for PPI failure is improper timing of doses.

If a bid PPI is ineffective, a pH probe on rx should be done to determine if the patient has inadequate pH control despite rx. For the small minority who will turn out to have inadequate pH control, a pH probe will be cheaper than increasing PPI doses for months on end. For those without good control by pH probe, a dx of ZE syndrome should be considered (p 145), and surgery or higher dose PPIs are the rx choices. Many pts on bid PPIs will have nocturnal periods of intragastric pH drops below 4.0 lasting more than an hour. This has been called nocturnal acid breakthrough (Aliment Pharmacol Ther 1998;12:1231). These pH drops in the stomach are associated with reflux events. The proportion of pts with refractory sx who have nocturnal acid breakthrough is unknown. The addition of ranitidine 300 mg qhs is effective in reducing nocturnal acid breakthrough (GE 1998;115:1335). This is more effective than a bedtime dose of omeprazole, perhaps because the meal-stimulated acid secretion necessary for omeprazole binding does not occur, or perhaps because histamine is more important in nocturnal acid secretion.

Some pts have persistent sx due to reflux of nonacidic gastric contents. Such pts may respond to metoclopramide in doses of 5-10 mg ac and qhs in addition to PPI rx. Long-term use should be avoided because of the risk of tardive dyskinesia. In some of these pts, gastroparesis has not been recognized as the major problem and a gastric emptying scan may be helpful (p 130).

In some pts with typical symptoms and normal endoscopies and pH probes, esophageal hypersensitivity may be the primary problem. When these pts are refractory to acid-blocking rx, there may be a role for other therapies (eg, antidepressants) to modulate the hypersensitivity, but this approach has not been well studied (Ann Intern Med 1996;124:950).

• *Surgical therapy for GERD:* While medical rx offers excellent relief of symptoms for the majority of pts, surgical rx is indicated in several circumstances. Surgery should be considered in (1) pts who would rather have surgery than take medications chronically and who are willing to accept the potential risks of surgery and (2) pts whose symptoms are not adequately controlled by medical rx.

The most common surgical approach has been the **Nissen fundoplication,** in which a portion of the mobilized gastric fundus is passed posteriorly to the esophagus and wrapped around the GE junction. The procedure was first performed by open laparotomy but is now widely being performed by the laparoscopic approach (World J Surg 1999;23:356). The laparoscopic method has a higher risk of dysphagia (by RCT [Lancet 2000;355:170]) but is associated with reduced morbidity and shorter hospital stay (Ann Surg 2004;239:325). In pts with poor motility, a 270-degree wrap (the Toupet fundoplication) can be used. In pts with foreshortened esophagus, the Collis gastroplasty (creating a tube of stomach as a neoesophagus) can be used. In pts with severe obesity, a transthoracic approach may be preferred. There is no single operation appropriate for all pts, and the choice of operation needs to be tailored to the anatomy of the patient (J Thorac Cardiovasc Surg 1995;110:141).

Based on a large series, the following results might be expected with laparoscopic Nissen fundoplication in expert hands (Ann Surg 1996;223:673): (1) relief of heartburn 93%; (2) elimination of atypical symptoms 87%; (3) minor complications 6%; (4) major complications 2%; (5) reoperation 2%; and (6) fundoplication failure 2%. Mortality in large series is about 0.2% (Surg Laparosc Endosc 1997;7:17). Data from 5-year follow-up indicates that the LES pressure drops over that period but that 86% of pts are satisfied with the outcome (J Am Coll Surg 2003;196:51).

Dysphagia is reported in 3-24% of pts undergoing fundoplication and can usually be treated by dilatation, except in those pts with a slipped fundoplication or in those pts who have had second operations (Am J Gastroenterol 1996;91:2318).

Upper endoscopy should be performed in all pts prior to fundoplication. If EGD shows erosive esophagitis, then surgery is one of the appropriate choices. A 24-hour pH probe is unnecessary if EGD shows erosions. If EGD is normal and the diagnosis is in doubt, then pH probe may be helpful in determining the certainty of the diagnosis and the appropriateness of surgery. Motility testing will change the operative approach in the 10% of pts in whom poor esophageal motility is found and an incomplete wrap is performed. Many experts use manometry in all pts prior to fundoplication.

There is a learning curve in laparoscopic fundoplication. This curve is at least 20 cases for an individual surgeon and 50 cases for a small group working together. The rates of complications, reoperation, and conversion to open procedures are all higher on the early portion of the learning curve (Ann Surg 1996;224:198). Causes of failure of antireflux procedures include disruption of initial repair (46%), repair around the stomach instead of esophagus (23%), a too-tight or too-long repair (10%), unrecognized esophageal motor disorder (9%), herniation (6%), and gastric denervation (6%) (Am J Surg 1996;171:36).

- *Endoscopic Treatment of GERD:* A variety of endoscopic methods are under development as alternatives to surgical fundoplication or medical therapy. Endoscopic injection of a nonresorbable polymer (Enteryx) into the region of the LES reduces reflux events and improves heartburn in 12-month follow-up (Am J Gastro 2003;98:1921). Endoscopic sewing or plicating methods that are modestly effective in short-term follow-up have been described (Gut 2003;52:34; Gastro Endosc 2004;59:163). Radiofrequency energy delivery to the LES (the Stretta procedure) reduces heartburn and improves quality of life, though it does not reduce esophageal acid exposure (GE 2003;125:668). Further study and long-term follow-up studies are needed.
- *Reflux during pregnancy:* First-line rx for symptomatic pts with GERD should include antacids or sucralfate. Cimetidine and ranitidine are the preferred H2RAs for pregnant pts (Gastroenterol Clin North Am 1998;27:153). There is limited experience with PPI use in pregnant pts, but omeprazole is probably safe (Am J Obgyn 1998;179:727).

2.2 Barrett's Esophagus

Am Fam Phys 2004;69:2113; Nejm 2002;346:836

Epidem: The mean onset of Barrett's is probably 40 years of age, the mean age of dx 55-60 years. M:F ratio is 4:1. It occurs 10-20 times more frequently in whites than blacks. It is more frequent in smokers and the obese. In pts having upper endoscopy for any reason, the prevalence is 1-2%. It is found in 8-12% of pts having endoscopy for GERD sx (Arch IM 1996;156:2174).

Pathophys:
- Barrett's esophagus is currently defined as a change in the esophageal epithelium of any length that is shown on bx to have intestinal metaplasia. Earlier definitions have required a

length of >3 cm without the necessity for intestinal meta-plasia. However, since intestinal metaplasia is the risk factor for adenocarcinoma, the new working definition makes this histologic feature the cornerstone (Am J Gastroenterol 1998;93:1028).

- There is convincing evidence that Barrett's is a consequence of GERD. Pts with Barrett's have high levels of acid exposure on pH probe, low resting LES pressures, and poor esophageal motility (Scand J Gastroenterol 1993;28:193). It is not clear which components of the refluxate are important in the devel-opment of Barrett's. Acid and pepsin are thought to be the most important, but biliary and pancreatic secretions, and per-haps saliva, may play a role in the metaplastic change (Arch IM 1996;156:2174).

- **Short segment Barrett's esophagus** is a length of intestinal metaplasia of less than 3 cm. Its prevalence on diagnostic EGD is an astounding 8-32%. It is associated with reflux symptoms, but pts have less severe acid exposure and better motility. The magnitude of the cancer risk associated with short segment Barrett's is unknown, but cancer is much less commonly seen in short segment than in long segment disease (metaplasia of greater than 3 cm in length) (J Clin Gastroenterol 1997;25:480).

- Barrett's is more common in pts with severe esophagitis on barium study (eg, stricture, ulcer, severe esophagitis), in those with GERD sx >5 years, and in those with scleroderma (Arch IM 1996;156:2174). EGD to detect Barrett's will have a higher yield in this group.

Sx: Sx are those of GERD, though pts with Barrett's tend to have a longer duration of sx, earlier age of onset of sx, and more fre-quently have GERD complications such as stricture (Am J Gastroenterol 1997;92:27). Up to 40% of pts who develop ade-nocarcinoma (presumably from Barrett's) have no GERD sx (Nejm 1999;340:825).

Cmplc: Adenocarcinoma complicates Barrett's in less than 0.5% of pts per yr (GE 2000;119:333). Prior overestimates due to publication bias fuel the current aggressive approach to screening. The RR of cancer in Barrett's is 30-125 compared to that of the general population. However, only a small proportion of pts with Barrett's esophagus will ultimately die of adenocarcinoma. In a series of 155 pts who did *not* undergo surveillance but who were followed up at a mean of 9.3 years, only 2.5% died of adenocarcinoma of the esophagus (Gut 1996;39:5). Survival in Barrett's pts is similar to that seen in age- and sex-matched controls (Gut 1989;30:14). Adenocarcinoma is more likely to develop in those with long segments of Barrett's, in those with hiatal hernia >3 cm, and perhaps in those with frank ulcers in Barrett's mucosa of the esophagus (Am J Gastroenterol 1999;94:3416).

Diff Dx: Intestinal metaplasia of the cardia of the stomach has an identical histologic appearance to that of Barrett's esophagus. Biopsies taken close to the apparent GE junction may actually be sampling stomach and be wrongly interpreted as showing Barrett's. Since short-segment Barrett's and intestinal metaplasia at the GE junction cannot always be distinguished, some experts offer surveillance to the pt with both conditions (GE 2004;126:567).

Endoscopy: Barrett's epithelium is suspected at endoscopy by the gross appearance of reddish to pink velvety mucosa in the distal esophagus, which generally stands out well against the more gray color of the squamous mucosa. Its presence, however, can only be proven by bx showing intestinal metaplasia. Active esophagitis can make Barrett's more difficult to detect.

Rx:

- Pts with Barrett's should have medical rx for their underlying GERD. PPIs are usually needed for adequate symptom control in these pts. However, control of symptoms is not synonymous with normalization of acid exposure. Some authors have gone so far as to suggest that proving adequate acid suppression by pH probe in Barrett's pts is necessary. However, current ACG guidelines call for control of sx alone (Am J Gastro 1999; 94:1434). Surgery is no more likely than medical rx to prevent progression of Barrett's to cancer (Am J Gastro 2003;98:2390)

- The compelling reason to consider endoscopic surveillance for Barrett's is the poor prognosis of adenocarcinoma found in symptomatic pts. Cancers found in surveillance programs do tend to be found at earlier stages and are thus more curable (Am J Gastroenterol 1998;93:1028; GE 2002;122:633). However, there are no convincing data to demonstrate that surveillance as currently practiced saves lives. Skeptics of the current approach to screening GERD pts for Barrett's and subsequent surveillance (Clin Gastroenterol Hepatol 2004;2:861) point out that (1) adenocarcinoma of the esophagus is uncommon while the number of GERD pts is enormous, (2) many pts with esophageal cancer never have GERD sx, and (3) surveillance is very costly.

    The first decision to be made with the patient is whether or not to begin a surveillance program. The data on cancer risk, the low chance of death from cancer, and the unknown benefit of surveillance should be discussed. Pts with significant comorbid illnesses are unlikely to have their lives improved by surveillance of unproven merit. Pts who are not surgical candidates are not likely to benefit from surveillance. Additional risk factors for cancer include a length of Barrett's >8-10 cm and presentation with esophageal ulcer (Arch IM 1996;156:2174; Gut 1996;39:5), and these pts may be more likely to benefit.

- Pts undergoing surveillance typically have biopsies taken from four quadrants of the esophagus, in intervals of less than 2 cm, for the entire length of the visibly abnormal epithelium. Where available, a jumbo bx forceps passed through a large-channel endoscope is preferred by some authors (GE 1993;105:40) so that larger samples can be obtained.

- Biopsies are obtained to look for dysplasia or cancer. Dysplasia is graded as negative, indefinite, low grade, high grade, and carcinoma. Interobserver agreement in the classification of dysplasia is a disappointing 72-85% among expert pathologists (Am J Gastroenterol 1998;93:1028). This makes decision-making more difficult, and a second pathological opinion is mandatory before major interventions.
- If no dysplasia is found, the ACG protocol is to use a 3-year interval of surveillance after 2 endoscopies (at unspecified intervals) are negative for dysplasia (Am J Gastro 2002;97:1888). Since ACG guidelines are based on overestimates of risk, some experts would extend the surveillance interval to 5 years (Nejm 2002;346:836).
- If low-grade dysplasia is found, then endoscopy is repeated in 3-6 months with intensive rx of the associated GERD. If dysplasia does not progress beyond low grade, endoscopy is then repeated yearly. In only 25% of pts surveyed does low-grade dysplasia persist (GE 2004;127:1233).
- The management of high-grade dysplasia is controversial. There are two choices of rx when high-grade dysplasia is found and confirmed by a second, expert pathologist. The first is esophagectomy. Surgical literature showing a 43% incidence of occult carcinoma in resection specimens of pts sent to surgery for high-grade dysplasia is cited as evidence to support surgery (Ann Surg 1996;224:66). In a recent series of 15 pts with high-grade dysplasia, 8 progressed and 7 regressed in endoscopic follow-up over 3 years (Am J Gastroenterol 2000;95:1888). In a series of 72 veterans followed for almost 20 years with yearly endoscopy because of high-grade dysplasia, adenocarcinoma developed in only 13 pts (GE 1998;114:1149). Ten of these 13 pts underwent curative surgery, and one who was not compliant with the yearly follow-up had metastatic disease and was not resected. In another series of 28 pts who had surgery for

cancer or high-grade dysplasia, endoscopic bx reliably separated the cancers from the high-grade dysplasias (GE 1993;105:40). On the basis of this experience, intensive surveillance is an alternative to esophagectomy. The ACG guidelines recommend surveillance every 3 months for these pts. The conventional 4 jumbo bx every 2 cm is not adequate for this group (missing half the cancers that develop) and 4 bx every cm is suggested (Am J Gastroenterol 2000;95:3089).

- Ablative therapies have long been under investigation as an alternative to surgical resection or watchful waiting. Ablation can be accomplished with laser, multipolar electrocoagulation, or photodynamic rx (Gastro Endosc 2003;58:760). Its use should be limited to selected pts with high-grade dysplasia who are unfit for surgery or to those in clinical trials. ✐

2.3 Benign Esophageal Strictures and Rings

J Clin Gastroenterol 1998;27:285

Pathophys: Esophageal strictures are a common problem and are generally due to acid reflux. Rings are less commonly a clinical problem. Some of the rings detected by barium swallow turn out to be GERD-related strictures. Rings and strictures are distinguished by their thickness. Narrowings with a thickness less than 3 mm are called rings, and those thicker than 3 mm are called strictures (J Clin Gastroenterol 1998;27:285). Most strictures are reflux-related, presumably due to cycles of acid-induced inflammation and healing with scar formation. Strictures can also be caused by pill esophagitis, caustic ingestion, radiation, sclerotherapy, and esophageal surgery. The cause of rings is unclear. Some of the lower rings are reflux-related and may evolve into frank strictures. They are unlikely to be congenital since they present after age 40 years. Lower esophageal rings (Schatzki's rings) are associated with hiatal hernia. It has been suggested that as reflux-related inflammation shortens the esophagus (and lengthens the hernia), the ring is formed from pleated esophageal mucosa (Dig Dis 1996;14:323).

Sx: Intermittent solid food dysphagia is the hallmark (see detailed sx description on p 9). Pts usually do not have dysphagia unless the luminal diameter of the stricture is less than 13 mm. Pts often do not report their dysphagia sx episodes unless specifically asked.

Crs: The typical pattern is one of an increasingly frequent, intermittent dysphagia to solids, which may progress over months to years. Strictures commonly recur, and repeated dilatation may be required.

Cmplc: Food impaction requiring endoscopy for removal (see Foreign Bodies, p 77).

Diff Dx: See diff dx of dysphagia in Table 1.3.

X-ray: Strictures can be demonstrated with a barium swallow using a 13-mm barium tablet. The tablet is helpful in reproducing symptoms and demonstrating more subtle strictures. Not all pts with dysphagia require barium studies. Pts with intermittent, mild to moderate dysphagia should undergo EGD without x-ray.

Endoscopy: Strictures and rings are visible at careful endoscopy if adequate care is taken to insufflate the esophagus. Bx are indicated to rule out malignancy in new strictures and may reveal histologic evidence of associated reflux.

Rx: The mainstay of rx is dilatation using mechanical dilators or balloons. A **mercury-filled dilator** (eg, the tapered Maloney dilator) passed blindly into the esophagus without aid of a guidewire is safe and effective for simple strictures or rings.

More commonly used are the polyvinyl **Savary dilators** that are passed over a guidewire placed endoscopically into the stomach. Fluoroscopy is used by some endoscopists but is often unnecessary, especially if the scope can be advanced to the antrum to deploy the wire and keep it in a fixed position (Am J Gastroenterol 1993;88:1381). Typically, three dilators are passed sequentially in a single session with an eventual goal of dilating to at least 15 mm (in multiple sessions if needed). Bx and dilation can be completed in the same session. For narrow strictures, several sessions spaced at intervals of 1-2 weeks are used until the target is reached.

Through the scope (TTS) balloons are the other popular method of dilatation. Balloon dilatation possesses the theoretical advantage of applying only radial force to the stricture, and balloons may be better tolerated by pts than the passage of three dilators. However, in practice, there is convincing evidence that the outcomes are the same no matter which method is chosen (Gastrointest Endosc 1999;50:13). Operator preference and expense (Savary dilators are reusable) are the major determinants of the method selected.

The most feared complication of dilatation is perforation, which occurs at a rate of 1 per 500 dilatations (Gastrointest Endosc Clin N Am 1996;6:323). Much higher rates have been reported for the dilatation of caustic strictures (Radiology 1998;209:741). Bleeding and bacteremia are very uncommon complications (Gastrointest Endosc Clin N Am 1996;6:323).

There are case series of using electrocautery to cut esophageal rings as an alternative to dilatation on refractory cases (Gastrointest Endosc 1993;39:616). In strictures that rapidly recur, injection of intralesional corticosteroids appears to be effective (Gastrointest Endosc 1995;41:596; Gastro Endosc 2002;56:829). In the past, monthly dilatations and self-dilatations were needed for those with severe disease. With the advent of PPIs, frequent dilatations are rare. It is clear that all pts with reflux-related strictures should have lifelong PPI rx (or surgery). Pts who receive PPIs after dilatation have better relief of dysphagia and need fewer dilatations than those placed on H2RAs (GE 1994;106:907). In pts whose strictures recur rapidly, high-dose PPI rx may be needed, and 24-hour pH probe may be cost effective in choosing an effective dose.

2.4 Eosinophilic Esophagitis and the Ringed Esophagus

Gastro Endosc 2002;56:260; Clin Gastroenterol Hepatol 2004;2:523

Epidem: Eosinophilic esophagitis (EE) is an uncommon disorder affecting children and adults for which limited epidemiologic data are available. The disease is often unrecognized though it is likely more prevalent in children than Crohn's disease (Nejm 2004;351:940). There is a strong male predominance.

Pathophys: Eosinophils infiltrate the mucosa and probably the muscle layers of the esophagus by both allergic (IgE dependent) and IgE independent mechanisms. The allergens are not clearly known, but pediatric pts have responded to elemental diets. Long-standing eosinophilic inflammation presumably leads to the gross changes seen at endoscopy in advanced cases.

Sx: Dysphagia to solids often presenting as food impaction. Most pediatric pts have associated allergic sx (asthma, food allergy, atopy) but these findings are less frequent in adult presentations.

Crs: In adults followed for >10 years, the illness is chronic with continued dysphagia (GE 2003;125:1660). The disease remains confined to the esophagus and is not associated with malignancy. The course in children (many of whom will outgrow their atopic/allergic conditions) is unknown.

Cmplc: Perforation occurs more frequently because the dx goes unrecognized and dilatation to large diameters is improperly attempted.

Diff Dx: See Dysphagia (p 9). Eosinophilia on esophageal bx can be seen in GERD (though typically it is in the distal esophagus and only a few eosinophils per high-powered field). A variety of other uncommon illnesses may be associated with esophageal eosinophils (J Clin Gastro 2000;30:242). Some cases presenting with rings and stenosis may be congenital stenosis (see Chapter 2.5) and some authors suggest that the ringed esophagus can result from GERD (Am J Gastro 2001;96:984).

X-ray: In advanced cases barium swallow may show a narrow caliber esophagus with rings or strictures.

Endoscopy: Subtle findings include loss of the vascular pattern, vertical furrows, a speckled pattern of whitish exudate that looks like candida but is actually eosinophilic infiltrations. More obvious findings include narrow caliber, the appearance of multiple rings, or a corrugated appearance. A dominant stricture in the distal esophagus may be seen.

Rx: Elimination diets may be useful, especially in children (Gastroenterol Clin North Am 2003;32:949). Oral steroids are effective but potentially toxic. Fluticasone proprionate 220 mcg/puff twice daily for 6 weeks provides relief for up to 4 months. The drug is swallowed, given without a spacer, and the mouth is rinsed with water after use (Mayo Clin Proc 2003;78:830). A minority of pts improve with PPIs given for what is likely secondary reflux. Dysphagia improves with dilatation but is risky with long linear tears frequently occurring. Reinspection with endoscopy after the passage of each dilator seems prudent.

2.5 Congenital Esophageal Stenosis and the Ringed Esophagus

Am J Gastroenterol 2000;95:32

Epidem: Some reputed adult cases of congenital esophageal stenosis are probably misdiagnosed ringed esophagus (see Chapter 2.4). The incidence is estimated to be 1 per 25,000 live births (Dig Dis Sci 1993;38:369).

Pathophys: Stenosis occurs due to tracheobronchial rings that presumably arise from sequestration of tracheobronchial precursor cells in the esophageal wall (Dig Dis Sci 1993;38:369).

Sx: Dysphagia to solids that usually goes back as far as the patient can remember. Pts usually have had multiple episodes of food impaction and are slow eaters.

Crs: Chronic dysphagia.

Cmplc: Perforation occurs more frequently because the dx goes unrecognized and dilatation to large diameters is improperly attempted.

Diff Dx: See Dysphagia (p 9) and Chapter 2.4.

X-ray: The proximal esophagus is dilated. In the upper esophagus, there is a long stenotic segment with multiple fine rings visible within in it. This appearance has been called "funnel esophagus."

Endoscopy: The proximal esophagus is dilated. In the stenotic segment, numerous cartilagenous rings, which have been described as having a coiled spring appearance, are seen (Dig Dis Sci 1993;38:369).

Rx: Treat esophagitis if present. Dilate with caution to a diameter the patient can live with and emphasize to the patient the need for careful chewing.

2.6   Foreign Bodies

Gastro Endosc 2002;55:802; Gastrointest Endosc 1995;41:33

Comment: This discussion does not cover FB above the cricopharyngeus. Guidelines for management of very young children may be different than guidelines presented here.

Epidem: Most FB ingestions occur in children from 6 months to 3 years. In adults, the majority of the FB are food impactions from esophageal pathology. Ingestions are also associated with psychiatric illness and mental retardation. Prisoners may ingest FB for secondary gain.

Pathophys: FB may impact in the esophagus in areas of stricturing and in normal anatomic areas of narrowing or angulation, such as cricopharyngeus, aortic arch, left mainstem bronchus, pylorus, duodenal sweep, ileocecal valve, and anus. Most objects pass spontaneously, but sharp objects create a risk of perforation.

Sx: Most pts will clearly describe the sensation of an FB in the esophagus, though their perception of the exact location may not be correct. A complete obstruction due to an esophageal FB usually presents as pain and the inability to handle oral secretions. Objects that pass beyond the esophagus are usually asymptomatic unless perforation or obstruction occur. The type of suspected FB (eg, food, pin, toothpick, etc) should be established.

Si: The exam is unhelpful unless perforation occurs, in which case there may be crepitus in the neck or findings of peritonitis.

Crs: About 80-90% of objects pass spontaneously, 10-20% require endoscopy, and less than 1% require surgery (Gastrointest Endosc 1995;41:39).

Cmplc: Perforation, obstruction.

X-ray: Radiopaque objects may be localized with plain films, but many ingested objects are not radiopaque. Contrast studies should be avoided because of the risk of aspiration.

Endoscopy: Endoscopy is indicated in some specific instances for FB removal (see Rx). A variety of instruments (snare, basket, retrieval nets, rat tooth forceps, alligator forceps, overtubes, endoscope hoods) may be required. Rigid endoscopy has a higher complication rate and should be used in the esophagus only if a flexible scope fails (Gastrointest Endosc 1993;39:626).

Rx: The characteristics of the object and its location in the GI tact determine management. **Food boluses** impacted in the esophagus should be removed promptly if there is evidence of distress or inability to handle secretions. If the patient is comfortable, the procedure can be delayed in case the bolus passes spontaneously, but it should be removed within 12-24 hours of ingestion. The bolus is usually removed with a snare or basket through a flexible scope with conscious sedation. An overtube can facilitate multiple passages of the scope and offers airway protection. Some experts blindly but gently push boluses into the stomach and fragment them with a snare if need be to promote passage (Gastro Endosc 2001;53:178). Barium studies should be avoided since they make endoscopy difficult. Glucagon can be given, but there are no controlled data to support its use (Emerg Med Clin N Am 1996;14:493). **Blunt objects** such as coins should be removed urgently if they are in the esophagus on plain film. However, if they reach the stomach, they are likely to pass spontaneously and should be managed conservatively (BMJ 1991;302:1321). These objects can be followed with weekly radiographs, and if they do not progress beyond the stomach, endoscopic removal is performed at 4 weeks. **Long objects** such as pens and toothbrushes should be removed since they will have difficulty passing the duodenal sweep. **Sharp, pointed objects** should be removed endoscopically. These dangerous objects often require the use of an overtube, or rubber hood over the endoscope, and in some circumstances endoscopy is done with general anesthesia. The sharp edge should be trailing to minimize the risk of puncture. Dry runs with similar objects can be helpful in selecting an instrument for grasping the object (Gastrointest Endosc 1995;41:39). **Button batteries** are managed differently because of the risk of damage from electric current or leak of alkali (Peds 1992;89:747). Batteries in the esophagus should be removed promptly, usually with a retrieval basket. If the battery is in the stomach, it should be removed only if it is large or if it fails to pass the pylorus within 48 hours. **Narcotic packets** should be left alone while the patient is observed in the hospital and should not be removed endoscopically because of the risk of rupture and fatal overdose. If packets fail to progress on radiographs, or if a toxic screen suggests leakage, they should be removed surgically (Post Grad Med J 1990;66:659).

2.7 Esophageal Cancer

Nejm 2003;349:2241; Ann Oncol 1998;9:951; Surg Oncol 1997;6:193

Epidem: The vast majority of esophageal cancers are either squamous cell or adenocarcinomas. There has been a dramatic rise in the proportion of adenocarcinomas to squamous cancers (33% adenocarcinoma in 1988 to 43% adenocarcinoma in 1993). Incidence varies widely through the world from a low of 4 per 100,000, to a high of 130 per 100,000 in endemic areas of China and Iran (Ann Oncol 1998;9:951; Semin Oncol 1994;21:403). There are a disproportionate number of (1) low socioeconomic status pts with this cancer (15% of esophageal cancer versus 10% for all other cancers), and (2) African Americans with this cancer (17% of esophageal cancers versus 8.2% for all other cancers).

Pathophys: The major risk factors for **squamous cell cancer** (see Brit J Surg 1996;83:1174; Semin Oncol 1994;21:403) are: (1) smoking (fivefold risk of smoker vs nonsmokers, tenfold risk for heavy smokers vs nonsmokers), (2) alcohol (20-50 times increased risk for heavy drinkers compared to nondrinkers), (3) nutritional deficiency (in endemic areas of China, Iran, and South Africa, diets are rich in wheat and corn and are low in carotene and vitamins), (4) dietary toxins (nitrosamines in pickled vegetables, barbecued food, and salted foods, and mycotoxins in moldy foods), (5) chronic irritation (from spicy and hot foods, achalasia, lye strictures), and possibly (6) infectious agents (papilloma virus, fungi, bacteria) (GE 1992;103:1336) and environmental factors and pollutants. The major risks for **adenocarcinoma** are: (1) Barrett's esophagus, (2) symptomatic GERD (Nejm 1999;340:825), (3) obesity (J Natl Cancer Inst 1998;90:150), (4) alcohol, and (5) the use of LES-relaxing drugs (Ann IM 2000;133:165). There may be **protective** benefits of aspirin and NSAIDs in both histologic types of esophageal cancer (GE 2003;124:47).

Sx: Dysphagia to solids, retrosternal discomfort, and weight loss.

Si: Cachexia, supraclavicular adenopathy.

Crs: The crs is similar for squamous and adenocarcinomas and depends on stage. Five-year survival for stage I disease is 42% and falls to 3% for stage IV disease. Only 25% of those with stage IV disease will survive a year (Cancer 1996;78:1820).

Tumors are divided into 4 stages based on a TNM system. Stage I tumors are limited to submucosa. Stage IIA tumors are deeper but have no evidence of local nodes. Stage IIB tumors have local nodes. Stage III lesions invade adventitia or local structures and have positive nodes. Stage IV lesions have distant mets.

Cmplc: Esophageal obstruction, tracheoesophageal fistula, blood loss, and malnutrition.

Diff Dx: Usually diagnosis is not difficult. Diagnostic confusion can arise in distinguishing benign from malignant strictures. Cancer needs to be considered if an apparently benign stricture rapidly recurs or is unusually difficult to dilate.

X-ray: Barium swallow generally reveals exophytic mass, nodularity, or stricture, all of which lead to endoscopy for diagnosis. CT scanning of chest and abdomen is useful for detecting distant metastatic disease but has an overall staging accuracy of only 67%. MRI is sensitive but not specific (Chest 1998;113:107S). PET scanning is superior to CT scanning in identifying distant disease and its use may prevent about 20% of pts from having surgery for unresectable disease (Ann Thorac Surg 1997;64:770).

Endoscopy: EGD reveals lesions that range from subtle nodularity to exophytic lesions that ulcerate. Dx is made by bx with at least 6 bx obtained. Cytology may pick up some lesions missed by bx, but a high degree of cytologic expertise is needed. EUS has a staging accuracy of about 80% in experienced hands, but is operator dependent. Overstaging occurs in about 14% and understaging occurs in up to 28% early on the learning curve and much less so (3%) with experience (Gastrointest Endosc 1996;44:58).

Rx:

- Surgical resection is the rx of choice for pts who are fit for surgical rx and who do not have evidence of distant disease. Lymphadenectomy and esophageal resection offer cure in about 20% of pts. Though cure is the goal for these pts, palliation is usually what is achieved. The choice of the surgical technique is based on location of the tumor and preference of the surgeon (Surg Clin N Am 1997;77:1169). En bloc esophagectomy may improve survival and certainly improves staging (Surg Oncol Clin N Am 1999;8:295). The data for lymphadenectomy involving cervical, mediastinal, and abdominal nodes (called three-field lymphadenectomy in the literature) also suggests improved survival compared with retrospective controls, and further prospective study seems warranted (Ann Oncol 1998;9:951). With esophagectomy, death occurs in 5%, MI in 1%, pulmonary embolus in 1%, arrhythmias in 10%, anastamotic leak in 7%, and vocal cord paralysis is seen in 4% of pts.
- Minimally invasive staging with thoracoscopy, mediastinoscopy, and laparoscopy are available, but their place in preoperative evaluation is not yet clear. However, minimally invasive surgical staging is more accurate than endoscopic ultrasound (J Thorac Cardiovasc Surg 1997;114:817).
- Because of the poor outcome with surgery alone or with radiation and chemotherapy given postoperatively, attention has turned to multimodality rx with preoperative chemotherapy and/or radiation rx (Surg Clin N Am 2002;82:729). Unfortunately, in pts with squamous carcinoma (despite more than 30 randomized controlled prospective trials with conflicting results), there is no increased resectability rate, and survival

rate and postoperative mortality rate appears higher (Brit J Surg 1999;86:727). The results are not convincingly different for adenocarcinoma (Gastroenterol Clin North Am 1997;26:635) despite some encouraging individual trials (Nejm 1996;335:462). A strong argument can be made to offer multimodality rx if at all possible in the setting of a clinical trial.

- Endoscopic palliation of dysphagia can be achieved with a variety of modalities: (1) esophageal dilatation, (2) self-expanding metal stents (SEMS), (3) Nd:YAG laser, (4) photo-dynamic therapy (application of laser light after administration of a photosensitizing material to create tumor-destroying oxygen free radicals), (5) BICAP tumor probe (which destroys tissue by direct heat), and (6) injection of ethanol or polido-canol to ablate tumor. Dilatation is inexpensive and techni-cally easy but a short duration of relief and a perforation rate of up to 5% limits its utility (Surg Clin N Am 1997;77:1197). SEMS have replaced plastic stents, which have unacceptable complication rates and limited efficacy. There are many types of stents, and technical evolutions are seemingly continuous. Immediate complications of stent placement are chest pain in 6%, bleeding in 0.2%, perforation in 1%, and stent migration in 2%. Late complications are expected in 10-30% and include bleeding (which can be fatal), stent migration, tumor ingrowth, and food impaction. Despite their limitations, SEMS have largely displaced the other techniques listed above for palliation of dysphagia. They are also rx of choice for tracheo-esophageal fistula (Chest Surg Clin N Am 1997;7:623).

2.8   Caustic Ingestion

J Clin Gastro 2003;37:119; Gastroenterol Clin North Am
    1991;20:847; Spechler S and Taylor M. Caustic Ingestions. In:
    Taylor M, ed. Gastrointestinal Emergencies. Baltimore: Williams
    Wilkins, 1997;19

Cause: Intentional ingestion of caustic substance by adults in suicide attempts and accidental ingestion of household caustics in children. Lye (a mixture of sodium and potassium hydroxide) is the most common ingestion. More dilute forms of lye, such as liquid drain cleaners that contain <10% lye, have replaced solid lye and highly concentrated liquid solutions, but are still strong enough to cause visceral perforation. Crystalline drain cleaners are 50% lye, but pain usually limits their ingestion. Most household ammonia solutions, household bleach, and detergents are weaker caustics, and catastrophic injury is uncommon. Strong acids may be encountered in swimming pool cleaners, toilet bowl cleaners, and batteries, but their accidental ingestion is much less common in the Western Hemisphere.

Epidem: Bimodal peak of incidence with children under 5 and adults 20-30, with about 80% of cases in children. About 5000-15,000 per yr in the U.S. (Am J Gastroenterol 1992;87:1).

Pathophys: Damage from lye has been experimentally studied and is divided into three phases. Initial injury occurs within seconds by a process of liquefactive necrosis accompanied over the next few days by vascular thrombosis and inflammation. Over the next 10 days, the necrosis sloughs and granulation tissue develops. Over the following months, reepithelialization occurs and strictures may develop. Ingestion of lye in concentrations of >25% is associated with gastric injury 95% of the time, but these concentrations are not readily available in the U.S. (Am J Gastroenterol 1992;87:337).

Acid produces coagulation necrosis, which may limit its depth of penetration. The esophagus is more resistant to acid injury than to alkali injury, but significant injury may occur to the esophagus and severe gastric injury may occur.

Sx: Caustic ingestion causes burning mouth pain. Cough, wheezing, and stridor are seen if aspiration occurs. In large ingestions, vomiting, chest pain, dysphagia, drooling, and epigastric pain may be seen.

Si: Oral burns (lack of oral burn does not rule out esophageal injury), wheezing, findings of peritonitis in advanced cases.

Crs: The acute phase is the initial 5 days, with si and sx described earlier. There is a latent phase of 10 days when patient may do deceptively well. Scarring occurs in third phase with 10-30% of pts developing strictures if esophageal injury occurred, and 80% of those becoming symptomatic within 8 weeks. During this phase strictures may progress rapidly and prompt evaluation, and rx are needed (Gastroenterol Clin North Am 1991;20:847). Gastric outlet obstruction can occur as a late finding 4-6 weeks or even years later. With Grade 2b injuries (See "Endoscopy") strictures develop in 70%. Grade 3a injuries are associated with complications requiring surgery in 25%. Grade 3b pts have a 70% incidence of acute complications with a mortality of 65%.

Cmplc: Esophageal or gastric perforation, esophageal stricture. Gastric outlet obstruction occurs as often in acid as in alkali ingestion, with a rate of about 5% in children requiring hospitalization (Pediatr Surg Int 1999;15:88). Squamous cancer of the esophagus is a late complication with a thousandfold relative risk of cancer. In a series of 63 pts, the mean latent period was 41 years (Cancer 1980;45:2655). These pts seem to have a better prognosis, perhaps because the cancer develops in the scar, preventing its dissemination. The ASGE recommends surveillance 15-20 years after ingestion at intervals of not more than 1-3 years, with prompt evaluation of sx.

Diff Dx: Usually the distinction between accidental and intentional ingestions is clear. Consider the ingestion of other substances in suicide attempts and consider that the patient may still be suicidal.

Lab: In suicide attempts, toxic screen for other ingested substances is indicated.

X-ray: CXR, abdominal series in suspected perforation or pneumonitis.

Endoscopy: EGD should be performed promptly if the pt is stable and without evidence of perforation or severe hypopharyngeal burns. The most risky period for EGD is 5-15 days after ingestion due to wound softening. The endoscope can be advanced until a circumferential ulceration is seen (J Clin Gastro 2003;37:119). Endoscopic findings are staged as follows. Grade 1: erythema, edema consistent with sloughing superficial mucosa. Grade 2a: friability, hemorrhage, blisters, erosions, shallow ulcers implying extension down to muscularis propria. Grade 2b: Grade 2 findings that are circumferential. Grade 3a: brown-black or gray discoloration with deep ulcers, implying possible transmural injury with erosion into adjacent structures. Grade 3b: severe involvement of 3a findings.

Rx: All pts should be brought to the emergency room. Emesis should *not* be induced. The airway should be assessed and endotracheal intubation performed if needed. There is no point to neutralizing alkali or acid in the stomach. If the patient is stable and there is no evidence of perforation clinically, EGD should be performed. Pts without injury may be discharged unless psychiatric or child safety concerns prevent it. Pts with Grade 1 or noncircumferential Grade 2 burns should be watched for 72 hours for evidence of perforation and then discharged with the assurance the strictures are unlikely. Circumferential burns need close follow-up for strictures that may develop and progress rapidly without rx. Steroids have been used to prevent stricture formation but are ineffective (Nejm 1990;323:637). Antibiotics do not appear to prevent strictures and should be used only for specific indications. Orally placed rigid esophageal stents have been used in pts who failed dilatation in the first 8 weeks with 70% success (J Pediatr Surg 1996;31:681). Symptomatic strictures are dilated, but perforation rates are higher and early recurrences are greater than with peptic strictures (Gut 1993;34:1498). Strictures with an esophageal wall thickness of greater than 9 mm by CT are very difficult to keep dilated and require multiple sessions (Gastrointest Endosc 1995;41:196). Surgical interposition may be required and carries significant mortality of 4-15% and high morbidity due to leaks and late stricturing (Pediatr Surg Int 1998;13:336).

2.9 Achalasia

Am J Gastro 1999;94:3406; Jama 1998;280:638; Gastroenterologist 1995;3:273

Cause: Unknown.

Epidem: Uncommon disorder with incidence of 0.5-1.2/100,000/yr. Incidence peaks at age 20-40 years, a with second peak in the 70s. Seen in all races and equally in the sexes.

Pathophys: The defining feature of achalasia is loss of esophageal peristalsis and failure of the LES to relax appropriately. The inhibitory neurons in Auerbach's that mediate LES relaxation are greatly reduced in number perhaps on an autoimmune or infectious basis. This results in unopposed cholinergic stimulation of the LES with inadequate relaxation.

Sx: Dysphagia, usually insidious in onset. Dysphagia is to liquids and solids, but the problems with solids may be more apparent to the patient than problems with liquids. Pts may describe a variety of maneuvers (drinking large volumes, raising arms over heads, jumping, straightening the back) to relieve sx (Jama 1998;280:638). Heartburn may occur due to fermenting, retained food in the esophagus. Chest pain is frequent and may be more prominent in younger pts. Weight loss is usually mild if present. Aspiration is uncommon.

Si: Usually none but cachexia and pneumonia may be seen.

Crs: Slow, progressive dysphagia.

Cmplc: Squamous cancer of esophagus due to stasis (RR=16) (Gut 1992;33:155). The NNT for annual surveillance EGD to detect one cancer is 406 for men and 2200 for women (Jama 1995;274:1359). Rx may lower risk.

Diff Dx: Pseudoachalasia due to destruction of neurons by cancers mimics achalasia. Other considerations are Chagas disease, non-specific motility disorders, and esophageal stricture.

Lab: Esophageal manometry is diagnostic when showing low amplitude, simultaneous contractions, and failure of the LES to relax. A variant with high amplitude, simultaneous contractions called vigorous achalasia can be identified at manometry.

X-ray: Plain films may show esophageal air fluid level. KUB may show absence of gastric air bubble. Barium swallow shows dilated esophagus, delayed passage of barium, and a bird beak of barium leading to the closed LES.

Endoscopy: May show retained food or esophagitis due to fermentation of retained debris. The sudden give of the endoscope as it pushes through the closed LES can also provide a clue, but often EGD is unrevealing.

Rx: The goal of rx is to reduce LES pressure and to allow gravity to empty the esophagus, because contractions are still not effective. There are four options for rx:

- Nifedipine and nitrates are 50-80% effective in relieving sx by lowering LES pressure. However, side effects limit their use, and long-term results are such that their use is reserved for those pts who are not candidates for more invasive rx (J Clin Gastroenterol 1999;28:202).
- Forceful disruption of the LES with a single session of pneumatic dilatation is effective for about 70% of pts over a period of 5 years of follow-up (Jama 1998;280:638). Additional dilatations improve that figure to about 80-90%. It is possible that there is lower morbidity in beginning with a 30-mm size and

increasing to 35 mm and then 40 mm for dilatations that fail at smaller diameters (Am J Gastroenterol 1993;88:34). The duration of inflation is not critical; a 6-second inflation is as effective as a 60-second inflation (Am J Gastroenterol 1998;93: 1064). The perforation rate should be in the range of 3%, though this figure varies widely in published studies. Gastrograffin swallow is sensitive for the detection of perforation. Pts treated surgically for a promptly recognized perforation undergo repair of the perforation and completion of the myotomy with a morbidity and outcome similar to morbidity and outcome of elective thoracotomy and Heller myotomy (Dig Dis Sci 1993;38:1409).

- Intrasphincteric injection of botulinum toxin results in inhibition of acetylcholine release from nerve endings. It is effective short-term rx for achalasia. About 60-70% of pts injected have a good response for 6 months (Gut 1997;41:87; Nejm 1995; 332:774). However, the response rate falls to 30% at one year (Gut 1999;44:231). This rx is an option for high-risk pts.
- Several surgical approaches to myotomy are available. The Heller myotomy, done through an abdominal incision, has been the most widely performed. Relief of dysphagia can be expected in more than 90% of pts, although reflux sx reduce the proportion of pts with an excellent result to 60% at 15-20 years (Ann Thorac Surg 1994;58:1343). Transthoracic and thoracoscopic approaches are no longer commonly used (Surg Clin N Am 2002;82:763). Currently, laparoscopic Heller myotomy with loose fundoplication is the favored surgical approach with excellent (90%) relief of dysphagia and a hospital stay of only 3-5 days (Am J Surg 1997;174:709; Ann Surg 1997;225:655). Surgery should be considered for: (1) very young pts given the likelihood of repeated dilatations over a lifetime; (2) failures of nonsurgical rx; (3) pts at high risk for dilatation due to tortuous esophagus, prior GE junction

surgery, or esophageal diverticula; and (4) pts who prefer a surgical approach given the better chance of long-term sx relief (J Clin Gastroenterol 1999;28:202).

2.10 Noncardiac Chest Pain

J Clin Gastro 2002;34:6; Am J Gastro 2001;96:958

Epidem: About 30% of pts who undergo cardiac catheterization have exams negative for coronary disease. This implies an annual U.S. incidence of noncardiac chest pain of about 180,000 cases (GE 1997;112:309).

Pathophys: Some of the pts with pain of esophageal origin will have structural esophageal disease, with perhaps 10-15% having esophagitis endoscopically (Am J Gastroenterol 1999;94:2310) and another 20-30% having nonerosive, occult GERD. The cause of pain for the remaining 60-70% is functional. Though many manometric abnormalities have been described in pts with noncardiac chest pain, no manometric pattern correlates well with sx (J Clin Gastroenterol 1999;28:189). Esophageal sensory function and CNS abnormalities are seen in pts with functional pain. These pts have lower pain thresholds with balloon distension (Ann Intern Med 1996;124:950) and a lower CNS threshold for perception of esophageal stimuli (Gut 1992;33:298).

Sx: Dysphagia, gross regurgitation, heartburn, and pain after meals may suggest GERD. Esophageal pain comes in frequent, long episodes usually without associated dyspnea, lightheadedness, palpitations, or diaphoresis. Pain radiation to the back is not uncommon. Be very cautious about implicating the esophagus in pain that radiates to the jaw, neck, or arms. Infrequent attacks of spontaneous pain are more suggestive of cardiac disease than esophageal disease (J Clin Gastroenterol 1985;7:477).

Si: Unhelpful, except to assess pt for signs of cardiac disease or musculoskeletal causes of pain.

Crs: Follow-up at a mean of 21 months shows that pts continue to have pain, though those with a specific esophageal diagnosis are less likely to require physician visits or be disabled by the pain (Am J Gastroenterol 1987;82:215). Pts with chest pain and a normal angiogram have 96% 7-year survival (J Am Coll Cardiol 1986;7:479).

Cmplc: Repeated medical evaluations, including repeat cardiac catheterization and emergency room visits. Disability secondary to pain and fear that pain is cardiac in origin.

Diff Dx: The differential diagnosis is broad, and most of these other disorders are readily excluded prior to GI evaluation. Angina is the most important differential point. Esophageal chest pain from GERD and angina frequently coexist. Chest wall pain may occur from costochondritis, rib fracture, arthritis, fibromyalgia, or zoster (prior to rash). Pulmonary causes include pulmonary embolus, pneumonia, and pneumothorax. Biliary pain, pancreatitis, and peptic disease usually are not sources of confusion. Psychiatric causes include anxiety disorders, panic attacks, depression, somatoform disorders, and fixed delusions. Psychiatric disorders are more common in pts with chest pain associated with motility disorders (Nejm 1983;309:1337).

Lab: A 24-hour pH probe is the most useful test for differentiating reflux-associated pain from other causes of pain. A 24-hour pH probe is more helpful than manometry, acid perfusion (Bernstein test), or edrophonium challenge test (trying to reproduce pain with a cholinesterase inhibitor that stimulates motility) (Am J Med 1991;90:576). The edrophonium test is considered positive when a patient's sx of chest pain is reproduced. This is a relatively specific test in that it rarely provokes pain in healthy controls or in those with irritable bowel (Dig Dis 1998;16:198). A strong argument can be made to use an empiric trial of a proton pump inhibitor (eg, omeprazole 40 mg qam and 20 mg qpm) just as would be done in other cases of clinically suspected reflux (GE 1998;115:42). This strategy is likely to reduce cost and to result in fewer diagnostic tests. Manometry is not routinely indicated in suspected esophageal chest pain (GE 1994;107:1865). It should be considered for pts with chest pain and dysphagia with a negative endoscopy (to identify those with true esophageal spasm or achalasia, for which there is specific rx). It may be of value in selected pts by establishing the presence of a nonspecific motility disorder. Pts who receive a specific dx are less likely to be disabled by their pain and less likely to have repeated physician evaluations. A 24-hour ambulatory esophageal manometry is technically possible but of uncertain value (Dig Dis 1995;13:145).

X-ray: Selective use of CXR, rib films.

Endoscopy: EGD reveals esophagitis in 10-15% of pts.

Rx: Therapy for GERD should be tried as outlined and continued if appropriate. Pts with initial responses and later relapses should be evaluated with pH probe rather than be committed to long-term GERD rx, because there might be an initial placebo response to any intervention. Trazodone 100-150 mg daily (GE 1987;92: 1027) or imipramine 50 mg po qhs (Nejm 1994;330:1411) may be effective treatment for those with visceral hypersensitivity. Oral nifedipine reduces contraction amplitude in pts with high-amplitude peristaltic contractions (the nutcracker esophagus), but it is no more effective than placebo at relieving sx (GE 1987; 93:21). Oral diltiazem decreased pain in one small study (Am J Gastroenterol 1991;86:272). Botulinum toxin injection has been associated with short-term benefit (Dig Dis Sci 1996;41:2025). Surgery to treat spastic conditions of the esophagus has been performed but seems unwarranted (Int Surg 1997;82:113).

2.11 Diffuse Esophageal Spasm and Related Spastic Disorders

Lancet 2001;358:823; Gastroenterologist 1997;5:112

There are 4 named disorders that are usually discovered in the evaluation of pts with chest pain or dysphagia. The clinical relevance of these diseases defined by manometry is unclear. These disorders are:

- *Diffuse esophageal spasm* (DES), a disorder dx in <2% of pts referred for manometry. It is defined by the presence of simultaneous (and therefore nonperistaltic) contractions in the body of the esophagus. This is the spastic disorder most likely to cause severe sx. Some pts with DES go on to develop achalasia.
- *Nutcracker esophagus*, defined manometrically as the presence of peristaltic contractions of high amplitude (>180 mm Hg).
- *Hypertensive lower esophageal sphincter*, defined as a resting LES pressure >45 mm Hg with normal LES relaxation and normal peristalsis.
- *Nonspecific esophageal motility disorder*, defined by nontransmitted contractions, low-amplitude contractions, prolonged contractions, triple peaked contractions, or nonperistaltic contractions (Am J Gastroenterol 1992;87:825).

2.12 Mallory-Weiss Tears

Am J Gastroenterol 1997;92:805; Am J Gastroenterol 1993;88:2056

Epidem: Mallory-Weiss tears represent about 5% of cases of UGI bleeding (Am J Gastroenterol 1993;88:2056).

Pathophys: These lesions are linear tears in the mucosa of the GE junction. They are often seen in association with vomiting, regurgitation, during endoscopy, during PEG lavage for colonoscopy (Am J Gastroenterol 1993;88:1292), or with other causes of increased abdominal pressure, but at times these tears occur without obvious cause. They were first described at autopsy in alcoholics with fatal hematemesis after an alcoholic debauch. Many tears are of little clinical consequence and go undiagnosed. However, massive bleeding can occur, especially in those with coagulopathies or portal HTN (Hepatology 1990;11:879).

Sx: Hematemesis, melena, or hematochezia, often after a vomiting illness.

Si: Volume depletion.

Crs: Rebleeding, usually within 24 hours, was seen in 7% of pts in a large series (Am J Gastroenterol 1997;92:805). Pts with coagulopathies, hematochezia, or hemodynamic instability at presentation were most likely to rebleed. Mortality has been reported at up to 12%, in association with multisystem organ failure (Am J Gastroenterol 1993;88:2056).

Endoscopy: Endoscopy excludes other causes of bleeding and helps to assess risk. Clean-based tears and tears with adherent clot are at low risk for rebleeding. Pts with bleeding at index EGD are most likely to rebleed (Am J Gastroenterol 1997;92:805).

Rx: General supportive measures for UGI bleeding are begun (p. 40). If there is active bleeding, endoscopic rx is appropriate, but there are limited data regarding the best technique. Multipolar cautery reduced the need for transfusion and surgery in a small RCT (Nejm 1987;316:1613). Sclerotherapy was effective in 13 pts with active bleeding from a tear, but was associated with a perforation (Am J Gastroenterol 1994;89:2147). Epinephrine injection and heater probe have been effective in small series (Am J Gastroenterol 1997;92:805).

2.13 Boerhaave's Syndrome

Post Grad Med J 1997;73:265; ANZ J Surg 2003;73:1008

This rare condition is spontaneous rupture of the esophagus. It is named after the physician who described a case of esophageal rupture that killed the Grand Admiral of Holland 18 hours after self-induced vomiting. The classic presentation is vomiting, severe lower chest pain, and subcutaneous emphysema. However, atypical presentations are the rule, and the diagnosis is frequently missed. Mortality climbs sharply if the dx is delayed more than 12 hours. The dx can usually be made with CXR, limited UGI series (starting with water-soluble contrast to try to keep large volumes of barium out of the chest), or CT scan in some cases. Treatment is surgical.

2.14 Zenker's (Hypopharyngeal) Diverticulum

Laryngoscope 1997;107:1436; Ann Otol Rhinol Laryngol 2003;112:583

Epidem: 50% of cases in 7th and 8th decades. More common in men.

Pathophys: The diverticulum forms in the Killian triangle, which is an area of scant muscular fibers between the horizontal fibers of the cricopharyngeal muscle and the oblique fibers of the inferior constrictor muscle in the dorsal wall of the most caudal part of the hypopharynx (Ann Otol Rhinol Laryngol 1994;103:178). The diverticulum forms in this weakness as a result of resistance to outflow from the pharynx (Gastrointest Endosc 1999;49:126).

Sx: Dysphagia (80%), regurgitation (50%), aspiration, coughing, throat clearing (30%), pneumonia (14%), hoarseness (5%), weight loss, halitosis, neck pain. Pts may describe coughing up food that is several hours old. GERD is frequently associated.

Si: A palpable mass may be felt in the neck.

Crs: Continued slow enlargement of the diverticulum with progressive sx.

Cmplc: Diverticular perforation may occur due to endoscopy, NG tube, or foreign bodies. Squamous cancer was observed in 0.5% in a series of 1249 pts (Hepatogastro 1992;39:109).

Diff Dx: Other causes of dysphagia need to be considered but barium swallow eliminates diagnostic doubt.

X-ray: Barium swallow most often reveals the diverticulum posteriorly and to the left of the esophagus.

Endoscopy: Generally not indicated and is risky due to possibility of perforation.

Rx: Therapy is surgical or endoscopic and the choice largely is determined by local expertise. Diverticulectomy with cricopharyngeal myotomy has been the standard rx in the U.S. This can be complicated by pharyngocutaneous fistula (3-13%), wound infection (3% or higher), mediastinitis, stenosis, bleeding, or death. Several procedures do not violate the esophageal mucosa and lead to fewer infections and more rapid recovery. These include diverticulopexy (where the tic is suspended by suturing it to the prevertebral fascia), imbrication (in which the tic is dissected free and inverted into the lumen of the esophagus), and myotomy alone (Laryngoscope 1997;107:1436). In the endoscopic method, the muscular bar that separates esophageal lumen from diverticulum is divided. In experienced hands, excellent patient satisfaction and low morbidity are seen (Ann Otol Rhinol Laryngol 1994;103:178). A technique with flexible endoscopy, conscious sedation, and a needle-knife papillotome has been recently described (Gastrointest Endosc 1999;49:93), but the safety requires further study (Gastrointest Endosc 1999;49:126).

2.15 Epiphrenic Diverticulum

World J Surg 1999;23:147; Ann Thorac Surg 1993;55:1109

Epiphrenic diverticula are found in the distal third of the esophagus and are associated with motility disorders (Ann Thorac Surg 1993;55:1109) or trauma (Am J Surg 1996;62:973). They present with regurgitation or dysphagia. They can be complicated by aspiration, squamous cancer from stasis, or candida

infection. Surgery can be considered for pts with severe sx, but
mortality is significant at 9% in some hands (Ann Thorac Surg
1993;55:1109), though not in others (World J Surg 1999;23:147).
Minimally invasive surgical treatments are being developed (Am
Surg 2003;69:465)

2.16 Rumination Syndrome

Peds 2003;111:158; Mayo Clin Proc 1997;72:646; GE 1995;
    108:1024

Epidem: This disorder is found in 6-10% of people who are institutionalized with mental retardation. It also occurs in pts of normal
intelligence, usually young adults, with a F:M ratio of 3:1.

Pathophys: The mechanism by which pts ruminate is unclear since
retrograde contraction does not occur in the human esophagus.
Not all episodes are associated with increased intra-abdominal
pressure. It is thought that rumination in adults of normal intelligence is a learned adaptation of the belch reflex, in which there
is prolonged LES relaxation (GE 1995;108:1024).

Sx: Repetitive regurgitation of partially undigested food, usually
within 10 minutes of eating and lasting 1-2 hours postprandially.
Weight loss is common, presumably because of spitting out the
regurgitated boluses. Bulimia nervosa is present in a subgroup
who spit out the refluxed boluses to control weight.

Crs: Over 3-year follow-up, most pts remain symptomatic. The
severity of sx decreases with time.

Diff Dx: GERD, gastroparesis, vomiting, obstruction, or pseudo-
obstruction. The early onset after eating is a clue to rumination
rather than gastroparesis, in which vomiting is delayed.

Lab: If performed, gastroduodenal manometry can show simultaneous
spikes in pressure at all recording levels (called R waves) as arti-
fact of a sudden increase in intra-abdominal pressure.

X-ray: UGI series, if done to exclude other causes, is normal. Gastric emptying scan may be needed to exclude gastroparesis.

Rx: Education, reassurance, or multidisciplinary rx as an eating disorder in adults of normal intelligence. Biofeedback has been used (J Clin Gastroenterol 1986;8:115). Behavior modification techniques have been used in the mentally retarded.

2.17 Candida Esophagitis

Curr Treat Options Gastroenterol 2003;6:55; GE 1994;106:509

Cause: *Candida albicans*, less commonly other *Candida* species.

Epidem: Most often a disease of the acutely or chronically immunocompromised pt; much less common in the population at large.

Pathophys: Defects in lymphocyte function (HIV pts), defects in granulocyte function (chemotherapy pts), altered microbial flora (such as after antibiotics), and structural (diverticula, strictures) or motility abnormalities (scleroderma) of the esophagus predispose to colonization followed by infection (GE 1994;106:509).

Sx: Dysphagia or odynophagia (see p 9) are the presenting sx in 60-80% of pts.

Si: Oral thrush may be present in one third, but the presence of thrush does not guarantee *Candida* in the esophagus and the absence of oral lesions does not rule it out.

Crs: Usually responds to rx but may become chronic or recurrent in the immunocompromised.

Cmplc: Esophageal stricture, disseminated candidiasis, esophageal perforation.

Diff Dx: See Dysphagia and Odynophagia (p 9).

Lab: Budding yeast, hyphae, and pseudohyphae are seen on histology, cytology, or KOH prep.

Endoscopy: *Candida* is suspected when discrete raised whitish lesions are seen. In mild cases they are small and discrete, but they increase in size and ultimately coalesce and ulcerate in more severe cases. The lesions should be brushed as well as biopsied, since bx alone has a substantial miss rate (Am J Clin Path 1995;103:295).

Rx: Clotrimazole troches, 10 mg, dissolved in the mouth 5 times daily for 7-10 days, are appropriate in an immunocompetent host with minimal sx. Fluconazole 100 mg po qd × 14 days should be used in those with moderate to severe sx or those with HIV infection or neutropenia. Fluconazole resistance is most likely in severely immunosuppressed pts and in pts who have long prior exposure to azole rx (J Infect Dis 1996;173:219). Those who fail fluconazole can be treated with itraconazole (200 mg po qd × 7-14 days). Systemic sx or disseminated infection may require amphotericin B with flucytosine (Curr Treat Options Gastroenterol 2003;6:55). Esophagectomy has been described for transmural necrosis with perforation (Ann Thorac Surg 1999;67:231).

2.18 Herpes Simplex Esophagitis

Curr Treat Options Gastroenterol 2003;6:55; GE 1994;106:509

Cause: *Herpes simplex* virus (HSV).

Epidem: Seen sporadically in healthy hosts, HSV esophagitis is largely a disease of the immunocompromised pt. Associated conditions include HIV infection, hematologic malignancy, transplantation, chronic steroid use, and diabetes (Am J Gastroenterol 1986; 81:246). Orogenital sexual transmission has been reported (Gastrointest Endosc 1999;50:845).

Pathophys: Primary HSV infection often occurs in childhood and is followed by a latent period of HSV infection of nerve ganglion cells. Reactivation is probably the dominant mechanism.

Sx: Classically, pts present with sudden onset of severely painful swallowing associated with retrosternal burning chest pain. Gastrointestinal bleeding, gross or occult, may also be a presenting sx (Am J Gastroenterol 1986;81:246). However, up to half of pts have neither odynophagia nor chest pain (Gastrointest Endosc 1991;37:600). Unexplained nausea and vomiting is a common presentation of HSV in bone marrow transplant pts (Transplantation 1986;42:602).

Si: Oral HSV lesion in approximately 30% of pts.

Crs: Self-limited infection with several days of sx in healthy host; may be prolonged or recurrent in immunocompromised pt.

Cmplc: Esophageal hemorrhage, herpes pneumonia, disseminated infection, tracheoesophageal fistula, and esophageal perforation.

Diff Dx: See Dysphagia and Odynophagia (p 9).

Lab: Viral culture from brushings and bx of ulcer edges. Histology shows multinucleated giant cells, intranuclear inclusions. Immunochemical staining is of value.

Endoscopy: 1-3 mm vesicles are the earliest lesion and are rarely seen. These develop into sharply demarcated ulcers with raised yellow edges. The ulcerations later coalesce and can develop inflammatory pseudomembranes. In a minority of cases, only inflammatory changes without discrete ulcers are seen (Gastrointest Endosc 1991;37:600).

Rx: Acyclovir 200-400 mg orally 5 times daily × 2-3 weeks. IV acyclovir (250 mg/m^2 iv q 8 h × 7-14 days) in moderate to severe cases or if pt is unable to take po. Foscarnet or famciclovir may be needed in pts with acyclovir resistance (Curr Treat Options Gastroenterol 2003;6:55). Small doses of 2% lidocaine provide sx relief.

2.19 Cytomegalovirus Esophagitis

Curr Treat Options Gastroenterol 2003;6:55; GE 1994;106:509

Cause: Cytomegalovirus.

Epidem: Peak ages of primary infection are preschool age and young adulthood.

Pathophys: CMV is typically acquired perinatally, in infancy, or through sexual contacts in adulthood. Primary infections are asymptomatic or present as a mild mononucleosis-type illness in adults without prominent GI effects. After primary infection, the virus enters a latent phase. Most symptomatic disease is reactivation that is seen in immunocompromised hosts (Ann IM 1993; 119:924).

Sx: Because CMV is systemic, sx of nausea, vomiting, diarrhea, weight loss, and fever are common. This distinguishes CMV from other viral causes of esophagitis. Odynophagia occurs in 60% of pts (GE 1994;106:509).

Si: Fever.

Crs: Self-limited in healthy hosts but can be chronic/relapsing in immunocompromised pts.

Cmplc: Stricture has been described (J Clin Gastroenterol 1991;13:678).

Diff Dx: See Dysphagia and Odynophagia (p 9).

Lab: Culture of bx of ulcer base is most sensitive. Histology shows large cells in subepithelial lining with intranuclear and cytoplasmic inclusions (the latter specific to CMV).

X-ray: Ba swallow is nonspecific; may be normal or show ulcerations or large flat ulcers several centimeters long.

Endoscopy: Early lesions are discrete ulcerations with raised borders. These progress to long, generally shallow ulcers. CMV infects the fibroblasts and endothelium, not squamous mucosa, so biopsies should be in base of ulcer.

Rx: Ganciclovir and foscarnet are the two equally effective drugs that inhibit CMV DNA polymerase. A randomized trial, in HIV-infected pts, of foscarnet (90 mg/kg iv bid) vs ganciclovir (5 mg/kg bid), (diluted in 750-1000 mL NS to reduce risk of renal toxicity) for 21 days, has shown symptomatic response in about 80% of pts, and endoscopic improvement in 70% of pts. Ganciclovir-resistant strains can often be treated with foscarnet (Am J Gastroenterol 1998;93:317).

2.20 Esophageal Manifestations of HIV Infection

Compr Ther 2000;26:163

Cause: The most common causes of dysphagia in HIV pts are: (1) *Candida*, (2) cytomegalovirus (CMV), (3) idiopathic esophageal ulcer (IEU), and (4) *Herpes simplex* (HSV). GERD is uncommon in these pts.

Pathophys: Opportunistic infection generally begins when CD4 counts drop below $100/\mu L$. The cause of IEU is unknown (Ann Intern Med 1995;123:143).

Sx: Dysphagia to solids more than liquids. Odynophagia suggests an esophageal ulcer. Nausea, vomiting, and systemic sx suggest CMV.

Si: Oral thrush is a helpful clue, but many pts may have more than one infection.

Crs: Prior to effective antiretroviral rx, relapses of candida were typical within 3 months (GE 1994;107:744). CMV esophagitis usually does well with rx (Am J Med 1995;98:169).

Diff Dx: See Cause. The broader differential of dysphagia should be considered if CD4 counts are $>200/\mu L$ (see Dysphagia and Odynophagia, p 9).

Lab: CD4 count.

Endoscopy: May show findings of candida, CMV, herpes, or IEU. Culture and histology should be obtained as described in earlier sections. IEU shows well-circumscribed ulcers similar to CMV.

Rx: Empiric fluconazole (200 mg po loading dose followed by 100 mg qd ×10 days) is a reasonable first step. In pts who do not respond, EGD is done to make a specific dx. CMV is treated with ganciclovir or foscarnet (J Infect Dis 1995;172:622), HSV with acyclovir, IEU with prednisone (Am J Med 1992;93:131) or thalidomide (AIDS Res Hum Retroviruses 1997;13:301).

2.21 Esophageal Leiomyoma

Chest Surg Clin N Am 1994;4:769

Cause: Esophageal leiomyoma is the most common benign tumor of the esophagus, but its frequency is only 1% of the frequency of esophageal malignancy. It is a smooth muscle tumor usually found as a submucosal mass in distal esophagus. It is usually asymptomatic but can cause dysphagia. Barium swallow shows a crescent-shaped filling defect that usually does not obstruct the lumen and that on EUS is a well-circumscribed, hypoechoic mass with fine internal echoes arising in muscularis propria (Gastrointest Endosc Clin N Am 1994;4:791). Surgery is considered when the patient is symptomatic or when malignancy is suspected. Enucleation is the safest approach for most lesions and can be done by a thoracoscopic approach (Surg Endosc 1997;11:280).

2.22 Esophageal Papilloma

Am J Gastroenterol 1994;89:245; Am J Surg Pathol 1993;17:803

This benign squamous epithelial tumor is typically found incidentally at EGD. It is usually <1.0 cm, and malignant degeneration is a rarity. It may form in response to mucosal irritation, but human papilloma virus is found by PCR in more than half the cases. It can be removed endoscopically, though it is not clear that this is necessary.

2.23 Esophageal Intramural Pseudodiverticulosis

J Clin Gastro 2001;33:378; Thorax 1985;40:849

This rare disorder is defined by the presence of numerous small diverticula (dilated mucous glands) contained within the wall of the esophagus. Ba swallow shows many 1-4 mm, flask-shaped (ie, narrow-necked) sacs projecting at right angles to the esophagus. There may be associated motor disorders, candidiasis, or esophagitis, and pts may present with dysphagia or, rarely, bleeding.

2.24 Esophageal Inlet Patch

Am J Gastro 2004;99:543

An inlet patch is a small area of heterotopic gastric mucosa in the cervical esophagus. It is thought to be congenital and is usually asymptomatic. It is a common finding (prevalence ~1%, often missed at EGD). Some pts develop dysphagia, hoarseness, cough, or strictures from acid produced in the patch. Malignant transformation is very rare.

Chapter 3
Stomach and Duodenum

3.1 Gastritis

Terminology for gastritis is difficult to follow and in its current state is of little clinical value. No satisfactory system that correlates endoscopic appearance, histologic findings, and clinical sx exists. What the endoscopist calls gastritis often bears no relationship to what the pathologist calls gastritis, which in turn often bears no relationship to the pt's clinical complaint. More than 80% of cases of histologic gastritis are caused by Hp (Endoscopy 1991;23:289). Other causes include autoimmune gastritis, drugs, allergy, Crohn's, sarcoid, vasculitis, and radiation, as well as other bacteria, viruses, or fungi. The Sydney system is currently the most widely used classification system for histologic gastritis. It was developed by European pathologists. It separates gastritis into 3 categories: (1) nonatrophic, (2) atrophic, and (3) special (Am J Surg Pathol 1996;20:1161). A second system that is frequently used in the literature classifies gastritis as: (1) type A (atrophic gastritis of the body, often autoimmune associated with pernicious anemia), (2) type B (diffuse antral gastritis usually associated with Hp), (3) type AB (atrophic gastritis involving body and antrum and a known risk for gastric cancer), and (4) type C (chemical gastritis). The term gastritis should probably be considered only a histologic dx given the lack of correlation between endoscopy, histology, and the pt's sx (Gut 1994;35:1172).

3.2   Helicobacter Pylori

Nejm 2002;347:1175; Am J Surg 1996;172:411; Jama 1995;274:1064

Cause: *Helicobacter pylori* (Hp). Humans are the major reservoir of
Hp, though human isolates can infect cats and cause gastritis
(Helicobacter 1998;3:225). Fecal–oral transmission has been
hypothesized but is difficult to prove (Am J Med 1996;100:12S).
Hp has been recovered from stool (BMJ 1997;315:1489) and
from drinking water (GE 1996;110:1031). Oral transmission from
stomach contents seems plausible. Oral–oral transmission from a
mouth reservoir in adults is not easy to demonstrate. Dentists (at
risk for oral exposures) do not have an increased prevalence
(Scand J Infect Dis 1995;27:149; Am J Gastro 1992; 87:1728),
but endoscopists do (presumably from infected endoscopes, pH
probes, etc) (Am J Gastro 1994;89:1987) and nurses do (at risk
for both oral and fecal exposure) (Arch IM 1993;153:708).

Epidem: Hp is found worldwide, but prevalence varies widely and is
greatest in developing countries. Risk factors for infection
include crowded or unsanitary conditions. In developing countries, the infection is probably acquired in childhood, and childhood prevalence is very high. In developed countries such as the
U.S., the prevalence is <20% in those under age 50, but rises
abruptly after that. This suggests that childhood acquisition was
likely in those infected prior to 1950 and that since 1950, the
infection has been slowly acquired through life (Jama 1995;
274:1064). In the U.S., the prevalence is greater in blacks and in
those with less education. However, there is a large geographical
variation that has not been well explained by socioeconomic
status alone (Am J Med 1996;100:12S). Smoking has little, if
any, effect on prevalence. A dose-dependent, protective effect of
alcohol has been observed. Drinking coffee is associated with a
greater prevalence (BMJ 1997;315:1489).

Pathophys: Hp survives in the acidic gastric environment by metabo-
lizing urea into ammonia. This creates an alkaline microenviron-
ment. The bug attaches to the surface mucus-secreting cells and
lives in the mucus layer, thereby escaping normal clearance by
the immune system (Jama 1995;274:1064). The organism produces toxins that damage the mucosa and induce the inflammatory mediators that cause the gastritis. More virulent strains
secrete vacuolating cytotoxin A (vacA), a cytotoxin that causes
vacuolization of gastric epithelium. Some of the same virulent
strains (about 60% of the total) possess the cytotoxin-associated
gene A (cagA) that is associated with more severe inflammation
and risk of subsequent development of ulcer, gastric cancer, and
atrophic gastritis (Nejm 1996;334:1018).

Sx: Acute infection (rarely diagnosed) causes dyspepsia or is asymptomatic. Chronic sx arise from complications of Hp infection.
These complications are DU, GU, MALToma, gastric cancer, and
possibly nonulcer dyspepsia.

Crs: Acute infection (documented by investigators intentionally
infecting themselves! [Am J Gastroenterol 1987;82:192]) causes a
dyspepsia-like illness, followed by achlorhydria, and a histologic
gastritis with neutrophils. A period of 10-15 years of chronic
active gastritis follows, during which there is inflammation, but
the stomach remains acidic. At the end stages, achlorhydria and
atrophic gastritis develop. Of those infected, DU occurs in <1%
per year. Only 20% of pts will ultimately develop a clinical consequence of infection (Lancet 1997;349:1020).

Cmplc: There have been four convincingly demonstrated consequences of Hp infection:
   • *Duodenal ulcer:* The most convincing evidence for the role of
     Hp as a cause of DU is the marked reduction in ulcer recur-
     rence following eradication of Hp with antibiotics (eg, Lancet
     1994;343:508; Nejm 1993;328:308). Until that evidence was
     available, causality was difficult to establish because of the lack

of an animal model and because of the high prevalence of Hp compared to DU. It was also difficult initially to establish why an infection that is predominantly in the antrum causes duodenal ulcer (Jama 1994;272:65). However, it is likely that the Hp resides in areas of gastric metaplasia in the duodenum and induces ulceration by the inflammation induced by Hp cytotoxins. Acid hypersecretion is also likely the result of Hp infection, which reduces the number of somatostatin-producing cells in the antrum. This in turn lessens negative feedback on gastrin secretion, resulting in higher gastrin levels and greater acid output (Jama 1995;274:1064).

- *Gastric ulcer:* The pathogenic role of Hp in GU is not as clear as its role in DU. However, Hp eradication speeds GU healing, reduces ulcer recurrence, and heals ulcers refractory to healing with acid suppression alone (Gut 1994;35:19).

- *Gastric cancer:* Gastric cancer is more common in pts infected with Hp. Data from case control studies nested within prospective cohorts suggest a RR=5.9 for noncardia gastric cancer in Hp infected pts (Gut 2001;49:347). In a large Japanese cohort, gastric cancer was seen only in those with Hp infection and was most likely in those with atrophy, corpus gastritis, or intestinal metaplasia (Nejm 2001;345:784). Long-term Hp infection in Mongolian gerbils causes adenocarcinoma, adding strong support to this connection (GE 1998;115:642). Screening and treating Hp might be cost effective in preventing gastric cancer (Lancet 1996;348:150).

- *Mucosa-associated lymphoid tissue (MALT) lymphoma:* Gastric mucosa does not ordinarily contain organized lymphoid tissue. However, in response to Hp infection, lymphoid follicles develop and may evolve into low-grade B cell lymphoma. About 90% of gastric MALTomas are associated with Hp infection, and Hp eradication cures the subset of pts with superficial and distal tumors (Ann IM 1999;131:88).

- *Nonulcer dyspepsia:* Between 30 and 60% of pts with NUD have Hp infection. However, properly performed population-based studies do not show a consistent association between Hp and NUD, and there is no convincing evidence of an effect of Hp on gastroduodenal motor or sensory function (GE 1997; 113:S67). The 2 best trials of rx have yielded conflicting results. One trial showed a benefit of Hp eradication (21% vs 7% sx relief at 1 year [Nejm 1998;339:1869]). The other trial showed no benefit (26% vs 31% sx relief at 1 year [Nejm 1998;339:1875]). However, the studies are similar in that the sx of NUD are not relieved in 75% of pts in whom Hp is eradicated, suggesting a limited role for Hp in NUD. Most clinicians treat Hp-positive pts with NUD.
- *Other questionable associations:* The ready availability of serologic tests seems to have inspired authors to search for non-GI associated manifestations of Hp infection. Preliminary associations have been made between Hp infection and CAD, cerebrovascular disease, HTN, Raynaud's phenomenon, migraine, sudden infant death syndrome, and ITP. However, the quality of the data is limited, and these associations remain speculative, and in some cases biologically implausible (Arch IM 1999;159:925).

Diff Dx: Most infections are asymptomatic; the clinical diff dx is usually that of dyspepsia (p 4).

Lab: (Am J Gastro 1998;93:2330)
- *Whom to test:* It only makes sense to test those pts who will be treated if the test is positive. Pts with DU, GU, and MALTomas should be tested. Gastric polyps in an Hp-infected stomach may disappear with Hp rx, so that group should be tested (Ann IM 1998;129:712). The data are conflicting on the utility of eradicating Hp in NUD, but most clinicians test and treat the positive pts. Some consider testing those with a family history of gastric cancer, but the value of that is

speculative. Testing may be considered prior to long-term NSAID use (p 120) or prior to long-term PPI use. No large group has yet endorsed screening and treating asymptomatic pts, but that day may come. The choice of test depends on the clinical circumstances.

- *Urease tests of bx specimens:* These tests depend on the urease activity in endoscopically obtained biopsies and show positive results by a color change in an indicator when the urease is present. The three U.S. FDA approved tests are Clotest, Pyloritek, and Hp-fast. Sensitivity is between 88 and 95%, specificity is 95-100%, and cost is $6-20. Sensitivity is reduced by prior use of PPIs (Aliment Pharmacol Ther 1996;10:289), H2RAs, bismuth, antibiotics, and alcohol consumption (Am J Gastroenterol 1997;92:1310). Bx from the antrum during active GI bleeding greatly reduces sensitivity of urease testing (Gastrointest Endosc 1999;49:302), so breath testing or serology should be used instead. Serology should also be used if testing is necessary in a pt who has been on antibiotics, PPIs, or H2RAs within the last month. Two antral bx are usually sufficient (Gastrointest Endosc 1994;40:342), but sensitivity can be improved using an additional bx from the body in pts on H2RAs or PPIs (Am J Gastro 1997;92:1310).

- *Histology:* With this method, both the presence of Hp and the inflammation can be detected. If there is no gastritis histologically, then Hp infection is reliably excluded. Specialized stains such as Giemsa can be used if H&E is negative and gastritis is present. The same conditions decrease sensitivity for histology as for urease bx testing (see previous bullet item). The sensitivity is 93-96%, specificity is 98-99%, and cost is $60-250, plus endoscopy. One strategy to reduce cost and maximize sensitivity is to run urease testing first and to proceed with histology only if urease is negative.

- *Urea breath tests:* (Am J Gastro 1998;93:2330; Gut 1994; 35:723) The pt swallows a small amount of ^{13}C (nonradioactive) or ^{14}C (radioactive) urea. Hp urease converts the urea to bicarbonate and ammonia. The bicarbonate is converted to CO_2, which is recovered in a breath sample and detected on mass spectroscopy (^{13}C) or scintillation counting (^{14}C). In the U.S., the FDA has approved a ^{13}C test (Meretek) and a ^{14}C test (Tri-Med). The ^{14}C has the advantage of lower expense ($20-65 vs $250-350) and the disadvantage that it cannot be given to children or pregnant women because of the radioactivity. Both tests perform well with sensitivity of 90-96% and specificity of 88-98%. Antibiotics lower sensitivity, and the test should be performed at least 4 weeks after completion of eradication rx. PPIs may reduce sensitivity for 2 weeks, and H2RAs do so for 5 days (Ann IM 1998;129:547).

- *Serology:* IgG for Hp by ELISA is 86-94% sensitive, 78-95% specific, and costs $40-100. It is readily available and is useful in detection when endoscopy is not being performed, but it does not distinguish remote from active infection. A fall in titer after rx is not consistent enough to be useful for determining response to rx, unless the titer falls to zero (Jama 1998;280:363).

- *Culture:* Culture is not readily available in many hospital labs and is not commonly used in clinical practice. It is 80-98% sensitive, 100% specific, and costs $150. Its major use would be for detecting resistant strains in pts who have failed rx. As a practical matter, an alternative rx is chosen without sensitivity information.

- *Whole blood tests:* These tests were designed for office use and have reduced sensitivity (67-88%), reduced specificity (75-91%), and reduced cost ($10-30) compared to serum-based ELISA testing. It does not seem worthwhile using them given the small cost savings at the expense of accuracy.

Endoscopy: There are no endoscopic features that identify Hp. A grossly normal stomach at endoscopy can be infected, and bx are mandatory if Hp infection is to be diagnosed or excluded.

Rx: (Curr Gastroenterol Rep 1999;1:518; Am J Gastroenterol 1998;93:2330; J Gastroenterol 1998;33:48; Gut 1997;41:8)

- Pts with a positive test should be treated if the test was obtained for an appropriate clinical reason. Since rx morbidity is minimal and the World Health Organization has called Hp a class 1 carcinogen, it becomes difficult not to treat the positives even if the test was obtained for inappropriate reasons. However, it has been argued that rx of all strains of Hp is premature since not all strains cause clinical disease (Lancet 1997;349:1020).

- *Characteristics of best therapies:* A bewildering 1409 Hp rx arms have been identified in a meta-analysis of Hp rx (GE 1997; 113:S131). In screening the literature for appropriate regimens, one needs to look for rx that is >80% effective in intent-to-treat analysis and >90% effective in per-protocol analysis, with reproducible results from different geographic areas. It should be well tolerated, simple, and cost effective. Regimens that are bid have greatly enhanced compliance.

- *Single agent rx:* Single drug rx is ineffective and should not be used.

- *Dual agent rx:* Dual agent rx combines a PPI with a single antibiotic, typically amoxicillin or clarithromycin. However, these regimens are not effective enough to be used as initial rx despite the fact that some of these are FDA-approved therapies.

- *PPI triple rx:* There is consensus in the current literature that PPI triple rx regimens are excellent regimens despite their cost. The regimens in the following list use omeprazole 20 mg bid or lansoprazole 30 mg bid, and all drugs are given twice daily for 2 weeks. Pantoprazole 40 mg po bid or rabeprazole 20 mg bid are probably equally effective (Aliment Pharmacol Ther 1999; 13:741).

  PPI + amoxicillin 1000 mg + clarithromycin 500 mg po bid × 2 weeks.

PPI + metronidazole 500 mg + clarithromycin 500 mg po bid × 2 weeks.

PPI + amoxicillin 1000 mg + metronidazole 500 mg po bid × 2 weeks.

Per-protocol eradication rates for these regimens exceed 90%. Some studies indicate that 1 week rx with such a regimen is highly effective (Aliment Pharmacol Ther 1999; 13:289), but data in the U.S. are lacking (Am J Gastroenterol 1998;93:2330). Meta-analysis suggests that a dose of clarithromycin 500 mg bid is superior to 250 mg bid (GE 1998;114:1169).

- *Ranitidine bismuth citrate (RBC) rx:* Bismuth citrate combined with ranitidine as a complex can be used in several highly effective regimens comparable to PPI triple rx. Suggested regimens include:

  RBC 400 mg (Tritec) + amoxicillin 1000 mg + clarithromycin 500 mg po bid for 2 weeks.

  RBC 400 mg + metronidazole 500 mg + clarithromycin 500 mg po bid for 2 weeks.

  Single week rx is also probably highly effective (Can J Gastroenterol 1999;13:213).

- *Bismuth + triple therapy:* Bismuth subsalicylate (Pepto Bismol) 525 mg qid + metronidazole 250 qid + tetracycline 500 mg qid for 2 weeks with H2RA bid for 4 weeks is highly effective, but compliance and tolerability are major problems.

- *Treatment failures:* (Nejm 2002;347:1175) Pt compliance and antibiotic resistance are likely important factors in treatment failures. Unfortunately, antibiotic susceptibility data are not readily available in most pts with treatment failure. Metronidazole resistance is common and clarithromycin resistance is growing. There are limited data to guide the choice of a second line of therapy. It is reasonable to try a PPI-based triple rx using metronidazole in those previously treated with clarithromycin or clarithromycin in those previously treated with metronidazole.

Other choices include bismuth plus triple therapy using a high dose of metronidazole (500 mg po tid) or regimens based on ranitidine bismuth citrate (RBC). A regimen of RBC 400 mg po bid + tinidazole 500 mg bid + clarithromycin 500 mg po bid for 14 days was effective in 81% of those who failed PPI-based triple rx (Aliment Pharmacol Ther 2001;15:1017). A 10-day regimen of levofloxacin 250 mg po bid + pantoprazole 40 mg bid + amoxicillin 1 gm po bid for 10 days was effective in 70% of treatment failures (Clin Gastroenterol Hepatol 2004;2:997).

- *Post-rx follow-up:* Confirmation of eradication 4 weeks after completion of rx is critical in pts with MALToma, ulcer complications such as bleeding, and early gastric cancer. Its importance in other pt groups is less well established. Breath testing is ideal unless endoscopy is needed for another reason (such as follow-up of GU).

3.3 Peptic Ulcer

Lancet 2002;360:933; Am J Gastro 1997;92:1255

Cause: Hp infection (see 3.2) and NSAIDs account for the vast majority of cases.

Epidem:

- *GU:* Incidence estimated at 0.1%/yr; much higher in NSAID users. About 3% of GUs turn out to harbor malignancy (Nejm 1995;333:32).
- *DU:* M:F incidence ratio is 2:1 (confounded by a higher smoking rate in men); higher in smokers $RR=2.2$ (J Clin Gastroenterol 1997;24:2), though not confirmed in a large prospective study (Epidemiology 1997;8:420); higher in those with an FH of DU (J Clin Gastroenterol 1995;20:104). It is unlikely that caffeine or alcohol are important risk factors (Epidemiology 1997;8:420). The literature on psychological

risks for DU is a quagmire, with purported risks ranging from life events stress (J Clin Gastroenterol 1995;21:185; GE 1986;91:1370) to a personality that prompts one to sport a half-mustache on the upper lip (J Clin Gastroenterol 1992;15:96). It seems unlikely that psychological factors are of major, definable, clinical relevance. Diet plays no clear role, and the traditional suggestion of a bland diet is not made on sound ground (especially with the suggestion that chili is protective for DU! [Dig Dis Sci 1995;40:576]).

Pathophys:

- *GU:* GU results when gastric mucosal defenses are overwhelmed by the harsh, intraluminal gastric environment rich in acid and pepsin. Gastric epithelium remains intact in the stomach by a series of prostaglandin-dependent defenses, including (1) the semipermeable mucus layer, (2) bicarbonate in an unstirred water layer, and (3) regeneration and repair (Gut 1997;41:425; Gut 1993;34:580). Hp infection causes epithelial injury by production of cytotoxins, urease, and other factors that cause cell injury and death, leading to ulceration. NSAIDs inhibit mucosal cyclooxygenase, thereby reducing prostaglandin production, inhibiting mucus and bicarbonate production, and decreasing mucosal blood flow. This prevents cell replication and leads to ulcer formation.
- *DU:* The initiating event in most DU is Hp infection. Antral gastritis from Hp infection results in a decrease in somatostatin-producing cells (D cells), whose role is to inhibit gastrin-producing G cells. This in turn leads to the increased parietal cell mass (perhaps also increased due to genetic or other environmental factors) that results in the increase in acid secretion seen in DU pts. Areas of intestinal metaplasia form, possibly in response to increased acid, and these are subsequently colonized by Hp. Duodenitis results from release of inflammatory mediators from Hp, and in the presence of acid, an ulcer forms.

NSAIDs presumably cause ulceration by reducing mucosal prostaglandin-mediated defenses. The foregoing theory does not account for DU that is seen in Hp-negative pts not taking NSAIDs. A meta-analysis of rigorously designed U.S. trials demonstrated 20% ulcer recurrence rate in pts cleared of Hp, suggesting that in a subset of DU pts, Hp infection is not the critical factor (Am J Gastroenterol 1998;93:1409). These so-called "idiopathic ulcers" may be more difficult to treat and may be more likely to result in complications (Am J Gastro 2002;97:2950).

Sx: There is no sx complex diagnostic for GU or DU, and sx do not reliably distinguish DU from GU or from nonulcer dyspepsia (GE 1993;105:1378). PUD often presents with epigastric pain, sometimes described as burning, aching, or as a hunger pain. Classically it is described as postprandial and may be relieved with antacids, but these features are highly variable. GU, especially NSAID-induced, can be asymptomatic or present with a complication such as bleeding or perforation in the absence of prior pain (Am Fam Phys 1997;55:1323). If the ulcer is near the pylorus, poor gastric emptying may result in reflux sx, vomiting, or early satiety. Sudden severe sx may indicate perforation, and constant pain may suggest penetration. Weight loss is more common with giant GU (>3 cm).

Si: Epigastric tenderness.

Crs:

- GU: The vast majority of GUs will heal with initial rx. A small subgroup refractory to H2RAs will heal with a PPI (Aliment Pharmacol Ther 1996;10:381). If NSAIDs are eliminated and Hp is cured, recurrence is low. Chronic GU should lead to investigation for a missed gastric malignancy (adenocarcinoma or lymphoma) or surreptitious NSAID use.
- DU: Before the advent of rx for H. pylori, DU was a chronic relapsing illness. With clearance of Hp, DU recurrence is

uncommon (eg, Lancet 1994;343:508; Nejm 1993;328:308). However, recent analysis of U.S. trials suggests that the proportion of pts who relapse after Hp eradication may be as high as 20% (Am J Gastroenterol 1998;93:1409). At one time it was thought that ulcer disease largely burned itself out, but long-term follow-up studies of pts dx in the pre-Hp era show that 50% remain symptomatic (Gut 1996;38:812).

Cmplc: Bleeding, gastric outlet obstruction, perforation, penetration into adjacent structures without free perforation.

Diff Dx: See dyspepsia (p 4). The diff dx of an endoscopically identified ulcer includes gastric adenocarcinoma, lymphoma, and Crohn's disease.

Lab: CBC, CMP, amylase, lipase aid in diff dx. Testing for Hp is usually done at EGD for GU but may be done by serology or breath testing if DU was diagnosed by UGI rather than EGD.

X-ray: UGI barium x-ray can establish dx but is highly operator dependent and is much less sensitive and specific than EGD. A variety of radiographic signs have been proposed to separate the benign from the malignant GU, but, if the pt is fit, EGD should be performed to rule out malignancy if UGI shows GU (Jama 1996;275:622). UGI should generally be discouraged in the evaluation of dyspepsia unless EGD is thought unsafe or unavailable. UGI should not be used to dx DU (because it is a poor negative). However, if a DU is found on UGI, then EGD is not mandatory since the cancer risk in typical DU is negligible.

Endoscopy: EGD is the gold standard for dx of ulcers. Ulcers are directly visualized, and features that predict risk for bleeding can be identified (p 126). A clean, punched-out appearance of a GU suggests that the ulcer is benign. At least 6 biopsies should be obtained to rule out malignancy. The endoscopic gross appearance is not a reliable negative, and 3 biopsies detect only 70% of cancers (GE 1982;82:228). All GUs should be followed to healing by EGD (not UGI) to prove benignity by healing. Some have advocated foregoing follow-up EGD because initial EGD and bx is 99% accurate (Dig Dis Sci 1993;38:284). However, the yield of finding a curable cancer at follow-up EGD is high enough (1 cancer per 250 endoscopies [Scand J Gastroenterol 1991; 26:1193]) that the practice is appropriate (Dig Dis Sci 1994; 39:442). DUs are usually identified in the first portion of the duodenum (often called the bulb or cap). Since they are at a very low risk for malignancy, follow-up EGD to document healing is rarely indicated.

Rx: (Jama 1996;275:622):

- *Suppress acid:* Though excess acid is not the primary cause of GU, acid suppression heals ulcers, and about 90% of ulcers will be healed in 12 weeks. Acid suppression relieves sx. Cimetidine (800 mg qhs) or ranitidine (300 qhs) are cheaper but not as rapidly effective as PPIs. Consider initial use of a PPI at a high dose (eg, omeprazole 40 mg daily) in large or complicated ulcers (Am J Gastro 1996;91:2516). About 90-95% of DUs heal by 8 weeks with acid suppression, and GUs typically take 12 weeks because healing is slower and GUs are often larger.
- *NSAID ulcer:* Stop NSAIDs. If NSAIDs are stopped, then an H2RA is appropriate rx unless the ulcer is very large. If NSAIDs cannot be stopped, the dosage might be reduced. If NSAIDs are continued, a PPI (eg, omeprazole 20-40 mg po qd) rather than an H2RA should be used to treat the ulcer (Nejm 1998;338:719).
- *Eradicate Helicobacter:* (p 106).
- *Refractory ulcer:* Consider malignancy, ongoing NSAID use (surreptitious or otherwise), and Zollinger-Ellison (p 145) as causes. High-dose lansoprazole (60 mg) results in >80% healing of GU not cured with 6 weeks of H2RA (Aliment Pharmacol Ther 1996;10:381), and cure can be maintained by 30 mg po qd. Consider surgery.

- *Giant GU:* Giant GU is defined as GU >3 cm. Historically, these were treated with early surgery because of perceived higher risk with medical rx. However, in the era after introduction of H2RAs, it became evident that these ulcers usually heal with medical rx. They more frequently present as emergencies, often relapse without maintenance (though data on Hp status is lacking), and are a marker for poor general health. The mortality rate from associated medical illness is high, though subsequent risk of cancer is low (Am J Gastro 1999;94:3478). A PPI would be appropriate medical rx.
- *Prevention of ulcer recurrence:* In uncomplicated Hp infected GU or DU, maintenance is not warranted. In Hp-infected pts with an ulcer complication, maintenance rx might be continued until Hp eradication is confirmed. In Hp-negative pts with a history of recurrent or morbid complications, maintenance rx with an H2RA is reasonable though data are limited. The typical maintenance dose of an H2RA is half the initial dose (eg, ranitidine 150 mg po qhs reduces endoscopic recurrence to 20-25%), but full dose may be warranted if the initial event was highly morbid.
- *Surgical rx:* Most surgery for PUD is now done emergently for complications. It becomes a matter of clinical judgment as to when to send a pt with a refractory ulcer to surgery. Indications for surgery include refractory sx, suspicion of malignancy, uncontrolled bleeding, and obstruction. Exclude ZE (p 145) prior to surgery. The need to exclude ongoing NSAID use by random salicylate or other NSAID levels (pts do lie sometimes!) is critical. Relatives should be questioned. A series of 30 pts from one center with postsurgical recurrence of ulcer due to aspirin use (half of it surreptitious) had a high incidence of stenosis, multiple operations, and a poor outcome (GE 1998;114:883).

    Surgery with wedge resection of GU is just as effective as more extensive resections with vagotomy to reduce acid, presumably because excess acid plays little role in the pathogenesis of the ulcer. Mortality in GU is substantial (6.9% all comers, lower electively, higher in those with cardiovascular disease), and ulcer recurrence is still 5% (Am Surg 1996;62:673).

For DU, the operation of choice for intractable pain and perforation is proximal gastric vagotomy (aka parietal cell vagotomy) (Surg Clin N Am 1992;72:335). This more limited vagotomy causes less postoperative morbidity than a truncal vagotomy. However, individual experience, the nature of the ulcer complication, and judgment are important factors in selecting the best operation. If a pt has an intractable DU, then medical noncompliance or NSAID use is likely, and operation should be approached with great caution.

- *Postgastrectomy syndromes:* (Surg Clin N Am 1992;72:445) About 20% of pts have postgastrectomy syndromes after ulcer operations. With a proximal gastric vagotomy, the incidence is only 5%. **Dumping syndrome** is one of the most common syndromes and is due to the rapid emptying of hyperosmolar, carbohydrate-rich food. Dumping syndrome causes GI sx of distension, cramping, nausea, vomiting, and explosive diarrhea. It causes vasomotor sx of diaphoresis, weakness, dizziness, flushing, and palpitations. It is treated by eating small meals, avoiding concentrated carbohydrates, and taking liquid 30 minutes after meals. Operative treatment is sometimes required. Other postgastrectomy syndromes include postvagotomy diarrhea, gastroparesis, problems with a small gastric remnant, alkaline reflux, and several syndromes related to the jejunostomy.

3.4 NSAID Gastropathy

GE 2001;120:594; Am J Gastro 1998;93:2037

Epidem: Of the U.S. population, 1.2% use NSAIDs on a daily basis (Am Fam Phys 1997;55:1323). Of these, 1-2% per year will be hospitalized for gi complications of bleeding or perforation, at an annual cost approaching $1 billion. Overprescribing of NSAIDs for pain rather than joint inflammation contributes greatly to the number of avoidable complications (Ann IM 1997; 127:429). The major **risk factors** for the development of serious complications are (Am J Gastro 1998;93:2037): (1) prior peptic ulcer or bleed (RR=2.74), (2) age >60 (RR=5.52), (3) high dosage— 2 times normal (RR=10.1), (4) concurrent corticosteroids (RR=4.4), and (5) concurrent anticoagulants (RR=12.7). Gender, smoking, and alcohol are *not* independent risks. Complications are more likely to occur within the first three months of rx. Use of multiple NSAIDs increases risk.

Pathophys: Prostaglandins protect the gastric mucosa by promoting secretion of gastric mucus and bicarbonate and by increasing mucosal blood flow and ultimately cell replication. NSAIDs inhibit prostaglandin production by inhibiting cyclooxygenase. Minor toxicity from NSAIDs occurs because of local effects of these weak acids on gastric mucosa that result in erosions (small, shallow mucosal breaks). More important are the systemic effects of these agents that can cause gastroduodenal injury even if given by the rectal or intravenous route.

There are two isoforms of cyclooxygenase that NSAIDs may inhibit. COX-I isoforms maintain mucosal integrity, and COX-II isoforms induce inflammation. A newer class of NSAIDs that selectively inhibits COX-II and thus does not reduce mucosal prostaglandins has become available. Two first-generation agents in this class, celecoxib (Celebrex) and rofecoxib (Vioxx), appear to be associated with a low risk of ulcer complications (Lancet 1999;353:307). Several more highly selective second-generation agents of this class have been developed, but there are significant concerns about cardiovascular events in drugs of this class (Lancet 2004;364:639). Rofecoxib was voluntarily withdrawn from the U.S. market when a randomized trial to examine the effect of this agent on adenomatous polyp recurrence showed an increased risk of stroke and myocardial infarction.

Of the older non–COX-II selective drugs, ketorolac and piroxicam have the highest toxicity; naproxen, indomethacin, ketoprofen, and diclofenac are intermediate in toxicity; ibuprofen is less toxic (Arch IM 1996;156:1623). Nabumetone is probably the least toxic of the older agents, but at the expense of reduced anti-inflammatory activity (Am J Gastro 1996;91:2080).

The role of Hp infection in the genesis of NSAID ulcers is unclear. A prior hx of ulcer is a risk factor for subsequent NSAID ulcers, and Hp is strongly associated with ulcers. It is tempting to hypothesize that Hp infection is a cofactor in NSAID ulcer rather than unrelated to NSAID ulcer development. Eradication of Hp does not seem to speed NSAID ulcer healing (Gut 1996; 39:22). While some studies suggest that Hp eradication prior to NSAID therapy lowers risk of ulcer (Lancet 1997;350:975) other studies show no benefit (Lancet 1998;352:1016). The data do not currently support testing for Hp prior to NSAID rx.

Sx: Dyspepsia may occur with NSAIDs but does not predict endoscopic ulcer. Most pts with NSAID gastropathy are asymptomatic. Up to 60% will remain so until they present with bleeding or perforation (Lancet 1986;1:462). Only about 1 in 10 NSAID-induced ulcers bleed.

Crs: Reversible illness upon withdrawal of NSAID, but mortality may occur.

Cmplc: Bleeding; perforation; death, especially in elderly women (Ann IM 1997;127:429).

Endoscopy: EGD is appropriate if there is suspicion of an ulcer complication. Erosions are common, especially early in a course of NSAID use.

Rx: Prevention of NSAID ulcer: Pts at high risk for NSAID gastroduodenal toxicity (as defined in "Epidem") should be considered for combination therapy with an NSAID and either misoprostol or a PPI (Am J Gastro 1998;93:2037). Alternatively such pts can be treated with a COX-II selective agent (a "coxib") (Arthritis Rheum 2000;43:1905). **Misoprostol** in a dose of 200 mg po qid reduces gi complications up to 40% compared with placebo (Ann IM 1995;123:241). Diarrhea is an intolerable problem in up to 20% of pts. This sx can be reduced by changing the dosage to bid or tid, but this approach is less effective in protecting against GU (Ann IM 1995;123:344). The drug may also be better tolerated if begun at a low-dose (100 mg) and slowly increased to the target dose. Omeprazole 20 mg po qd is more effective than ranitidine (Nejm 1998;338:719) or low-dose misoprostol (200 mg po bid) (Nejm 1998;338:727) in prevention of NSAID ulcer, and omeprazole is better tolerated than misoprostol. Lansoprazole 30 mg po qd also appears effective. Conventional dose H2RAs are ineffective as prophylaxis against GU and therefore should not be used for prevention.

The use of **COX-II selective agents** (coxibs) is an effective way to reduce NSAID ulcer toxicity. However, there are concerns about the cardiovascular risk for agents in this class. In addition, the total burden of NSAID complications may paradoxically increase with use of these agents as more pts are placed on them because of their lower toxicity and aggressive marketing. Recent evidence suggests that as NSAID use in the population increases because of coxibs, the total number of NSAID bleeds increases because of the greater number of at-risk pts. It is important to note that several studies demonstrate that the combination of low-dose aspirin and a coxib has similar gastroduodenal toxicity to that of a conventional NSAID alone (eg, GE 2004;127:395).

Data comparing the use of a coxib to a PPI with a conventional NSAID are very limited but suggest similar efficacy (Nejm 2002;347:2104). Unfortunately neither strategy is highly effective in high-risk pts. In a study of coxib versus NSAID + PPI in pts with previous ulcer bleeding, the risk of ulcer recurrence or bleeding was about 30% at 6 months with either rx (GE 2004; 127:1038). Given these poor outcomes, a study of the combination of a coxib with a PPI might be of value.

3.5 Stress Ulcer

Drugs 1997;54:581

Epidem: In the modern ICU, the incidence of bleeding from stress ulcer steadily declined from 20-30% in the 1970s to 1.5-14% in 1995 (Am J Gastro 1995;90:708).

Pathophys: (Am J Gastro 1995;90:708) Stress ulcer is a term used to refer to gastroduodenal ulcers or diffuse erosive disease that occurs in critically ill pts in an ICU setting. Erosions and superficial mucosal hemorrhage are seen in 70-90% of critically ill pts and progress to confluent ulcers in a smaller subgroup. Ulcers in pts with burns and head injury are probably due to gastrin-stimulated acid production. Mucosal ischemia is probably important in many other groups at risk. In a large study weighted to cardiac surgery pts, the two major risks for bleeding were mechanical ventilation for more than 48 hours (15 times risk) and coagulopathy (fourfold risk) (Nejm 1994;330:377). Other risk factors include shock of any cause, multiple trauma, major organ failure, burns of >35% body surface area, head trauma, sepsis, and quadriplegia. The risk of bleeding rises markedly if there are 3 or more risk factors.

Sx: Hematemesis, melena, NG aspirate with coffee grounds or frank blood.

Si: Hypotension.

Crs: Usually dictated by the underlying medical illness rather than stress ulcer itself.

Cmplc: Bleeding. Perforation is much less common than bleeding in stress ulcer.

Diff Dx: Acute bleeding from preexisting upper tract lesions, including PUD and malignancy (see gi Bleeding, p 32).

Lab: Hgb (look for drop of >2 gm to suspect important bleeding). PT/INR, PTT, platelets; DIC screen if DIC is suspected clinically on basis of initial labs or multiple bleeding sites.

Endoscopy: EGD is performed in these critically ill pts if there is ongoing bleeding for which endoscopic rx may be needed. Usually EGD is unnecessary in pts with evidence of bleeding (ie, coffee grounds in NGT) without hemodynamic consequences.

Rx: The rx of stress ulcer is that of bleeding peptic ulcer (p 126). The greatest focus has been on prevention. The cornerstone of prevention is the optimal management of the underlying illness. Improvements in ICU care are probably responsible for some of the decline in stress ulcer bleeding. Several agents can be considered to prevent bleeding:

- *H2RAs:* These agents have been shown in meta-analysis to reduce risk of clinically important bleeding, and a trend suggests that they are more effective than sucralfate. This reduction in bleeding may come at the risk of a trend toward increased risk of nosocomial pneumonia (Jama 1996;275:308). However, a prospective study of 1200 ventilated pts confirmed the benefit of ranitidine over sucralfate in prevention of clinically important bleeding (1.7% vs 3.8%) but did not show a higher pneumonia risk in the ranitidine group (Nejm 1998; 338:791). While continuous infusion of H2RAs results in better acid suppression, it does not translate into less bleeding and is not necessary (Am J Gastro 1995;90:708).

- *Sucralfate:* The argument for using sucralfate has been the apparent lower pneumonia rate and a reduced mortality rate (Jama 1996;275:308). This may be especially important in pts undergoing prolonged mechanical ventilation who are not enterally fed (Drugs 1997;54:581). In such pts the apparent lower efficacy of sucralfate in preventing bleeding may be offset by a lower risk of pneumonia.

- *Other drugs:* While antacids appear to lower the risk of bleeding, they must be given q 1-2 hr with close monitoring of gastric pH and dosage titration. Thus, they are infrequently used for stress ulcer prophylaxis. Data are very limited on the use of misoprostol and PPIs.

3.6 Treatment of Bleeding Peptic Ulcer

Surg Clin N Am 1996;76:83; Nejm 1994;331:717

Endoscopy: Endoscopy identifies the cause of bleeding and predicts risk of rebleeding in the first week. Endoscopy is performed after volume resuscitation and stabilization of the pt. If the endoscopist identifies active arterial spurting from the ulcer, the chance of rebleeding in the first week is 80% without rx. If a nonbleeding visible vessel is seen (generally a red or bluish lesion of a few mm sticking up in the ulcer bed), the rebleed rate is 50%. An adherent clot has a 30% risk, a flat black spot carries a 10% risk, and a clean, exudate-covered ulcer base has a risk of less than 5%.

Rx: Endoscopic rx reduces the risk of rebleeding by 40%, the need for surgery by at least 60%, and mortality in acute bleeding by 60% (GE 1992;102:139). Bleeding can be treated by direct application of thermal energy to coagulate blood vessels, by application of hemostatic clips or by injection of various substances into the vessel and surrounding tissues. Endoscopic rx is clearly indicated for active bleeding and ulcers with visible vessels. Endoscopic therapy is also appropriate for ulcers with adherent clots after epinephrine injection and careful removal of the clot (GE 2002; 123:407).

    Thermal energy is applied with a bipolar electrocautery probe or a heater probe. Pressure is applied directly onto the vessel until bleeding stops. This squeezes the opposite walls of the vessel together and allows highly effective coagulation. There is no convincing evidence that one device is better than another. The difficulty can be getting *en face* to the vessel so that pressure can be directly applied, because many ulcers can only be approached tangentially. Long, low energy bursts of current are applied (Surg Clin N Am 1996;76:83).

Injection rx can be carried out with 1:10,000 diluted epinephrine, alcohol, thrombin, or other sclerosants. The beauty of injection rx is that the device is inexpensive, the technique easy to master, and it can be used to treat an ulcer that can only be approached tangentially. Epinephrine is safe, simple, and effective. Generally 10-20 mL total are injected in several sites. The vasoconstriction and tamponade effect of the large volume stop bleeding. The initial success rate is >90% (BMJ 1997;314:1307). The addition of sclerosant to epinephrine adds nothing. The disadvantage of sclerosants and alcohol is the perforation risk, because extensive tissue necrosis may occur (Brit J Surg 1996; 83:461).

Combination therapy with injection of epinephrine followed by a thermal method is currently popular among experts following a trial from a respected center showing increased effectiveness (BMJ 1997;314:1307). The concept is that epinephrine controls immediate bleeding, and thermal rx prevents late rebleeding. Endoscopic application of metal clips to bleeding ulcers is a new approach but results of trials comparing it to thermal methods are conflicting (compare Am J Gastro 2002;97:2250 to Gastro Endosc 2001;53:147).

Failures of endoscopic rx are best managed with a second attempt at endoscopic rx (Nejm 1999;340:751). Endoscopic retreatment reduces the need for surgery without increasing the risk of death and has fewer complications than surgery. **Pharmacologic rx** might be considered when endoscopy is not available or fails. A meta-analysis suggests that somatostatin or octreotide may reduce the risk of continued bleeding and may be useful prior to endoscopy or if endoscopy fails (Ann IM 1997; 127:1062). There is no evidence that H2RAs alter the early rebleeding rate in bleeding ulcers (Endoscopy 1995;27:308). Very high-dose omeprazole added to endoscopic therapy appears beneficial (Nejm 2000;343:310) but is not available in the U.S. Surgery is needed for those who fail endoscopic and medical rx.

3.7 Nonulcer Dyspepsia

GE 2004;127:1239; Nejm 1998;339:1376; GE 1997;112:1448

Epidem: The prevalence of dyspepsia is about 15% in the adult population. The majority of these pts have normal endoscopies and could potentially be labeled as having nonulcer dyspepsia (NUD).

Pathophys: (Mayo Clin Proc 1999;74:1011) NUD is defined as persistent or recurrent pain centered in the upper abdomen that lasts more than 3 months and is not associated with a biochemical or anatomic abnormality. A variety of causes of NUD have been proposed, including (1) Hp infection, (2) histologic gastritis or duodenitis, (3) GERD with a negative EGD, (4) heightened visceral sensitivity, (5) gastroparesis, (6) impaired gastric accommodation to a meal, (7) other motility abnormalities, or (8) a psychiatric disorder. None of the data are convincing for a single etiology. Clinicians should not think of this as a single disease, for it is really a sx with multiple elusive causes.

Sx: By definition, NUD is pain in the upper abdomen. There can be associated nausea, bloating, early satiety, or postprandial fullness. Subtypes have been identified (reflux-like, dysmotility-like, ulcer-like, and nonspecific) but are not helpful in choosing empiric rx (GE 1992;102:1259).

Cmplc: None by definition.

Diff Dx: The diff dx is that of dyspepsia (p 4). To truly make a dx of NUD, there is a large number of exclusions that must theoretically be made. However, exhaustive testing is often unnecessary, and testing should be tailored to the severity and persistence of the complaint.

Lab: Normal by definition.

X-ray: Normal by definition.

Endoscopy: Normal by definition.

Rx:

- *Treat Helicobacter:* Between 30 and 60% of pts with nonulcer dyspepsia have Hp infection. The 2 best trials of rx in NUD with Hp infection have yielded conflicting results. One showed a benefit of Hp eradication (21% vs 7% sx relief at 1 year [Nejm 1998;339:1869]). The other showed no benefit (26% vs 31% sx relief at one year [Nejm 1998;339:1875]). However, the studies are similar in that sx of NUD are relieved in 25% of pts in whom Hp is eradicated. Since rx is quite benign, and since Hp is a risk for gastric cancer and future peptic disease, it is reasonable to treat Hp in the setting of dyspepsia.

- *Trial of a PPI:* Since a large number of pts with GERD have a normal EGD and not all pts with GERD have typical retrosternal sx, a trial of a PPI is warranted (p 61). If the pt has a good response, an attempt to taper rx to an H2RA or stopping it entirely is reasonable. If sx relapse, a dx of GERD may be entertained. If confirmation is felt mandatory, a pH probe could be considered.

- *Trial of a prokinetic agent:* It has been common practice to try a promotility agent, especially if pts have sx of bloating or postprandial fullness. These agents appear to be about 40% better than placebo. The withdrawal of cisapride from the U.S. market has made this approach less desirable. Metoclopramide, an alternative agent, is often poorly tolerated. Domperidone is not available in the U.S. but may be a useful trial where available. In a pt with troublesome sx, an evaluation for gastroparesis (next section) may replace empiric promotility agents until safer drugs are found.

- *Psychotropic drugs and psychotherapy:* In the absence of a specific psychiatric diagnosis, there are no data to support the use of psychotropic agents in NUD. However, because anxiety and other psychiatric disorders may coexist with dyspepsia and make the sx less tolerable, many clinicians offer pts rx for the psychiatric disorder. There is insufficient evidence to conclude that psychological rx is effective (Am J Gastro 2004;99:1817), though data on the possible benefits of hypnotherapy are intriguing (GE 2002;123:1778).

3.8 Gastroparesis

GE 2004;127:1592; Scand J Gastroenterol (suppl) 1995;213:7

Cause: Acute gastroparesis (<3 months) can be seen postoperatively. It can also be caused by viral agents, hyperglycemia, hypokalemia, hypothyroidism, and drugs including narcotics and anticholinergics.

Chronic gastroparesis is most commonly caused by diabetes or is idiopathic. It can also be caused by gastric surgery (Am J Surg 1996;172:24), cancer (especially lung and pancreas), anorexia nervosa, scleroderma, amyloid, polymyositis/dermatomyositis, chronic pseudo-obstruction, porphyria, and CNS disease.

Pathophys: The stomach stores ingested food, mixes it with digestive juice, grinds it, and releases it in a controlled fashion into the small intestine. Emptying of solids occurs after a lag phase during which food is moved from proximal stomach to the antrum, where it is ground up. After this initial lag phase, emptying of solids is linear, with about half of solids emptying in 60-100 minutes. A wide variety of motor abnormalities with poor coordination and hypomotility result in poor emptying.

Sx: Early satiety, nausea, and vomiting are the hallmarks of gastroparesis. Gastroparesis is probably an overlooked cause of postprandial abdominal pain and heartburn (Am J Gastro 1999; 94:1029). Diabetics may exhibit sx of poor glycemic control. Sx do not correlate well with emptying times.

Si: Rarely, a succussion splash is heard from retained gastric contents. This is demonstrated by placing the stethoscope over the stomach and rocking the pt side to side.

Crs: The course is generally chronic, but pts whose illness is associated with features suggesting a viral illness (sudden onset, fever, vomiting, cramps, and diarrhea) seem to improve with time (Am J Gastro 1997;92:1501).

Cmplc: Malnutrition, aspiration, GERD.

Diff Dx: The sx of gastroparesis are nonspecific, so the differential is broad and includes GERD, PUD, nonulcer dyspepsia, gastric cancer, and other causes of upper abdominal pain (p 1) and nausea (p 11).

Lab: Appropriate labs include CBC, CMP, Hgb A_1c, and TSH to look for correctable causes or clues to other disorders in the diff dx.

X-ray: Scintigraphic gastric emptying studies are the gold standard for the dx of gastroparesis. Pts are given a meal of solids, typically eggs, laced with a radioisotope. Studies are typically reported as the time to empty half the isotope (normal is 60-100 minutes), or as proportion emptied at 100 minutes. The variation for repeat studies in individuals is about 15% (GE 1998;115:747).

Endoscopy: EGD is generally indicated to make sure that there is no mechanical cause of poor emptying (gastric outlet obstruction due to PUD or tumor).

Rx: General measures include rx of electrolyte disorders, small frequent meals, low-fat meals, and avoidance of high fiber and nondigestible solids (peels, fruit pulp, etc). It may be helpful to replace solids with liquids. Glycemic control in diabetics should be optimized. Drugs for symptomatic pts include cisapride, metoclopramide, erythromycin, and domperidone. Response is highly variable. Cisapride 10-20 mg po qid was the drug of choice until it was withdrawn from the U.S. market for its association with cardiac arrhythmias. Metoclopramide 5-10 mg po ac and qhs is effective but is often poorly tolerated because of CNS side effects such as anxiety, restlessness, somnolence, and depression. In addition, tardive dyskinesia is an important long-term risk. Erythromycin, a motilin agonist, can be helpful but is not always well tolerated (Dig Dis Sci 1998;43:1690). Domperidone 40-80 mg daily in divided doses is effective in diabetic gastropathy (Drugs 1998;56:429) but is not available in the U.S. In refractory cases, jejunal tube feeding may be needed. Surgery (gastrostomy, jejunostomy, gastrectomy) or gastric pacemakers may have a role in refractory pts, but data showing benefit are very limited (Am J Gastro 2003;98:2122). A pilot study suggests possible benefit of botulinum toxin injection into the pylorus (Am J Gastro 2002;97:1653).

3.9 Hiatal Hernia

Postgrad Med 1990;88:113

Epidem: Prevalence rate of 0.8-2.9% of all pts undergoing barium studies.

Pathophys: There are 3 commonly recognized types of hiatal hernia. In the **sliding hiatus hernia,** the GE junction is in the chest above the diaphragmatic hiatus, and the GE junction is the lead point of the hernia. This is by far the most common type of hernia. It is strongly associated with endoscopic esophagitis (Dig Dis Sci 1979;24:311) and sx of reflux. The diaphragmatic crus contributes substantially to the antireflux barrier at the normal

GE junction, and this benefit is lost when the GE junction is displaced into the chest. In a **paraesophageal hernia,** the GE junction stays fixed and the fundus and sometimes the body of the stomach migrate into the posterior mediastinum. The stomach may later rotate in the chest, causing obstruction (Arch Surg 1986;121:416). Very rarely the stomach may herniate through an entirely separate defect in the crus. In **mixed hernias** the GE junction is in the chest and a large portion of the stomach slides up to be beside the esophagus in the chest. Linear gastric erosions in the portion of stomach at or near the diaphragm commonly occur in pts with substantial sliding hernias. These ulcerations are often multiple, are seen on the crests of the folds, and may be blood covered (GE 1986;91:338). They are a well recognized cause of iron deficiency and are referred to as Cameron ulcers (Gastrointest Endosc Clin N Am 1996;6:671).

Sx: Most pts with small or moderate sliding hiatal hernia are asymptomatic or have sx of GERD. In massive hernias and paraesophageal hernias, mechanical sx predominate and include the sudden onset of chest or epigastric pain, vomiting, and dysphagia (J Thorac Cardiovasc Surg 1998;115:828). Chronic reflux sx are also present in over half of pts. A sense of dyspnea may develop in massive hernias. In paraesophageal hernia sx of postprandial chest pain dominate complaints of heartburn (Dig Dis Sci 1992;37:537). Acute incarceration can present as a surgical emergency with severe pain, fever, and sx of esophageal or gastric obstruction.

Si: None except in those presenting with incarceration who may be febrile and appear toxic.

Crs: Most pts with hiatal hernias have a benign course. There are no adequate data on the course of untreated massive hernias or paraesophageal hernias. The published series come from academic surgical centers where pts with severe disease are likely overrepresented and where operative intervention is the norm.

Cmplc: Bleeding, usually occult, is common in large hernias. Incarceration, strangulation, and perforation are feared but rare except in massive and paraesophageal hernias.

X-ray: UGI series shows gastric mucosa above the diaphragm.

Endoscopy: The diaphragm can be seen endoscopically and moves with respiration. Hernia is diagnosed when the end of the tubular esophagus and apparent GE junction is above the diaphragm. The retroflexed view often makes the defect more obvious.

Rx:

- *Surgery:* (Semin Thorac Cardiovasc Surg 1997;9:163) Absolute indications for surgery include (1) severe obstruction that occurs when a large amount of stomach is in the chest and a volvulus results, (2) necrosis from incarceration, and (3) malignancy in the hernia. Other indications for operations are less clear cut. Some experts operate on all pts with paraesophageal hernia because of the perception that these pts are at high risk of dangerous complications (Arch Surg 1986;121:416). However, watchful waiting is reasonable since the mortality of emergent operation is not as high as previously thought (Ann Surg 2002;236:492). Some pts may have surgery for chronic iron deficiency though most such pts respond to medical rx. Symptoms from intermittent volvulus of the herniated stomach or symptomatic incarceration manifest by postprandial chest pain or fullness are relative indications for surgery. In surgery the distal esophagus is restored to an intra-abdominal position, a fundoplication is usually created, and the defect in the diaphragmatic hernia is fixed. Laparoscopic repair can be carried out in experienced hands (J Am Coll Surg 1998; 186:428).
- *Medical therapy:* Most hernias require no specific medical rx except when associated with GERD or iron deficiency. In pts with iron deficiency, the blood loss is so slow that often iron supplementation alone is adequate. When iron is stopped

anemia recurs. The lesions do not heal with iron rx alone but do frequently heal with short courses of H2RAs. Maintenance with H2RAs has not been well studied. It seems reasonable to treat with H2RAs and iron and attempt to stop iron after stores are repleted. This is the preferred course if pts have associated reflux sx. However, long-term iron supplementation alone is usually effective (Am J Gastro 1992;87:622).

3.10 Gastric Volvulus

Gastroenterologist 1997;5:41

Epidem: Seen in young pts with congenital defects and in older pts associated with hiatal hernia.

Pathophys: A gastric volvulus is a 180-degree or greater rotation of the stomach out of its normal position. This occurs when the ligaments that hold the stomach in place are disrupted. This is associated with paraesophageal hernias in adults, congenital hernias in children, or it may be a primary event without any other evident defects. An **organoaxial volvulus** is created when the body of the stomach rotates on its long axis (a line connecting cardia and pylorus). Think of the stomach as a washcloth being wrung out. Twists occur in the proximal and distal stomach where the blood supply becomes compromised, and the clinical presentation is acute. There is also a chronic presentation in which the twist is not severe enough to obstruct or compromise the vasculature. A **mesenteroaxial volvulus** is created when the stomach folds upon itself around a line drawn from the mid-lesser to the mid-greater curve. There is no highly obstructing twist and no immediate threat to the vascular supply, so the clinical presentation is chronic.

Sx: **Acute** volvulus presents with the triad of sudden onset pain, vomiting followed by retching, and inability to pass an NG tube.

Chronic volvulus has a nonspecific presentation with vague upper abdominal pain, bloating, and early satiety.

Cmplc: Perforation or bleeding in the acute presentation.

Diff Dx: For **acute** volvulus, the other differential points are the causes of sudden acute severe epigastric pain, notably perforated ulcer disease, pancreatitis, and, less likely, cholecystitis or other intra-abdominal catastrophe. For **chronic** volvulus, the differential is even broader given the vague sx and includes peptic disease, gastric malignancy, gastroparesis, GERD, chronic pancreatitis, chronic mesenteric ischemia, and biliary colic (see p 4).

X-ray: Barium studies are diagnostic and this is one of the situations in which x-ray is more informative than EGD (shudder!). In organoaxial volvulus, the stomach looks upside down with the greater curve above the lesser curve and the cardia and pylorus on the same plane. Mesenteroaxial volvulus is harder to visualize. The stomach may just be a distended sphere, or the antrum may be seen above the body. There are usually 2 gastric bubbles on plain film, one for the fundus and one for the antrum, with nothing in between where the fold is located.

Endoscopy: EGD may show the twist of organoaxial volvulus and the inability to intubate the pylorus. Otherwise the endoscopist just notes the odd anatomy and orders the barium study!

Rx: Acute volvulus is a surgical emergency. The volvulus is reduced, resection may be needed if there is necrosis, and the predisposing defects are fixed. In chronic volvulus, rx can also be surgical, but endoscopic reduction of the volvulus (Am J Gastro 1990;85:1486) and placement of 2 PEG tubes to anchor the stomach in place is an alternative (Am J Surg 1998;64:711).

3.11 Gastric Cancer

Lancet 2003;362:305; Am Fam Phys 2004;69:1133; Nejm
    1995;333:32

Epidem: Wide variation of rates throughout the world with high inci-
    dence areas in Japan, China, South America, and eastern Europe
    (30-80 cases/100,000/yr), and much lower incidence in western
    Europe and the U.S. (10 cases/100,000/yr). M:F ratio is approxi-
    mately 2:1. In the U.S., incidence is more frequent in nonwhites
    than whites. Incidence declined steadily from 1930 to the 1970s.
    The incidence of adenocarcinoma of GE junction is rising
    rapidly. In the U.S., the mean age at diagnosis is 70 years (Ann
    Surg 1993;218:583).

Pathophys: Two types of adenocarcinoma are seen. The **intestinal
    type** is made up of gland forming epithelium that results in dis-
    crete masses that ulcerate and are most often found in the distal
    stomach. This type of adenocarcinoma accounts for the greatest
    percentage of cases in high-incidence countries. In the **diffuse
    type,** cells have minimal cohesion and infiltrate the gastric wall
    without forming a discrete mass. This is more often seen in the
    proximal stomach, more often in younger pts, and has constant
    incidence throughout the world.

   Early gastric cancer (EGC) is a cancer confined to the
    mucosa or submucosa regardless of lymph node involvement. In
    Japan, EGC has a 90% 5-year survival rate, which makes
    screening more attractive. Perhaps 40% of Japanese cancers are
    EGC, but the rate is much lower in the West. For unknown rea-
    sons, survival is much better in Japanese pts with EGC than in
    Western pts (Gut 1997;41:142).

   Conditions predisposing pts to gastric cancer include
    (1) chronic atrophic gastritis with intestinal metaplasia,
    (2) gastritis associated with pernicious anemia or gastric resec-
    tion, (3) Hp infection (see p 108), (4) hypertrophic gastritis, and

(5) adenomatous gastric polyps. DU lowers risk (Nejm 1996; 335:242). **Genetic factors** may be important since gastric cancer clusters in families, in HNPCC pts, and in FAP pts, and is more common in blood group A pts. **Environmental factors** that are associated with increased risk include smoking and diets rich in salted, smoked, pickled, or poorly preserved food. Lower risk is seen in people with diets rich in fresh fruits and vegetables. The role of nitrates and nitrites is unclear.

Sx: Only half of pts have abdominal pain. Other sx include weight loss (62%), nausea (34%), anorexia (32%), and less often dysphagia, melena, and early satiety. It can be difficult to distinguish GU from cancer in the elderly pt by hx. Twenty-five percent of gastric cancer pts have a history of GU (Ann Surg 1993; 218:583).

Si: Abdominal mass, supraclavicular node (Virchow's node), periumbilical nodules from peritoneal spread (Sister Mary Joseph's node), enlarged ovary (Krukenberg tumor), mass in the cul-de-sac, and ascites.

Crs: The disease is staged by a complex TNM system into 4 stages based on tumor penetration, regional nodes, and distant mets. Involvement of intra-abdominal lymph nodes other than perigastric nodes puts pts into the unresectable stage IV. For all stages combined, 5-year survival is 18% (CA Cancer J Clin 1995;45:8). In the U.S., 5-year survivals are 50% for stage I, 29% for stage II, 13% for stage III, and 3% for stage IV. Survival is 40% higher for stage I and II tumors in Japan.

Diff Dx: Gastric lymphoma, leiomyosarcoma, PUD.

Lab: Anemia (40%), hypoproteinemia (26%), abnormal LFTs (26%), and positive FOBT (40%). Tumor markers (CEA, AFP, CA19-9) not helpful in early dx.

X-ray: If malignancy is suspected, endoscopy rather than UGI should be done. If UGI is done and shows questionable cancer or ulcer, EGD should be done.

Endoscopy: EGD may reveal an ulcer, a mass, or a diffuse infiltrative appearance in a nondistensible stomach. Multiple bx and brushings should be performed.

Rx: **Preoperative staging** is crucial, since pts with stage IV disease do not benefit from surgery in the absence of a sx to palliate such as bleeding or obstruction. Laparoscopy prevents laparotomy in up to one fourth of pts by finding intra-abdominal lymph nodes or other mets not seen on CT (Nejm 1995;333:1426). Laparoscopic ultrasound may provide additional data on T and N staging. EUS is useful in initial T staging. Those with apparent T1 or T2 tumors should have resection, but those with T3 or T4 tumors should have laparoscopy (with possible laparoscopic ultrasound) to look for advanced nodal disease which would place the pt in the unresectable stage IV (Semin Oncol 1996;23:347).

Resection of the primary tumor and the adjacent lymph nodes is the only chance for cure. Unfortunately, most pts in the West present with relatively advanced disease. If preoperative staging reveals no distant disease, surgery is undertaken. At operation, lymph node dissection can be of varying degrees. A D1 resection removes lymph nodes within 3 cm of the tumor en bloc with the stomach and greater omentum. A D2 resection additionally requires the resection of celiac nodes to the aorta, hepatoduodenal and retroduodenal nodes, splenic, and retroperitoneal nodes. In practice, D2 operations often require distal pancreatectomy and splenectomy and dissection of the major vascular pedicles down to the aorta. In Japan, D2 resections are typically carried out except in the very elderly (Brit J Surg 1996;83:836), with survival about 30% better in stage II and III disease than in Western pts (Cancer 1999;86:1657). However, in Western countries, increased morbidity and mortality after D2 resections seems to negate any survival benefits of more extensive lymphadenectomy (Lancet 1996;347:995). It is not clear if this is due to differences in disease biology, pt age, or surgical skill between the two regions. Adjuvant **chemotherapy** is of so little benefit that its use should be confined to clinical trials.

Enthusiasm for chemotherapy is higher in Asia (Cancer 1999;86:1657). Tumor-antigen-specific immunochemotherapy is a new investigational approach (Semin Surg Oncol 1999;17:139).

3.12 MALT and Other Gastric Lymphomas

Am J Gastro 2003;98:975; Br J Haematol 1998;100:3; Gastroenterologist 1996;4:54

Epidem: Gastric lymphoma is an uncommon disease. Lymphoma represents 3% of all gastric malignancies and up to half may be of the MALT type (J Clin Gastroenterol 1999;29:133).

Pathophys: The stomach does not ordinarily have lymphoid tissue. Mucosa-associated lymphoid tissue (MALT) in the stomach is made up of nonneoplastic lymphoid follicles. These follicles arise in response to chronic antigenic stimulation, typically due to Hp infection. **MALT lymphoma** (MALToma) arises from malignant transformation of a clone of B cells. The B cells respond to signals from Hp-specific T cells (Lancet 1993;342:571), and the tumor tends to stay localized in the stomach by virtue of a homing mechanism in the B cells. However, MALTomas can transform into higher grade lesions and disseminate into lymph nodes and bone marrow (Br J Haematol 1998;100:3). Most other primary gastric, **non-Hodgkin's lymphomas** are diffuse, large cell lymphomas of B cell origin. About 60% of gastric lymphomas arise in chronic gastritis.

Sx: Epigastric pain, weight loss, anorexia, vomiting, melena, hematemesis, back pain, and nausea.

Si: Epigastric tenderness, positive FOBT.

Crs: MALT lymphoma is generally an indolent disease, often remaining localized for years without rx, with a 5-year survival of 82% (Br J Haematol 1998;100:3). For other gastric lymphomas, 5-year survivals vary widely but overall survival runs about 40% (Gut 1995;36:679). Five-year survival is closer to 88% in pts whose disease does not spread into other intra-abdominal organs or outside the abdomen (Eur J Surg Oncol 1994;20:525).

Cmplc: Bleeding and perforation may occur, especially with chemotherapy, but are not as common as once feared.

Diff Dx: Gastric cancer, benign gastric ulcer, gastric Crohn's, gastric TB, gastric sarcoid, syphilis (Nejm 1995;332:1153), and the broad diff dx of dyspepsia (p 4).

Lab: Histologically, MALTomas appear as lesions in which gastric glands and crypts are invaded and partially destroyed by abnormal lymphocytes (Br J Haematol 1998;100:3). Confusion with Hp gastritis can be a problem for the pathologist, and sampling error may be a problem.

X-ray: CT scan may show thickening of the stomach or nodal involvement.

Endoscopy: EGD may demonstrate a malignant appearing mass or ulcer, thickened folds, or nonspecific gastritis. EUS can identify disease that is beyond the submucosa.

Rx: For **MALT lymphoma,** a trial of Hp rx (p 112) should be the first line for pts with disease confined to mucosa and submucosa. A response rate of 60% is expected but may take months to occur (Ann IM 1995;122:767). Pts with disease beyond the mucosa and submucosa at EUS do not respond to antibiotic rx alone (GE 1997;113:1087), but elimination of Hp is still worthwhile. Chemotherapy and radiation are considerations for pts who do not respond or relapse after antibiotics. Surgery is now generally reserved for those with localized residual disease or complications after medical therapy.

For **non-MALT lymphomas,** gastric resection was once the mainstay of rx. This operation was performed to make a tissue dx, to stage, and to cure the cases in which the disease was confined to the stomach. It was thought that gastric resection would prevent future hemorrhage or perforation when pts received chemotherapy. However, surgery is usually not needed for dx, understaging is a moot point if systemic chemotherapy is used, and the incidence of perforation and bleeding may be lower than the morbidity of surgery. Therefore, as in MALT lymphoma, surgery is largely reserved for disease persisting after medical rx (Ann Surg 2004;240:28).

3.13 Gastric Polyps

Endoscopy 1995;27:32

Epidem: Autopsy prevalence of gastric polyps is 0.12-0.8% (Am J Gastro 1995;90:2152). Adenomatous gastric polyps are uncommon under the age of 50; fundic gland polyps, hyperplastic polyps, and inflammatory polyps are more common in women (Endoscopy 1994;26:659).

Pathophys: A large series of studies on gastric polyps (Endoscopy 1994;26:659) showed several histologies. **Fundic gland polyps** were seen in 47%. Histologically they are nonneoplastic, glandular cysts found in body and fundus, and endoscopically they are small and hemispherical. They are of no clinical consequence unless they are associated with FAP or attenuated FAP (GE 2003;125:1462). They are often seen as a consequence of PPI rx. **Hyperplastic polyps** were seen in 28%. Hp infection may be etiologic in that clearance of Hp causes regression of polyps (Ann IM 1998;129:712). There are reports of large hyperplastic polyps harboring carcinoma (Gastrointest Endosc 1993;39:830) and reports of the development of focal carcinoma in hyperplastic polyps (Am J Gastro 1995;90:2152). However, this is rare enough that most practitioners consider them harmless (Endoscopy 1995;27:32) unless they bleed or obstruct the pylorus. **Adenomatous polyps** (10% of the total) are neoplastic lesions in which malignant transformation occurs about 10% of the time (Am J Gastroenterol 1998;93:2559). Other less frequent lesions include **polypoid adenocarcinoma** (7%), **inflammatory polyps** (3%), **carcinoid** (2%), and, rarely, Brunner's gland heterotopia, pancreatic rests, Peutz-Jeghers, Cronkite-Canada, and juvenile polyps.

Sx: Usually none unless they bleed or prolapse through pylorus and cause pain and vomiting (Endoscopy 1996;28:452).

Cmplc: Bleeding, malignant transformation, obstruction of pylorus.

Diff Dx: Gastric epithelial polyps may be confused with submucosal lesions such as GIST, leiomyoma or lipoma. However, in these entities, bx of the overlying mucosa is normal.

Endoscopy: Fundic gland polyps are shiny and generally small (mean 4 mm) so that they can be plucked like grapes with a bx forceps. Hyperplastic polyps are soft and often have an eroded surface. Eroded surfaces can also be seen in inflammatory polyps and polypoid cancers. Because endoscopic appearance is not diagnostic, a forceps bx is always indicated (Endoscopy 1994;26:659).

Rx: All gastric polyps should undergo bx. If an adenoma is detected, the polyp should be excised and follow-up should be done. The American Society for Gastrointestinal Endoscopy (ASGE) recommends repeat EGD in a year and every 3-5 years thereafter. If hyperplastic polyps are found, Hp should be sought and eliminated (Ann IM 1998;129:712). Routine follow-up EGD thereafter seems like overkill. However, some authors recommend excision of large hyperplastic lesions (because they are more likely to harbor cancer), and a minority excise all such polyps and perform follow-up endoscopy (Am J Gastro 1998;93:2559). Consider FAP or attenuated FAP (see p 246) if a large number of fundic gland polyps are found. Bleeding or obstructing lesions should be excised.

3.14 Submucosal Gastric Lesions

Gastro Endosc 2002;56:S43; GE 2004;126:301

Cause: Most submucosal lesions of the stomach are found incidentally at upper endoscopy and may arise from any of the layers of the stomach (not just the submucosa). The most common of these is the gastrointestinal stromal tumor (GIST) (Gastro Endosc 2003;58:80). Older literature is confusing because GISTs were previously thought to be leiomyomas, leiomyoblastomas or sarcomas. Lipomas are the second most common submucosal tumor. Other causes of submucosal gastric lesions include extrinsic compression, varices, pancreatic rests (ectopic pancreatic tissue), true leiomyomas, carcinoids, cysts, lymphoma, and metastatic disease.

Epidem: GISTs typically present in pts over 50. The incidence is unknown with estimates of up to 6,000 new cases/yr in the U.S. with up to 30% of these malignant in behavior.

Pathophys: GISTs are believed to arise from the interstitial cells of Cajal which are pacemaker cells important in normal motility (Hum Pathol 2002;33:456). They are defined by immunohistochemical staining for CD-117 (aka KIT protein), a cell membrane receptor with tyrosine kinase activity. All GISTs appear to have malignant potential and it is not possible to classify them as simply benign or malignant. Recent classification schemes use size and mitotic count of excised specimens to define risks (Hum Pathol 2002;33:459). Lesions under 1 cm are almost always benign in behavior and those under 2 cm with low mitotic counts are very low risk. Risk increases with size and lesions >5 cm are very high risk. Lipomas are almost always unimportant except in rare instances where they cause bleeding or obstruction.

Sx: Usually none unless they bleed, obstruct, or metastasize.

Cmplc: Bleeding, malignant transformation, obstruction of pylorus.

Diff Dx: The cause of a submucosal lesion is determined by EGD, EUS, or other imaging modalities.

Endoscopy: (GE 2004;126:301) Submucosal lesions are evaluated for size, consistency, color, and shape. The overlying mucosa is biopsied and some submucosal elements may be sampled. GISTs are usually firm and immobile. Lipomas are often yellowish, compress like a pillow with a forceps, and are usually mobile. Varices are usually bluish in color. Pancreatic rests are often antral and may have a central umbilication. Changing pt position may help to define extrinsic compression.

Lesions that are <1 cm undergo follow-up EGD in a year to ensure stability. Lesions >1 cm that do not appear to be lipomas at EGD should be evaluated with EUS, which can determine the size, the layer of origin, identify features suggestive of malignancy, and typically establish a dx. Fine-needle aspiration (FNA) may identify a GIST by immunohistochemical staining for CD-117, but mitotic activity can only be evaluated in excised specimens. Endoscopic submucosal resection and core needle biopsy are evolving approaches to dx and rx.

Rx: Lipomas require no specific management. Extrinsic compression, metastatic disease, lymphoma, and varices are evaluated and treated as clinically appropriate. GISTs under 1 cm can be safely followed. For lesions >3 cm surgical excision is warranted. The management of lesions from 1-3 cm should be individualized in discussion with the pt since even these lesions can become malignant. Options include surgery or yearly follow-up with EUS. Metastatic GIST can now be treated with imatinib, a tyrosine kinase inhibitor that targets the specific molecular abnormality seen in GISTs (Lancet 2001;358:1421).

3.15 Zollinger-Ellison Syndrome

Annu Rev Med 1995;46:395

Cause: Gastrin secreting tumor.

Epidem: Incidence about 0.1-3/million/yr. Mean age of onset is 50 with a range of age 7-90. Incidence greater in men than in women.

Pathophys: Gastrinomas secrete gastrin, which causes gastric acid hypersecretion. The hyperacidity results in PUD in most cases or in sx of severe GERD. Diarrhea is caused by direct damage to small intestinal mucosa, inactivation of lipase by acid, and precipitation of bile salts (Nejm 1987;317:1200). The tumors (which can be multiple) can be difficult to find. They are usually located in the gastrinoma triangle, bounded by the junction of cystic duct with common bile duct superiorly, the junction of 2nd and 3rd portions of duodenum inferiorly, and the junction of the body and head of pancreas medially. Metastatic disease most often involves the liver and is the usual cause of death.

Sx: Epigastric pain is the usual presenting sx, and 90% of pts will have PUD at some point. Up to 60% of pts will have sx of GERD, often severe. Diarrhea can be the sole sx in 20% of pts.

Crs: The growth of the tumor can be very slow and the course protracted. The survival of all pts with gastrinoma is about 60% at 5 years and 50% at 10 years. Ten-year survival is very high (90-100%) when no tumor is found at surgery and much lower (20-40%) in pts with unresectable metastatic disease.

Cmplc: Complications of ulcer disease with bleeding, perforation, or obstruction may occur.

Diff Dx: ZE must be distinguished from simple recurrent PUD. The latter is quite uncommon in the setting of rx for Hp and cessation of NSAIDs. ZE should be ruled out when pts present with recurrent ulcers despite rx. Severe diarrhea, especially if associated with PUD, should raise consideration of ZE. A strong family hx of ulcer or the combination of ulcer with hyperparathyroidism raises the question of ZE and multiple endocrine neoplasia (MEN type 1 [Ann IM 1998;129:484]). MEN type 1 is present in 10-50% of pts with ZE and ZE occurs in 20-70% of MEN type 1 pts (Medicine 2004;83:43).

ZE is not the only cause of a high gastrin. High gastrin can be caused by achlorhydria (due to pernicious anemia, PPIs, or atrophic gastritis), G-cell hyperplasia, postvagotomy state, renal failure, gastric outlet obstruction, and retained gastric antrum after surgery. These can be distinguished by provocative lab tests.

Lab: Serum gastrin is highly sensitive and is typically obtained by fasting pts for 3 days, because serum levels can fluctuate. A value of >100 pg/mL raises the question of ZE, but typically levels are much higher. Achlorhydria as a cause of elevated gastrin is excluded by verifying that the stomach produces acid by gastric sampling. A variety of provocative tests in which tumors are stimulated to produce gastrin by the infusion of secretin, calcium, or other substances have been used. The secretin test is preferred. An increase in the gastrin levels of >200 pg/mL within 2-15 minutes of secretin infusion is diagnostic (Surg Clin N Am 1995;75:511).

X-ray: Localizing the tumor is difficult, but it is crucial to the outcome. Multiple imaging tests (combinations of CT, MRI, angiograms, portal venous gastrin sampling, and labeled octreotide analog scans) are typically required since no single test is sensitive for both the primary lesion and metastatic disease (Clin Radiol 1994;49:295). The purpose of imaging is to identify lesions for a cure, to identify multiple lesions if present, and to find hepatic or other metastases which may preclude surgery or require resection (Surg Clin N Am 1995;75:511).

Endoscopy: EUS may reduce the need for angiograms and portal venous sampling (Gastrointest Endosc 1999;49:19).

Rx: PPIs are the drugs of choice for suppression of acid in the pts who are not cured by surgery. The drug dosage is titrated to lower the basal acid output (BAO) to <5 mmol/hr for pts with intact stomachs and to <1 mmol/hr for postgastrectomy pts who need higher levels of acid suppression (Aliment Pharmacol Ther 1996; 10:507).

All pts should undergo laparotomy unless substantial hepatic mets are found. In expert hands, short-term cure is 80% and long-term cure is 30% (Ann Surg 1992;215:8). In pts with persistent or recurrent disease after a first operation, a reoperation cures 30% of pts and should be considered if imaging studies show the tumor (Surgery 1996;120:1055). Pts with MEN type 1 have tumors that are small and multifocal, and cure is rare. Some experts suggest operation only if tumor is found on preoperative imaging studies (Surg Clin N Am 1995;75:511).

3.16 Bezoars

Gastrointest Endosc Clin N Am 1996;6:605

Epidem: Trichobezoars are typically found in girls. Phytobezoars are more common in middle-aged men.

Pathophys: A bezoar is swallowed material that fails to clear from the stomach and forms into a mass or concretion. Most bezoars form in pts with prior gastric surgery, gastroparesis, or unusual ingestions on a psychiatric or behavioral basis. The most common type is a vegetable matter bezoar **(phytobezoar).** Excessive vegetable fiber intake and poor mastication may be important, but prior gastric surgery seems to be the biggest risk (Brit J Surg 1994;81:1000). Unripened persimmons frequently cause bezoars from a coagulum caused when the fruit pulp is exposed to acid. Less common are hair bezoars **(trichobezoars)** typically found in children who compulsively pull and eat their hair (Mayo Clin Proc 1998;73:653). A large number of foreign substances, such as cement, shellac, cotton, paper, and a variety of pills can develop into bezoars. These foreign substance bezoars are most frequently found in psychiatric or institutionalized pts with pica.

Sx: Abdominal pain, nausea, bloating, early satiety, halitosis, and weight loss.

Crs: Because the underlying disease is usually still present, bezoars frequently recur.

Cmplc: Gastric ulcer, perforation, bleeding.

Diff Dx: Diagnosis is usually not a problem when the investigation of a nonspecific sx leads to a diagnostic UGI, CT, or EGD.

X-ray: UGI or CT shows a freely mobile mass.

Endoscopy: Needed for definitive dx. Phytobezoars are amorphous masses. Trichobezoars are usually black, slimy, and have visible hairs.

Rx: A few days of a liquid, low-residue diet may be sufficient in mild cases. Papain (a proteolytic enzyme) or cellulase are 80% successful in dissolving phytobezoars (Am J Gastro 1993;88:1663). Underlying gastroparesis should be treated to prevent recurrence, and foods high in fruit pulp and vegetable fiber need to be avoided. Trichobezoars are challenging to remove endoscopically (Gastrointest Endosc 1993;39:698). Surgery may be needed if bezoars have caused perforation or are too large for endoscopy (Mayo Clin Proc 1998;73:653).

3.17 Gastric Antral Vascular Ectasias

Gut 2001;49:866; J Clin Gastroenterol 1992;15:256

Epidem: Uncommon disorder, true incidence unknown. Predominance in women, with age range of 50-90 years in most series (Am J Clin Pathol 1998;109:558).

Pathophys: The dx of gastric antral vascular ectasia (GAVE) is made when intensely red stripes of mucosa are seen in the antrum radiating from the pylorus in a pt with evidence of chronic gi bleeding. Biopsies, if done, show features of vascular ectasia, intravascular thrombi, and vascular hyperplasia, but are not specific or diagnostic. This disorder is more frequent in pts with chronic liver disease and in pts who have undergone bone marrow transplant (Gastrointest Endosc 1996;44:223). The pathogenesis is unknown, and theories have postulated roles for portal HTN, antral motility disorders, and humoral factors (Gastrointest Endosc 1996;44:355).

Sx: Those of the anemia associated with chronic gi blood loss and intermittent melena.

Crs: Chronic gi blood loss without rx.

Diff Dx: Two areas of confusion may arise. The first is distinguishing GAVE in pts with liver disease from severe portal hypertensive gastropathy (p 430). This distinction usually is made on the basis of the endoscopic appearance, with the latter involving the more proximal stomach and being more diffuse. Histology may aid in the distinction. The other endoscopic confusion might be in separating mild GAVE from stripes of antral inflammation.

Lab: Iron deficiency.

Endoscopy: As described in "Diff Dx."

Rx: Laser photocoagulation (J Clin Gastroenterol 1992;15:256), thermal methods (such as heater probe and bipolar electrocautery) (Gastrointest Endosc 1989;35:324) and argon plasma coagulation (Endoscopy 2002;34:407) are effective though several sessions may be needed. Antrectomy is effective but is not generally necessary if endoscopic rx is available (GE 1984; 87:1165).

3.18 Dieulafoy's Ulcer

Gastrointest Endosc Clin N Am 1996;6:739; Am J Gastro 2001; 96:1688

Epidem: An uncommon cause of UGI bleeding representing 1.5-2% of all cases of massive upper bleeding. Mean age of incidence is 60, with a large age range and predominance in men.

Pathophys: A Dieulafoy's ulcer is a tiny mucosal ulcer that forms over a very large submucosal blood vessel. It has been proposed that the ulcer forms because the mucosa is compromised by mechanical effects of the large blood vessel close to the surface. Dieulafoy's ulcers are most often seen in the proximal stomach

(75%), distal stomach (13%), or proximal duodenum (12%), but have also been reported elsewhere in the small intestine and colon (J Clin Gastroenterol 1998;27:169).

Sx and Si: The sx and si are those of acute massive upper GI bleeding (p 32).

Crs: After initial hemostasis is achieved by endoscopic means, recurrent bleeding is uncommon (Endoscopy 1997;29:834). Episodes of rebleeding years later have been recorded (Gastrointest Endosc 1999;50:762).

Cmplc: Perforation due to endoscopic rx is uncommon.

Diff Dx: The diff dx is that of UGI bleeding (p 32). However, the lesion should be listed high on the differential when there is a substantial acute bleed and the initial EGD shows no cause or shows minor abnormalities that do not adequately explain a massive bleed.

X-ray: Arteriography cannot make a dx unless there is active bleeding, and it is of little value.

Endoscopy: EGD shows the tiny ulcer, sometimes with the tip of a protruding vessel poking out. There is little if any surrounding inflammatory reaction. Good air insufflation is needed. The dx is made at initial EGD only half the time, and multiple EGDs may be needed. Sometimes if an exam is done within a few hours of the bleeding, some clot remains in the ulcer, which makes it easier to spot.

Rx: Endoscopic rx is successful on the first attempt in about 85% of cases. In other cases, a second endoscopic attempt or surgery is needed. There is no science to guide the selection of the method of endoscopic rx. Heater probe, bipolar electrocautery, sclerotherapy, hemoclipping, band ligation, and laser all seem effective (Endoscopy 1997;29:834). When endoscopic rx fails, surgery with limited wedge resection using intraoperative endoscopic guidance is appropriate (J Am Coll Surg 1994;179:182).

3.19 Ménétrier's Disease

This is a rare condition characterized clinically by giant gastric folds, usually in body and fundus, by low gastric acid secretion even when stimulated, and by protein loss from hyperplastic gastric mucosa (Ann Surg 1988;208:694). Pathologically, there is hyperplasia of the surface of the mucosa and atrophy of the glandular component in the body. Surgery is the definitive rx (Ann Surg 1988;208:694), but response to medical rx including anticholinergics, acid blockers, and prednisone have been reported (J Clin Gastroenterol 1991;13:436). Response to rx with a monoclonal ab to epidermal growth factor receptor has been reported (Nejm 2000;343:1697). Gastric carcinoma may complicate the illness.

CHECK SERUM ALBUMIN
SERUM GASTRIN (FASTING)
CMV serology
H. PYLORI

Chapter 4

Inflammatory, Functional, and Other Intestinal Disorders

4.1 Irritable Bowel Syndrome

GE 2002;123:2105; Nejm 2003;349:2136; Am J Gastro 2002;97:S1

Epidem: In a large U.S. householder survey, the prevalence of irritable
bowel syndrome (IBS) sx was 9.4% (Dig Dis Sci 1993;38:1569).
In a large U.S. county survey, the prevalence of IBS sx was 17%
(GE 1991;101:927). In contrast, only 2.9% of the population
reports a medical dx of IBS, because most people with sx of IBS
do not become *pts* with IBS (GE 1990;99:409). Women are more
than twice as likely to have IBS sx and even more likely to seek
care for IBS sx (GE 1991;100:998). Sx reporting decreases with
age, suggesting the benign course of these sx (Scand J
Gastroenterol 1994;29:102). There are no differences between
the physical or psychological sx of men and women, but there are
few studies of sx in men (Am J Gastro 2000;95:11). The economic cost is huge. Pts with IBS lose twice as many work days
due to illness, require greater numbers of physician visits for gi
and non-gi sx (Dig Dis Sci 1993;38:1569), and undergo many
more appendectomies, cholecystectomies, hysterectomies, and
back surgeries (GE 2004;126:1665).

Pathophys:

- *Definition of IBS:* A working definition of IBS is needed to conduct sound clinical studies. This has proved to be difficult. The most widely used criteria to define IBS are referred to as the Rome criteria, which were published in 1992 and then substantially revised (Gut 1999;45 [suppl 2]:II43). Given the limited number of gi sx possible with any gut disorder, it is impossible to develop a definition, based on clinical sx, that will distinguish IBS from other bowel diseases (Am J Med 1999;107:5S). As a practical matter, IBS is considered when a pt presents with abdominal pain and disordered defecation in the absence of structural disease.

- *Abnormal motility and IBS:* Resting motility is similar in IBS and non-IBS pts, but IBS pts have increased motility in response to stimuli such as food or psychological stress. The severity of pain does not correlate with abnormal motility (Gastroenterologist 1994;2:315).

- *Abnormal visceral perception and IBS:* (Gut 2002;51 [suppl 1]: i67) There is a growing body of evidence suggesting that enhanced visceral sensitivity is a major factor in IBS pathophysiology. IBS pts perceive pain from balloon distension of the rectum or ileum at pressures and volumes much lower than controls do. The mechanisms of enhanced sensitivity are unclear. It is thought that multiple inciting factors (genetic factors, chronic inflammation, psychological stresses, peripheral nerve irritation) alter afferent pain pathways to the brain and leave them permanently revved up long after the inciting stimulus goes away. In a sense, the IBS pt develops a pain memory that causes stimuli, which an ordinary subject would not perceive, to be experienced as pain. These stimuli are further modulated by the CNS in ways that might further enhance the perception of pain.

- *Psychosocial factors and IBS:* Up to 60% of IBS pts have psychosocial difficulties, including major psychiatric disorders, personality disorders, stressful life events, a history of physical or sexual abuse, and chronic pain behaviors. These psychosocial factors distinguish IBS pts from pts with IBS sx who do not seek medical attention. Psychosocial factors play a major role in explaining why the IBS pt experiences symptoms as being more severe than the individual who has the same IBS sx and copes without medical evaluation. These psychosocial problems translate into worse outcomes (measured by more disability days, more physician visits, and more medicines). A history of sexual or physical abuse is one of the strongest predictors of poor outcome. Those with the most severe IBS have the greatest psychosocial stressors (Am J Med 1999;107:41S).

- *Food intolerance:* A subgroup of pts have sx of IBS in response to specific foods. These intolerances have been verified with blinded administration of the offending foods through an NG tube. The mechanism does not appear to be allergic, but it does provide a rational basis for the use of food and sx diaries in pts with moderate sx. Some clinicians have pts pursue strict exclusion diets to find the offending food (Lancet 1982;2:1115).

Sx: Since IBS cannot be defined by any test or structural abnormality, it is recognized by its sx. Three sx patterns are recognized. The patterns require different diagnostic workups and respond differently to rx (Am J Med 1999;107:20S). Common to all three subtypes are that: (1) the pts have pain or closely related noxious sx; (2) the sx are chronic, typically lasting years; (3) the sx typically begin insidiously in young adulthood; and (4) there is no evidence of structural diseases (ie, no weight loss, bleeding, fever, etc). Sudden onset sx, especially in older pts, are usually not IBS. Sx that awaken pts from sleep are less common but do not rule out IBS. The three recognized symptom patterns are:

- *Diarrhea predominant IBS:* The pts have pain associated with loose, watery BMs and great urgency. Pts often describe the stools as explosive, and typically several will be passed in a short period requiring several trips to the toilet. The BMs often cluster in the morning. Pts are usually well once the flurry of activity passes. Sometimes bouts are directly related to stressful events (taking tests, job related stress, Monday morning).

- *Constipation predominant IBS:* These pts have crampy lower abdominal pain associated with infrequent BMs. The stool is hard and looks like it is composed of individual pellets packed together. There is a sense of incomplete evacuation and straining at stool. Pain is relieved by passage of a BM. After the initial hard, dry stool has passed, a number of looser BMs may follow and the pt may complain of diarrhea. The pt then may be without sx for a day or two. Interestingly, such constipation predominant pts are more likely to have dyspepsia, musculoskeletal pain, poor sleep, and sexual dysfunction (Am J Med 1999;107:20S).

- *Pain/discomfort predominant IBS:* This group presents with complaints of generalized discomfort/pain, usually associated with bloating, a perception of abdominal distension, and a sensation of gas. Their sx may or may not be related to meals, and the relief with bowel movements is variable. They tend to experience sx over a greater part of the day. The distension is often thought by physicians to be imaginary, but increases in abdominal girth are seen in IBS pts compared to controls without a clearly defined mechanism (Gut 1991;32:662).

Si: PE is useful only for detecting structural diseases by palpation of masses, detection of blood, and identification of abdominal wall pain. No positive finding on physical exam makes IBS more likely or predicts clinical outcome or response to rx (Am J Med 1999;107:33S).

Crs: Combining results of observational studies, it is evident that more than 50% of pts have improvement in their sx over the course of years. Complaints vary in severity over time, but tend not to change in their quality. Psychological distress and a long duration of complaints correlate with poorer outcome (Scand J Gastroenterol 1998;33:561).

Diff Dx: One approach to differential diagnosis in IBS is to list all disorders known to humankind that cause diarrhea, constipation, or abdominal pain. This can lead to a lengthy list and the compulsion to rule out each dx on the list with a specific test. In practice, such a complete diff dx and subsequent workup is unnecessary. It is more fruitful to consider a short diff dx for the specific set of pt complaints, taking into account the age of the pt and the duration and severity of sx.

For pts with **diarrhea** as a predominant sx, consider lactose intolerance, drug-induced diarrhea, sorbitol ingestion (p 16), surreptitious laxative use, and IBD. Infections are uncommon if the sx are long standing, except in areas endemic for parasitic infections. The malabsorptive diseases, such as pancreatic insufficiency, rarely present with the crampy lower abdominal pain typical of diarrhea predominant IBS. Celiac disease (p 200) should be considered if pain is midabdominal rather than lower abdominal or if there is weight loss. Uncommonly, collagenous colitis and selective bile salt malabsorption are considerations. Only in refractory cases does a more extensive diff dx for chronic diarrhea need to be considered (p26).

For pts with **constipation** predominant sx, age and duration of sx guide testing. In those with a short duration sx and in those >40 years of age, colonic obstruction due to malignancy is a consideration. The reader should review the discussion of constipation (p 17).

The diff dx for pts with **pain/discomfort** predominant IBS is more complex. Consider lactose intolerance (p 172), sorbitol ingestion (p 16), partial mechanical obstruction (p 206), Crohn's disease (p 177), pseudo-obstruction (p 212), malabsorption (p 30), gastroparesis (p 130), and bacterial overgrowth (p 283).

Lab: A CBC and CMP are commonly performed to find clues to more serious illness. Stool testing for FOBT is reasonable. TSH should be done for specific reasons such as diarrhea or constipation. Stool studies for infectious causes are of very low yield if the sx are long standing and not recently changed. Stool testing can be considered in areas endemic for parasitic infection or in pts with recent exacerbation of diarrheal sx. In refractory diarrhea, a 72-hour stool collection for weight and fat can help identify those with a structural cause of diarrhea by demonstrating stool weight >300 gm/day or malabsorption of fat (p 30).

X-ray: SBFT is indicated if Crohn's disease is suspected or if there are other clues to mechanical obstruction. Air contrast BE can be used in combination with sigmoidoscopy in the small number of pts in whom obstructing neoplasm must be ruled out. However, colonoscopy would be the test of choice in pts over the age of 50, who might have the secondary benefit of screening for polyps.

Endoscopy: Endoscopy is not indicated in the vast majority of pts with IBS. The threshold to perform colonoscopy to evaluate possible IBS sx should be lower in older pts, in pts with sudden onset sx, and in pts with refractory diarrhea. The yield will be higher in these pts, and they gain the additional benefit of clearing the colon of polyps as a means of preventing future CRC. Sigmoid-oscopy should not be part of the routine workup of IBS but should be done for specific clues that pathology is within reach of the sigmoidoscope.

Rx:

Initial Approach:

- *Evaluation of the pt's complaints can be therapeutic:* Pts with long-standing complaints seek care for a variety of reasons. Many are concerned that they may have a dangerous underlying illness while others simply seek relief of sx. It is important to know the pt's reason for seeking care. A detailed history, obtained with empathy, is crucial to demonstrate to the pt that you take the complaints seriously and to establish your competence to evaluate them. A cursory history and blind reassurance on that basis can be destructive even if the physician is entirely correct with the dx. Explain to the pt the diff dx being considered and the planned evaluation to rule out structural illness. Reassure the pt that if they fail to respond to the initial rx approach and the initial testing is unrevealing that further testing and rx will be carefully considered. However, it is important to not create unrealistic expectations about the goals of rx or the extent of diagnostic testing needed.

- *Dietary fiber:* Establish the importance of diet in the pt's sx with a detailed dietary history. Estimate the pt's daily fiber intake in grams by determining the pt's intake of whole-grain bread, cereal, beans, fruits, and vegetables (Am Fam Phys 1995;51:419). A fiber intake of 25 gms will generally improve pts with constipation and helps some with diarrhea predominant IBS. Its use in diarrhea predominant pts is controversial, given limited evidence of efficacy (Am J Med 1999;107:27S). Some pts will experience bloating as fiber is increased due to fermentation/degradation, so the amount of fiber should be increased gradually. Fluid intake should be increased as dietary fiber is increased. As an alternative, fiber supplements containing psyllium seed, methylcellulose, or polycarbophil can be used (p 21), but diet should be tried first in those who are willing.

- *Trial of lactose exclusion:* Establish the daily intake of lactose-containing products. In pts with diarrhea or bloating, a therapeutic trial of exclusion of lactose (for 7-14 days) is worthwhile. Some authors do breath testing for lactose intolerance instead. This spares some pts an unneeded trial but does not answer the question as to whether lactose intolerance is responsible for sx (p 172).

- *Exclude excessive sorbitol:* In pts with diarrhea or bloating, determine the intake of sorbitol. Sorbitol is not absorbed and is then fermented by bacteria, causing distress or diarrhea. It can be found in sugarless gum, breath mints, some hard candy, apples, pears, peaches, prunes, and foods sweetened for diabetics.

- *Legumes:* Determine the intake of beans, cabbage, broccoli, and cauliflower. For pts with bloating and gas, consider a trial of exclusion or of an alpha-galactosidase preparation such as Beano (J Fam Pract 1994;39:441).
- *Fatty foods:* In IBS there can be abnormal motility in response to a variety of triggers, and for some pts this includes fatty foods.

In Pts without a Good Response to the Initial Approach Consider:

- *Rethink the dx:* If pts do not improve with initial management, the physician should rethink the diagnosis and workup. For example, failure of constipation to respond to high fiber diet might prompt excluding obstruction. Failure of diarrhea to improve after excluding milk and sorbitol may cause reconsideration of other causes of chronic diarrhea (p 26) especially celiac disease or IBD.
- *Antidiarrheal agents:* Loperamide is effective in treating chronic diarrhea due to IBS. It reduces diarrhea and diminishes urgency. The dosage should be gradually increased from 2 mg to a max of 16 mg daily in 4 divided doses. Pts should be cautioned about the risk of impaction with excessive loperamide. A second-line agent is cholestyramine, which may relieve the diarrhea due to the malabsorption of bile salts that occurs frequently in pts with functional diarrhea and treats those with the uncommon disease of idiopathic bile salt malabsorption (Am J Med 1999;107:27S). A dosage of 4 gm tid can be used as a trial. Some pts prefer 1 gm colestipol hydrochloride tablets when low doses are required.
- *Smooth muscle relaxants:* In the U.S., dicyclomine (10-20 mg po qid prn) and hyoscyamine (0.125-0.25 mg po qid prn or as a

timed release preparation [eg, Levsinex] 0.375 mg po q 12) are widely used for relief of pain in IBS. There are limited data to support their use due to methodological limitations in the available trials. A meta-analysis of smooth muscle relaxants in IBS showed that they achieved some benefit in control of pain and resulted in global improvement (Aliment Pharmacol Ther 1994;8:499). A meta-analysis of peppermint oil did not show convincing benefit (Am J Gastro 1998;93:1131).

- *Antidepressants:* Tricyclic antidepressants are appropriate for pts whose sx are persistent over months, especially if there is associated depression or anxiety. They probably work centrally as analgesics. Doses needed for IBS are often lower than doses needed for depression (10-25 mg of amitriptyline, 50 mg of desipramine). Trials of 2-3 months seem appropriate, and a second agent should be tried if the first fails, as success will be seen about 50% of the time on a second trial (Aliment Pharmacol Ther 1994;8:409).
- *Tegaserod:* Agonists of the $5\text{-}HT_4$ receptors appear beneficial in **constipation predominant IBS.** Tegaserod (2-6 mg po bid) improves sx of pain and constipation and is well tolerated (Aliment Pharmacol Ther 2001;15:1655).
- *Alosetron:* Alosetron is a $5\text{-}HT_3$ receptor antagonist that improves pain and bowel movement frequency in pts with **diarrhea predominant IBS** (Lancet 2000;355:1035). Unfortunately, it was withdrawn from the U.S. market because of a possible association with cases of ischemic colitis. The $5\text{-}HT_3$ receptors are extensively present in the enteric nervous system, and further attempts to develop agents based on blockade of these and other nervous system receptors is inevitable.
- *Chinese herbs:* Chinese herbal remedies reduce sx but are not readily available or standardized (Jama 1998;280:1585; Jama 1998;280:1569).

If Pts Are Refractory to Anything on the Preceding List:

- *Reconsider the diagnosis:* At this point if the pt has refractory sx, especially if they are long standing and constant, the dx is likely secure. Additional testing is unlikely to be needed. However, pts with IBS are not prevented from coming down with serious unrelated illnesses, and the physician should guard against failing to listen to the pt's sx.

- *Review the abuse history:* Hopefully, long before this point in rx, the physician will be able to establish whether there is a history of verbal, physical, or sexual abuse. However, because this history is so depressingly common in pts with refractory sx (Ann Intern Med 1995;123:782), the physician must reexplore this area.

- *Psychological rx:* (Arch IM 2003;163:265) A variety of modalities are available, which may be of benefit to pts whose sx are more severe and result in substantial effects on their quality of life (Ann IM 1995;123:688). These include stress management, psychotherapy, behavioral rx, hypnotherapy, and biofeedback/relaxation training. Choice of rx is usually made by the mental health professional on the basis of pt's needs and resources.

4.2 Physical and Sexual Abuse and GI

Ann IM 1995;123:782

Pts with chronic, functional gi complaints have a distressingly high (44%) incidence of prior physical or sexual abuse (Int J Colorectal Dis 1995;10:200; Ann IM 1990;113:828). Most of these pts never report these tragic life experiences to their physicians. A large number of factors that suggest a history of abuse have been identified (Ann IM 1995;123:782). The link between abuse hx and gi symptoms may be that chronic or traumatic stimulation increases sensitivity of visceral afferent receptors (Am J Med 1994;97:105). As a simple rule of thumb, always consider physical or sexual abuse in pts with functional complaints that do not respond readily to routine measures and in pts who have seen multiple providers for the same complaint. Eliciting a hx of abuse can be easily done in the routine office setting. Sometimes the pt may make a veiled reference to prior difficulties in life that open a door of inquiry. At other times a supportively phrased question is most helpful. For example, say, "Many pts I have seen with difficult or long-lasting belly pain have told me that they have been sexually or physically abused in their lifetimes—has that ever happened to you?" Most pts are surprised at the question, and most have never been previously asked about abuse by a physician. Most pts will respond well to a supportive inquiry. In an academic center only 3% of pts required urgent counseling after the inquiry (Ann IM 1995;123:782). It is then useful to go on to explain the possible connection between chronic gi complaints and the abuse history and to reassure pts that many others have had similar difficult experiences. For pts who answer affirmatively to an abuse history, it is often sensible to limit testing and to try to work with dietary and other therapies while the process of counseling is initiated. The pt is followed along with mental health clinicians until the picture improves. Occasionally, the inquiry throws a schedule into disarray but there is greater satisfaction in steering such a pt to expert help than in being on time for the next endoscopy.

4.3 Food Allergy

Am J Gastro 2003;98:740; Lancet 2002;360:701; BMJ 1998;316:1299

Cause: The most common causes of true food allergy are cow's milk, hen's eggs, cod (and other fish), shrimp (and other shellfish), peanuts (and other nuts), soybeans, wheat, and food additives. Those allergic to pollen may have reactions with a variety of foods.

Epidem: The confirmed prevalence of food allergy in adults is only 1.4-2.4% compared with a 20% pt perceived prevalence (Lancet 1994;343:1127). Rates of true allergy are higher in children.

Pathophys: Adverse reactions to food can be (1) IgE-mediated allergy (involving basophils and mast cells [GE 1992;103:1075]); (2) delayed non-IgE-mediated immunologic reactions (eg, eczema from milk); (3) nonallergic food intolerance (eg, scromboid fish poisoning due to high histamine levels, reaction to monosodium glutamate in Chinese food); and (4) food aversion. The last category is the most common, and sx are nonspecific and cannot be confirmed by blinded food challenge. Food additives (benzoates, sulfites, tartrazine, food colorings, and salicylates) may cause a nonimmunologic, harmless, contact urticaria.

Sx: Pts develop specific and reproducible sx or si involving the mouth, gut, skin, and respiratory systems. At least two of these systems should be involved. Sx include oral itching and swelling, nausea, vomiting, abdominal pain, diarrhea, asthma, cough, rhinitis, atopic dermatitis, or anaphylaxis. In a subgroup, sx develop only after exercise.

Si: Angioedema, urticaria.

Crs: About one third of children and adults lose clinical reactivity to food allergens, though lab testing can remain positive for years.

Cmplc: Anaphylaxis.

Diff Dx: Food aversion is the major differential point and is much more common than allergy. Reactions to additives and other intolerances can be difficult to separate from allergy. When symptoms suggest allergy, the dx is confirmed by lab testing followed by eliminating and then rechallenging (under medical supervision) with the offending food.

Lab: Antigen-specific IgE to water-soluble extracts of food antigens can be evaluated in serum. Many clinically insignificant cross-reactivities create false positives. Skin prick testing with food extracts is the alternative.

Rx: Rx is food avoidance. Epinephrine should be available to the pt at home, along with a user-friendly delivery device (eg, EpiPen). Anti-IgE and immunomodulatory therapies are being developed.

4.4 Colonic Diverticulosis and Diverticulitis

Lancet 2004;363:631; Am J Gastro 1999;94:3110

Epidem: Rare in children. In Western countries, the prevalence of diverticula is <10% in those under age 40, 20-30% in those over age 50, and >50% in those over age 80. Rare in rural Africa and Asia. Based on prevalence of data and hospitalization data, only 0.5% of pts are hospitalized for diverticular disease.

Pathophys: (Gastroenterologist 1994;2:299) Left-sided diverticula are pseudodiverticula that contain only mucosa and submucosa rather than all layers of bowel. They form in between the longitudinal muscle layers of the colon that are present in three bands called the tenia coli. Diverticula form in between the mesenteric and the 2 antimesenteric tenia, where the nutrient arteries pierce the circular muscle layers. These arteries create weak points where herniation can occur. The association of each diverticulum with a nutrient artery predisposes to diverticular hemorrhage.

In Western countries, 90% of pts have left-sided disease, and in Asia, right-sided disease dominates. The number of diverticula can range from a few to hundreds and are usually 5-10 mm in diameter. Resected specimens with diverticular disease show a shortening of the tenia, thickening of the colon wall, and deposition of elastin in teniae, though not true muscular hypertrophy. The thickening of the circular muscle folds is due to shortening of the tenia (Gastroenterologist 1994;2:299). The colon in pts with diverticular disease appears to be less elastic and pliable.

New diverticula may be formed when dysmotility causes high pressure segments to develop within the sigmoid.

Because of the epidemiology, it was hypothesized that diverticulosis was a fiber deficiency disease. Fiber increases the bulk of stool, increases luminal diameter, and decreases intraluminal pressure. A high-fiber diet reduced the risk of symptomatic diverticular disease (RR=0.63) in the prospective U.S. Health Professionals Study (J Nutr 1998;128:714). A study of 1800 rats also demonstrated a protective effect of a high-fiber diet (Am J Clin Nutr 1985;42:788).

Diverticulitis is the result of a small perforation of a diverticulum. This is thought to occur when undigested food debris blocks the neck of the diverticulum. This results in bacterial fermentation and mucus secretion in a closed space, which increases pressure in the diverticulum. The vascular supply becomes compromised and perforation occurs. Most of these perforations are walled off by the mesocolon or appendices epiploicae (Nejm 1998;338:1521). The walled abscess (stage I) may lead to other intra-abdominal or pelvic abscesses (stage II), or to peritonitis from rupture of the abscess (stage III). Bowel contents do not spill into the abdomen in stage III because the diverticulum is swollen shut at its neck. In stage IV disease there is a large hole in the colon that allows free spillage of stool into the abdomen with its attendant morbidity and mortality.

Diverticular bleeding is arterial. Thus, it tends to be fairly large volume and abrupt in onset. Bleeding occurs from the rupture of the artery in the diverticulum as it courses over the dome of the diverticulum. Inflammation is not part of the picture histologically (GE 1976;71:577). It is not clear what predisposes an artery to thinning. NSAID use is associated with diverticular hemorrhage (Dig Dis Sci 1997;42:990).

Sx: Most pts with diverticular disease have no sx. A subgroup will present with abdominal pain without evidence of diverticulitis. It is not clear if the pain is related to the diverticulosis. The pain is typically crampy, LLQ, associated with bloating, and has features similar to IBS, though in many cases the history is of recent onset pain (Am J Clin Nutr 1985;42:788). **Diverticulitis** typically presents as sudden onset of LLQ pain and fever, usually associated with a change in bowels. There may be minor bleeding or pain elsewhere in the belly. Pneumaturia suggests colovesical fistula, and feculent vaginal discharge may indicate colovaginal fistula. Dysuria and frequency may occur from inflammation of the bladder. **Diverticular bleeding** presents as a sudden, large volume bleed, usually reddish bloody stool with clot, as would be expected from rupture of an artery. Intermittent, chronic, small volume hematochezia should not be attributed to diverticular bleeding. Melena from bleeding right-sided diverticula is rare.

Si: Tenderness to palpation is almost universal in diverticulitis and is usually in the LLQ. Percussion tenderness and localized or diffuse peritoneal signs are variably present and reflect the severity of the episode. Fever is usually present. A palpable mass may be evident in more severe cases. FOBT may be positive but gross bleeding is rare in diverticulitis.

Crs:

- *Diverticulitis:* The risk of recurrence after a first attack of diverticulitis managed medically is about 25%, but the rate reported in the literature does vary widely (Am J Gastro 1999;94:3110). About 15-30% of pts sick enough to be hospitalized undergo surgery during that admission. About a third of pts who recover from a first attack continue to have mild intermittent sx of abdominal pain without frank diverticulitis, a third have recurrent diverticulitis, and a third remain asymptomatic (BMJ 1969;4:639). If a second attack occurs, it is much less likely to respond to medical rx, more likely to have complications such as abscess, and more likely to require surgery in two stages. The response to medical rx after a third attack is only 6%

(Dis Colon Rectum 1995;38:125). Diverticulitis recurs in 10% of pts treated surgically and requires reoperation in 3%, especially if the anastomosis is to distal sigmoid rather than rectum.

- *Diverticular hemorrhage:* Bleeding stops spontaneously in 80% of pts. It recurs in 22-38% of pts, and the chance of a third bleed after a second bleed may be as high as 50% (Am J Gastro 1999;94:3110). Pts who require less than 4 units of blood per 24 hours usually stop spontaneously (Ann Surg 1994;220:653).

Cmplc: Pylephlebitis (inflammation or infection of the portal vein and/or its tributaries); fistulae to bladder, vagina, or skin; intra-abdominal abscess.

Diff Dx: Many causes of acute abdominal pain need to be considered (p 1). The most important differential considerations for diverticulitis are: (1) ischemic colitis (in which there is usually prominent bloody stool and dx is made at sigmoidoscopy); (2) CRC (where the hx of sx is usually longer); (3) Crohn's or ulcerative colitis (where extraintestinal manifestations and chronic diarrhea may be a clue); (4) appendicitis (especially if diverticulitis is right sided); (5) pain from an ovarian source (cyst, abscess, or torsion); (6) ectopic pregnancy; (7) bacterial colitis, including C. *diff* (where diarrhea is prominent); and (8) perforated ulcer disease. The diff dx for diverticular hemorrhage includes brisk upper gi bleeding, bleeding from AVMs, cancer, or ischemia (p 32).

Lab: In diverticulitis severe enough for hospitalization, the wbc is usually elevated, but may be normal (Surgery 1994;115:546).

X-ray: An abdominal series to look for free air under the diaphragm is indicated in pts in whom perforation is suspected. However, since diverticulitis is really an extraluminal disease, the best imaging test is CT scan. CT with oral and, if needed, rectal contrast can reveal thickening of the colon, infiltration of the pericolonic fat (so-called "greying" of the fat), abscess, or air or contrast outside the bowel wall. If abscess is seen, CT can be used for percutaneous drainage. In addition, CT may show an alternative diagnosis. False-negative rates for CT vary widely and are reported in 2-21% of pts (Nejm 1998;338:1521). Contrast enemas are often nondiagnostic (since the disease is outside the bowel), but force the dx to be reconsidered if there are no diverticula seen. Ultrasound has its advocates but is very operator dependent, and studies on its use have been small (Am J Gastro 1999;94:3110).

Endoscopy: Endoscopy should be avoided in acute diverticulitis for fear of creating free perforation from the air or the instrument. Limited sigmoidoscopy is appropriate acutely if there is strong diagnostic concern for IBD or infectious colitis and stool studies are negative. After the pt recovers from a clinically diagnosed bout of diverticulitis, the entire colon should be evaluated (generally with colonoscopy, but the combination of BE and sigmoidoscopy is a reasonable alternative). This is typically done several weeks after recovery from the acute bout. Diverticular inflammation can be an incidental finding in asymptomatic pts that does not require treatment (Am J Gastro 2003;98:802).

Rx: (Am J Gastro 1999;94:3110; Dis Colon Rectum 1995;38:125)
- *Medical rx of diverticulitis:* Mild to moderate episodes in otherwise healthy pts can be treated on an outpatient basis with oral antibiotics. Severity is judged by fever, wbc count, physical exam, and reported sx severity. Pts must be well enough to be hydrated orally and be in a safe setting in case they become more ill. A 10-day course of oral antibiotics with aerobic and anaerobic coverage is prescribed. There are many acceptable choices, including amoxicillin-clavulanate (500 1 po tid × 10 days); trimethoprim-sulfamethoxazole (1 DS tab po bid) plus metronidazole (500 mg po tid); or ciprofloxacin (500 mg po bid) plus metronidazole. Because the majority of pts who recover from their first attack of diverticulitis never have a recurrence, surgery should not be offered after a single uncomplicated bout.

- *Surgical rx of recurrent uncomplicated diverticulitis:* Because each attack of diverticulitis makes it more likely that another attack will occur and less likely that the next attack will respond to medical rx, surgery is a consideration after a second bout of diverticulitis. There are no hard-and-fast rules, and the decision should be individualized. The medical fitness of the pt for an operation, the severity of the attack, the response to medical rx, and the desires of the pt all factor into the decision. In general, fit young pts should be considered for surgery after a second, uncomplicated attack. If pts are treated while not acutely ill and have a good preoperative bowel prep, they can undergo resection of the diseased segment and anastomosis in a single operation (primary anastomosis). A one-stage operation may not be possible in complicated disease.

- *Complicated diverticulitis:* Abscess, fistula, free perforation, and obstruction define complicated diverticulitis. All pts with complicated diverticulitis should be offered surgery unless the medical risk is prohibitive. Small pericolic abscesses may resolve with antibiotics (Surgery 1994;115:546). Larger abscesses can be drained with CT-guided drainage or surgery. If CT drainage is successful, the pt can usually have a one-stage operation with primary anastomosis. If CT drainage is not possible or is unsuccessful, laparotomy with resection is done. If contamination is substantial, a Hartmann procedure is done. In this operation, the diseased segment is resected, an ostomy is created for the portion of bowel still in the fecal stream, and the free end of the defunctionalized bowel is closed. In the fit pt who makes a good recovery, a reanastomosis can be performed (a two-stage operation). Pts with obstruction often respond to medical rx initially and can undergo resection with primary anastomosis electively. Pts with free perforation should have resection with colostomy. This group has high morbidity and mortality (6-35%).

- *Diverticulitis in the young:* Some authors have suggested that diverticulitis in young pts is a more virulent disease that requires surgery more than 70% of the time (Am J Surg 1994;167:562). Others have argued that the emergent surgery is often done for the wrong indication, such as a question of appendicitis (Dis Colon Rectum 1997;40:570), and that the disease is no more virulent in the young. On balance, it seems reasonable to offer young pts surgery after a first, well-documented, and significant bout because their surgical risk is very low and they have a long life over which to develop recurrent disease.
- *Diverticular hemorrhage:* The approach to suspected lower gi bleeding is outlined on p 36. In suspected diverticular bleeding, an anorectal cause should be excluded by anoscopy. If the pt is bleeding actively, a tagged rbc scan is obtained to try to localize the bleeding site. If the site is localized and bleeding does not stop, a **resection** is performed. Upper endoscopy may be needed to exclude an upper source. If bleeding stops, the pt should undergo colonoscopy to look for a treatable cause of the bleeding. Some centers offer urgent **angiography** with selective embolization as therapy. Angiography can be diagnostic and therapeutic but is associated with a high incidence of complications, requires more vigorous bleeding than a rbc scan requires for visualization (≥ 0.5 mL/min), and surgery is still frequently required (GE 2000;118:978). Some authors advocate urgent colonoscopy following vigorous bowel prep with polyethylene glycol lavage (eg, Colyte, GoLytely). The purpose is to stratify the pt's risk of rebleeding (by identifying those with active bleeding, visible vessels, and adherent clots) and to treat high-risk lesions endoscopically. **Endoscopic rx** includes injection of the base of the actively bleeding diverticulum with 1-2 mL of 1:20,000 epinephrine in 4 quadrants and bipolar electrocoagulation for visible vessels. Endoscopic clips can be

used (Gastro Endosc 2004;59:433). A recent nonrandomized trial suggests benefit (Nejm 2000;342:78), but a large, randomized, multicenter trial is needed to assess safety and efficacy of this approach. Retrospective data suggest a high risk of recurrence for those treated endoscopically (Am J Gastro 2001;96:2367).

4.5   Lactose Intolerance

Am Fam Phys 2002;65:1845; Postgrad Med 1998;104:109

Cause: Deficiency of lactase, a small intestinal enzyme.

Epidem: The prevalence of adult lactase deficiency is low in northern Europeans (2-7%) and U.S. Caucasians (6-22%) and is higher in Hispanics (50-80%), African Americans (60-80%), Native Americans (80-100%), and Asians (98-100%). The prevalence rises with age (Dig Dis Sci 1994;39:1519).

Pathophys: Lactase is normally present in the brush border of small intestinal epithelial cells. At birth, levels of the enzyme are high but decline up to 90% by age 20. In some cases, lactase deficiency is acquired due to infection (eg, *Giardia*), drugs, or other diseases of the bowel. When dietary lactose is not appropriately broken down into glucose and galactose, it passes unabsorbed into the colon. In the colon, bacteria ferment lactose, producing gas and other metabolites that cause net fluid secretion into the colon. Not all pts who maldigest lactose become symptomatic; some live blissfully with their deficiency. Most of the sx are associated with the gas production. Sx from less than 12 gm lactose (1 cup of milk) are minimal to nonexistent, and sx increase in a dose-related fashion thereafter (Aliment Pharmacol Ther 1995;9:589).

Sx: Abdominal pain, bloating, flatulence, and diarrhea after the consumption of lactose.

Si: Distension is usually not detectable clinically.

Crs: Surprisingly, sx can improve with continued lactose exposure in pts who are lactase deficient. This occurs not by improved lactose digestion but by colonic adaptation (Am J Clin Nutr 1993;58:879).

Diff Dx: Since the sx of lactose intolerance are similar to those of IBS, the two conditions are easily confused. Lactose intolerance is as common in IBS as in the general population.

Lab: Several tests are available for the diagnosis of lactase deficiency. The most widely used is the breath hydrogen test that measures the amount of hydrogen produced after the ingestion of 25 gm of lactose. If breath hydrogen rises more than 20 ppm, lactase deficiency is diagnosed. Small bowel bx is the gold standard but is largely a research tool. Other serum tests have been described (Scand J Gastroenterol [suppl] 1994;202:26). There is controversy regarding which pts to test for lactase deficiency. Since not all pts with lactose maldigestion have sx and some pts have sx without proven maldigestion, it seems reasonable to do a trial of exclusion of lactose without a diagnostic test. However, this approach risks making a diagnosis of a lifelong condition with a trial of questionable validity (Aliment Pharmacol Ther 1995;9:589). If this approach is taken, a rechallenge with lactose should be considered after the pt has been asymptomatic for some time.

Rx: (Postgrad Med 1998;104:109) Rx is for the control of sx. The mainstay is the avoidance of lactose-containing foods. Most pts tolerate the amount of lactose in less than 1 cup of milk daily. Foods highest in lactose include milk, ice cream, cottage cheese, and yogurt. Yogurt is often well tolerated because of the lactase found in live cultures. Calcium supplements may be needed in those who avoid dairy products. In pts who do not respond to exclusion of the obviously offending foods, it is possible that lactose added to other foods or used as a carrier in pills is causing sx. However, it is more likely that the pt's sx are not related to lactose. A variety of oral lactase supplements are available (eg, Lactrase, Dairy Ease, LactAid), and they are helpful for most pts who wish to use milk products moderately. Different preparations may have different efficacies (Am J Gastro 1994;89:566), but large comparative studies are lacking. Reduced lactose milk is available but has a sweet taste not acceptable to many. Calcium supplements may be needed to maintain adequate intake if dairy products are avoided.

4.6 Appendicitis

Nejm 2003;348:236; Am Fam Phys 1999;60:2027

Epidem: (Am J Epidemiol 1990;132:910) This common illness affects 8.6% of men and 6.7% of women over a lifetime, though 12% of men and 23% of women have appendectomy! The peak incidence is in pts aged 10-20, but it can occur at extremes of age where diagnosis is more difficult. It is 1.5 times more likely to occur in whites, and incidence peaks in summer. For unknown reasons the incidence declined 15% between 1970 and 1984.

Pathophys: The appendix is long, tubular, and lined with lymphoid follicles. It can be up to 20 cm long and thus cause pain anywhere in the abdomen. Most often it is behind the cecum (60%), but it may lie below, in the pelvis, anteriorly or posteriorly to the ileum, or up in the RUQ behind the liver. These variations result in varied sx and physical findings. Appendicitis results from luminal obstruction that is most commonly caused by lymphoid hyperplasia (due to any number of infectious illnesses), fecaliths, or more rarely by parasites, tumors, or Crohn's.

Sx: (Jama 1996;276:1589) Abdominal pain is the cardinal sx of appendicitis and is usually of less than 36 hours duration on presentation. It is usually RLQ in location but may occur in the flank, RUQ, or elsewhere depending on appendiceal anatomy. About half the time pain begins diffusely in a periumbilical location before localizing. Anorexia and nausea are common but do not help much in the diff dx. Vomiting is a clue if it occurs after the pain, but if it precedes the pain, an alternative dx should be sought.

Si: (Am Fam Phys 1999;60:2027) Tenderness occurs in the RLQ unless the appendix is in an unusual location. Tenderness is to direct palpation and often to percussion. Suggestive positive signs include percussion in the LLQ causing RLQ pain and localizing pain with cough. A positive psoas sign (pain on extension of the right thigh with the pt lying on the left side) may occur when the appendix is retroperitoneal. A tender rectal exam may occur in a pelvic appendix. A positive obturator sign (pain on internal rotation of the flexed right thigh) may also indicate a pelvic appendix. Low-grade fever is common. A pelvic exam should be done since this is the major differential point in women.

Crs: Appendicitis is usually an acute illness, but there are data to suggest that about 6% of pts who come to appendectomy have had recurrent bouts of a similar pain, and that the pain is relieved by appendectomy (recurrent appendicitis) (Brit J Surg 1997;84:110). My sister was convinced of this when her "murmuring appendix" was removed in her 30s with good relief after years of recurrent attacks (so much for evidence-based medicine).

Cmplc: Perforation, with resultant intra-abdominal sepsis, is the most important complication and is seen in 18% of cases (Am J Epidemiol 1990;132:910). The perforation rate climbs to 50% in those over 65 years of age, indicating the greater difficulty of diagnosis in this age group.

Diff Dx: (Emerg Med Clin N Am 1996;14:653) It is possible to draw up an exhaustive differential for this common illness. In women, ruptured ovarian cyst, ectopic pregnancy, pelvic inflammatory disease, endometriosis, ovarian torsion, and tubo-ovarian abscess are important considerations. Diverticulitis, Crohn's, perforated viscus, Meckel's diverticulitis, gastroenteritis, and a plain old bad tummy ache are the gi considerations. Renal stones, pyelonephritis, UTI, psoas abscess, and rectus sheath hematoma are only a partial list of remaining considerations.

Lab: (Emerg Med Clin N Am 1996;14:653) The wbc is elevated in 80% of pts, often with a left shift, but this finding is nonspecific. An elevated C-reactive protein (>0.8 mg/dL) is also common. The absence of all 3 of these lab parameters (an elevated wbc, a left shift, and elevated C-reactive protein) argues strongly against appendicitis. A pregnancy test should be obtained in females. A urinalysis may be helpful in the diff dx.

X-ray: (Am Fam Phys 1999;60:2027) **Plain films** of the abdomen are useful in ruling out obstruction or free air but of little specific value in diagnosing appendicitis. **Ultrasound** is helpful in pts with equivocal clinical findings. It is most helpful in female pts to look for pelvic pathology and in pediatric or pregnant pts to avoid radiation. A negative ultrasound is one in which the appendix is seen and is less than 6 mm. Ultrasound is less sensitive, less specific, and more operator dependent than CT, but is less expensive. **Helical CT scan** (Radiol Clin North Am 1999;37:895) is the most sensitive and specific test for equivocal cases. Best results are reported when a gastrograffin-saline enema is given, but even standard CT is probably better than ultrasound. It is superior in its ability to assess the inflammatory process around the appendix. Some have advocated the routine use of appendiceal CT after a prospective trial showed that it lowered cost for pts admitted to hospital for suspected appendicitis by preventing unnecessary appendectomy and unnecessary observation days (Nejm 1998;338:141).

Rx: Appendectomy is the rx of choice and negative appendectomy rates of 22% for women and 9% for men can be expected (Can J Surg 1999;42:377). There is a need for a large, randomized controlled trial to determine if laparoscopic appendectomy is superior to the open approach. A meta-analysis suggests that by using the open approach, operating time is shorter, hospital stay is unaffected, but return to normal activity takes longer (Can J Surg 1999;42:377).

4.7 Crohn's Disease

Nejm 2002;347:417; Am J Gastro 2001;96:635; BMJ 1999;319:1480

Cause: No causative agent has been identified.

Epidem: The incidence of Crohn's disease has a bimodal distribution. The first peak occurs in the early 20s and a second peak occurs in the 50s. The incidence in women is about 20% higher. U.S. blacks and whites have similar incidences and disease courses (Am J Gastro 2000;95:479), but African blacks have a lower incidence, suggesting an environmental influence. Jews have a higher incidence, and U.S. Hispanics have a low incidence (GE 1992;102:1940). The disease is more frequent in higher socioeconomic status populations, urban populations, and in those with sedentary occupations. The annual incidence varies greatly with location, with high rates in Scandinavia and northern Europe (3.6-9.8/100,000), and in North America (up to 15/100,000), and with low rates in southern Europe (0.3-3/100,000), Asia, and Africa (GE 1999;116:1503). Great variation in incidence within regions suggests the importance of local environmental factors. For obscure reasons, the incidence has rapidly risen in the last 30 years. Smoking doubles risk of developing disease (Dig Dis Sci 1989;34:1841) and worsens the clinical course (Gut 1992; 33:779). First-degree relatives of Crohn's pts have 15 times the risk.

Pathophys: Crohn's disease represents a failure of the immune system to control or down-regulate an inappropriate inflammatory process in the intestinal mucosa. The ongoing immune response is probably driven by the normal intestinal flora and defects in the intestinal mucosal barrier and mucosal immune system

(Nejm 2002;347:417). There is strong evidence for a genetic predisposition (GE 2003;124:521). The high concordance in twins, the increased risk of a family history, ethnic and racial variations, and the association of Crohn's with other rare genetic illnesses all suggest a genetic predisposition. Unlike the case in simple Mendelian disorders, where a single mutation causes disease, multiple gene defects are required in Crohn's disease. There is also a large environmental component (suggested by the epidemiology) that any model of Crohn's pathogenesis must explain.

The inflammatory mediators produced in Crohn's disease are presumably a response to antigenic stimulation and result in mucosal inflammation, ulceration, and ultimately fibrosis. The structural abnormalities created result in the diarrhea, obstruction, bleeding, and fistula formation seen in the disease. To produce these effects, the inflammatory process must be initiated and then be inappropriately perpetuated. Environmental factors such as viral or bacterial infections or toxins could be the antigens that act as initiators. Some data implicate *Mycobacterium paratuberculosis*, measles, or *Listeria* infections, but a single-agent cause is unlikely. Chronic antigen stimulation in the gut from other bacterial antigens or toxins or from a leaky mucosal barrier may be important. There are differences in the presentation of antigens to the immune system by intestinal epithelial cells in normal versus diseased individuals (GE 2000;118:S68). The role of exogenous factors such as excess dietary sugar and cigarettes, both associated with increased risk, is not yet defined (J Clin Gastroenterol 1992;14:216). No matter what the underlying events turn out to be, there is an imbalance created between proinflammatory and anti-inflammatory mediators.

Many of the important proinflammatory and anti-inflammatory mediators have been identified in animal models of IBD, and drug rx can be targeted to those mediators (see "Rx"). The interleukins (especially IL-1), the leukotrienes, and tumor necrosis factor (TNF) are important mediators of inflammation that can be targeted by drugs. Autoimmunity (the failure to recognize normal host antigens as self) is probably not a major factor in Crohn's disease, though a variety of autoantibodies have been described (Inflamm Bowel Dis 1999;5:61).

Sx:

- *Gut sx:* Crohn's disease can present clinically in many ways since it can involve the gut from esophagus to anus and has many extraintestinal manifestations. Disease is limited to the distal ileum in 30% of pts, is limited to the colon in 20% of pts, and is seen in large and small bowel in 50% of pts. Sx vary with disease location. The nature of the sx will be different depending on whether the pt has fistulizing disease, fixed obstruction due to fibrosis, or primarily inflammatory changes of the mucosa. Pts with distal ileal disease commonly present with RLQ pain, diarrhea, and weight loss. Gross bleeding is uncommon. Sometimes, obstruction from the inflamed ileum is more prominent, and pts have crampy, postprandial pain, and bloating and diarrhea may not be prominent. A subgroup will have minimal sx until they present with near complete small bowel obstruction. Crampy lower abdominal pain, diarrhea, minor bleeding, and weight loss are common in colonic disease. Pts with gastric and/or duodenal involvement present with epigastric pain that may be suggestive of PUD. Diffuse jejunoileal Crohn's is uncommon, but such pts are usually quite ill with pain, weight loss, and diarrhea (Gut 1993;34:1374).
- *Perianal disease:* About one third of pts will have perianal sx of fissures, fistulas, or abscess that may be the dominant sx or may precede the bowel sx by years. A hx of perianal disease can be an important clue in diagnosis.
- *Extraintestinal disease:* (Gastroenterol Clin North Am 1999;28:255) Joint sx are common, especially arthritis. A nondestructive peripheral arthritis involving large joints (15-20%), ankylosing spondylitis (3-5%) or sacroiliitis (9-11%) may be

seen. In the skin, erythema nodosum presents as red, painful nodules, especially on the shins (in up to 15%). Pyoderma gangrenosum is a skin lesion that causes deep sterile ulcers and is usually seen on the legs or on the abdomen near stomas after colectomy (1-2%). Iritis may present as a red, painful eye with a halo of erythema outside the cornea. Sclerosing cholangitis (1%) is the important hepatic manifestation (p 391). Aphthous ulcerations of the mouth are common. Gallstones and renal diseases are extraintestinal manifestations seen in Crohn's but not in UC. Fistulas, ureteral obstruction, oxalate stones, amyloid, and other urologic abnormalities may complicate Crohn's (Am J Gastro 1998;93:504). A variety of uncommon, steroid responsive lung diseases have been reported (Medicine [Baltimore] 1993;72:151).

- *Fistulas:* Fistulas may develop because Crohn's is a disease of the entire thickness of bowel, not just the mucosal surface. Fistulas may develop from bowel to bladder (enterovesical) and cause multiorganism UTIs or pneumaturia. Fistulas between loops of bowel (enteroenteric) can present as masses or abscesses. Fistulas to skin (enterocutaneous) present as feculent drainage and are most common around the anus. Rectovaginal fistula is an uncommon event.

Si: Low-grade fever is common, but temps >101°F usually represent a complication such as abscess. There may be findings of cachexia. A mass may be palpable, either because of inflamed loops of bowel matted together or because of abscess. FOBT may be positive. Skin findings as in the previous list.

Crs: Dx is delayed an average of 3 years in small intestinal disease (Digestion 1985;31:97). The course is unpredictable. Based on the placebo arm of 2 drug trials, it can be expected that 30-60% of placebo-treated pts with active disease enter remission within 4-5 months and half of these will stay in remission for 2 years (Digestion 1985;31:97; GE 1979;77:898). Postoperative recurrence is common, with endoscopic recurrence rates of >70% at 3 years. Thirty percent of surgically treated pts ultimately require a second resection (see "Rx").

Cmplc:

- *Colorectal cancer:* Pts with Crohn's colitis are at increased risk for CRC, but the magnitude risk is not as well defined as it is in ulcerative colitis. A well-performed, population-based study showed an absolute cancer risk of 8% at 22 years and an RR of 18 in pts with more than a decade of extensive colitis (Gut 1994;35:651). Many of the prior studies that failed to show an association were flawed because they failed to account for the cancer-preventing effects of resective surgery and failed to examine cancer rates in those still at risk (Gut 1994;35:1507). Malignancy is most likely in long-standing extensive disease, strictures, and fistulizing disease. Surveillance strategies for Crohn's and ulcerative colitis should probably be similar since the risks are of the same magnitude (Am J Gastro 1996; 91:434).

- *Other malignancies:* Small intestinal malignancy is more common in Crohn's pts than in the general population, but the magnitude of the risk is unclear and surveillance does not seem justified. Lymphoma appears to be associated with Crohn's, but the association is not clear cut (Am J Gastro 1996;91:434).

- *Osteoporosis:* Pts with Crohn's disease commonly have osteopenia or osteoporosis. Malabsorption, inflammation, and corticosteroid rx all contribute, and specific strategies for prevention and rx have been proposed (Am J Gastro 1999; 94:878).

Diff Dx: The differential varies with the major presenting sx. Usually, chronic diarrhea is the predominant sx, and Crohn's must be distinguished from IBS, ischemic colitis, ulcerative colitis, infectious diarrhea, and other dietary and drug causes of chronic diarrhea (p 26). Short duration and abrupt onset of diarrhea usually argues against IBD as the cause. When disease is confined to the ileum, appendicitis and other causes of bowel obstruction may be the major differential points. Gastroduodenal Crohn's is confused with PUD.

Often the major diagnostic problem is determining whether pts have Crohn's colitis or ulcerative colitis. Crohn's is diagnosed by the presence of small bowel involvement, by its tendency to spare segments of bowel (skip areas), especially sparing the rectum, by its endoscopic features, and by histology (see "Endoscopy"). In 5-10% of cases of colitis, a convincing dx cannot be made (indeterminate colitis).

Lab: A CBC should be obtained to look for anemia and leukocytosis. Sometimes pts with active inflammation can have very high wbc counts (above 20,000/mm³) due to the inflammatory process and steroid rx, even in the absence of abscess. CRP is another useful marker of inflammation. CMP is appropriate to assess electrolytes, renal function, and liver function. Elevations of alk phos may be a clue to sclerosing cholangitis as a complication. There has been recent interest in the use of antineutrophil cytoplasmic antibodies (ANCA) and antisaccharomyces cerevisiae antibodies (ASCA) in screening pts with sx suggestive of IBD and in distinguishing subgroups of IBD, but their role is not yet well defined (Inflamm Bowel Dis 1999;5:61).

X-ray: SBFT is appropriate in all cases to assess the extent and activity of small bowel disease. Findings are most often positive for disease in the distal ileum where narrowing of the bowel lumen, mucosal ulceration, and fistula might be detected. Barium enema can demonstrate mucosal abnormalities or strictures in Crohn's and can be used to visualize strictures that cannot be traversed with an endoscope. However, where Crohn's is suspected, colonoscopy is preferred for more certain diagnosis. CT scanning is helpful to identify abscess, can often detect bowel wall thickening indicative of inflammation, and can help distinguish Crohn's from appendicitis in some cases. CT scanning is not as sensitive as endoscopy or barium radiography. Indium leukocyte scanning, which can detect Crohn's lesions (Dig Dis Sci 1993;38:1601), is of limited value.

Endoscopy: Colonoscopy is used for initial diagnosis, to look for recurrence in symptomatic postoperative pts, and to survey for dysplasia. It is also used to assess disease activity and distribution in pts with established Crohn's disease in situations where knowledge of the endoscopic findings would change the drug or surgical rx. It should not be used to assess response to steroid rx, because it adds nothing to clinical sx in determining when a steroid taper can begin or in predicting outcome (GE 1992;102:1647).

In Crohn's colitis the rectum is often normal. The involvement with the inflammatory process is usually discontinuous. Aphthous ulcers in a background of normal mucosa, linear ulcers, and cobblestoning are common. The diffuse friability and granularity of UC is uncommon in Crohn's (Med Clin N Am 1990;74:51).

Biopsies are useful in establishing the dx. Biopsies may show evidence of inflammation with lymphocytes and plasma cells and distorted crypt architecture. Granulomata, often not seen in endoscopic biopsies, help distinguish Crohn's from ulcerative colitis when present. Histologic features help distinguish acute self-limited colitis due to infection from a first presentation of IBD (Scand J Gastroenterol 1994;29:318).

Rx: (Am J Gastro 1997;92:559; GE 2000;118:S68)
- *Assess disease severity and distribution:* In order to choose rx, it is essential to know the severity and distribution of the disease. Colonoscopy and SBFT are generally performed to determine which segments of bowel are affected. Severity is assessed by the clinical features, diarrhea, weight loss, abdominal findings, ability to maintain nutrition, and laboratory parameters such as

anemia, hypoalbuminemia, and functional status. Based on severity of illness, rx is chosen as indicated.

- *Mild to moderate disease:* These pts are ambulatory, carry out most of their usual activities, tolerate an oral diet, and do not have severely disruptive symptoms or signs. The 5-aminosalicylates (5-ASA) compounds are initial rx for most pts. **Sulfasalazine** is less effective in Crohn's disease than the newer mesalamine-containing preparations. Two agents available in the U.S. are **Asacol** (which releases mesalamine in the distal small bowel and colon), and **Pentasa** (which releases mesalamine more proximally in the small intestine). Asacol 0.8-1.6 gm po tid for ileocolonic disease or Pentasa 1 gm po qid for small bowel disease will achieve remission in about 40% of pts (Aliment Pharmacol Ther 1996;10:1). **Metronidazole** is an alternative regimen and is given in doses of 250-500 mg po tid for 12 weeks, with about a 50% response rate (Gut 1991;32: 1071). **Ciprofloxacin** with or without metronidazole (Can J Gastroenterol 1998;12:53) appears to be effective in 50-70% of pts, though adverse reactions to long courses of antibiotics are common. Often antibiotics are added in pts who are not doing well with 5-ASA products alone but who are not ill enough for steroids.

- *Moderate to severe disease:* These pts have often failed 5-ASA and antibiotics or have more severe disease at presentation with fever, malnutrition, and sx of diarrhea and pain preventing normal activities. These pts are usually treated with corticosteroids, which are effective in about 70% of pts within 4 weeks (BMJ 1999;319:1480). **Prednisone** 40-60 mg po qd is used initially and is tapered by 5 mg a week after substantial improvement occurs. Sometimes in tapering, a flare of sx will occur and the dose is boosted by 10-15 mg until sx improve. It is often necessary to taper more slowly (2.5 mg per week) once the dose is below 20 mg or if a flare occurred with the taper. When the prednisone dose is down to 20 mg, 5-ASAs are often resumed. The major concern with steroid rx is toxicity. Side effects include hyperglycemia, hypertension, adrenal suppression, osteoporosis, aseptic necrosis of the hips, sweats, proximal myopathy, depression, insomnia, impaired wound healing, and growth retardation. **Budesonide,** a steroid with high topical potency and rapid first pass metabolism in the liver, is as effective as prednisone for disease in the ileum and proximal colon but with less toxicity (GE 1998;115:835; Nejm 1994;331:836). Some experts use budesonide as initial rx instead of 5-ASA compounds. In addition to the concerns about side effects, about half of pts will be unable to stop steroids or will become steroid resistant (Gut 1994;35:360).

The immune modulators **azathioprine** or **6-mercaptopurine (6-MP)** should be used if a pt is ill enough to have required a course of steroids. Azathioprine is a prodrug that is metabolized to 6-MP and ultimately to the active metabolite, 6-thioguanine, which is cytotoxic to lymphocytes. These agents take a median of 4 months before the benefits are fully evident, and steroids are often needed as a bridge. Azathioprine doses are usually 2-3 mg/kg, and 6-MP is dosed at 1-1.5 mg/kg. Typically, 50 mg of either agent is used to start and if tolerated, the dose is increased to the weight-based target dose a couple of weeks later. Metabolism of these drugs requires the enzyme thiopurine methyltransferase (TPMT). About 90% of pts have high levels of TPMT, but 10% have reduced levels and 0.3% have little or no activity. Measurement of TPMT levels prior to beginning rx guides dosing and identifies the rare pt with absent activity who will certainly develop toxicity (Ann IM 1998;129:716). The correlation between 6-TG levels and remission is weak. However, measurement of 6-TG levels in nonresponders can identify pts who are noncompliant and those who preferentially metabolize 6-MP to the inactive 6-methylmercaptopurine (6-MMP) metabolite (Am J Gastro 2004;99:1744). Side effects of these agents include nausea, rash, pancreatitis, hepatitis, and bone marrow suppression. CBC is typically monitored weekly for 4-8 weeks and every 1-3 months thereafter. LFTs are also periodically checked, but the optimal frequency has not been established.

- *Severe disease:* These pts are unable to tolerate oral feeding and medicines and require hospitalization. They often have evidence of obstruction, malnutrition, and fever. They are treated with intravenous steroids (eg, methylprednisolone 60-80 mg iv daily in divided doses or by continuous infusion) or infliximab (see next bullet). Infectious causes of diarrhea, especially C. *difficile*, are sought, and CT scanning is considered to look for abscess. Antibiotics such as metronidazole or ciprofloxacin are added empirically. Surgery is considered depending on the clinical course and response to steroids.

- *Infliximab:* (Am J Gastro 2002;97:2962) **Infliximab** is a wildly expensive and novel biologic rx. It is a mouse-human chimeric antibody to tumor necrosis factor α, an important mediator of inflammation in Crohn's. It is indicated to induce remission in moderate to severe disease unresponsive to conventional rx and in fistulizing disease with enterocutaneous or perianal fistulas. Because of its potency and rapid onset of action, it may also be beneficial in hospitalized pts with severe disease who have not failed all conventional rx. It also appears beneficial in pts with extraintestinal manifestations such as ankylosing spondylitis, sacroiliitis, arthritis, and pyoderma gangrenosum.

    A single infusion of 5 mg/kg in pts with disease resistant to other modalities results in remission in 65% (Nejm 1997; 337:1029). The commonly used (and FDA approved) method of inducing remission is to infuse 5 mg/kg at 0, 2, and 6 weeks because it appears to be more effective and may reduce subsequent infusion reactions (Am J Gastro 2002;97:2962). Repeated infusions of 5-10 mg/kg every 8 weeks help maintain remission and maximize the chance of discontinuing steroids (Lancet 2002;359:1541). However, some experts advocate reserving scheduled infusion for those who fail to be maintained with 6-MP/AZA, given the great cost and side effects of therapy (GE 2004;126:598).

Infusion reactions and loss of efficacy are associated with the development of antibodies to infliximab (Nejm 2003; 348:601). The concomitant use of 6-MP/AZA reduces that risk, as does the use of hydrocortisone 200 mg iv prior to infliximab infusion (GE 2003;124:917). Loss of efficacy in maintenance rx can be treated by dose escalation from 5 up to 10 mg/kg. Infusion reactions are not decreased by scheduled infusions (GE 2004;126:598).

Infliximab is costly and is associated with serious side effects. The cost of a single 5 mg/kg infusion for a 70-kg pt is upwards of $3200. In a reported series of 500 pts, 6% had a serious adverse reaction. These include acute infusion reactions (3.8%), serum sickness illness (2.8%), drug-induced lupus, multiple sclerosis, serious infection, and death (0.8%). Serious infection and demyelinating diseases are contraindications to rx. A causal relationship between infliximab and malignancy (seen in 1%) is unproven. A variety of opportunistic infections have been described. The incidence of tuberculosis is much higher than that of other opportunistic infections and screening for latent tuberculosis is indicated prior to rx (Nejm 2001;345: 1098). PPD testing is limited by the high incidence of anergy; obtaining a history of tuberculosis risks and CXR may be of great importance (Clin Gastroenterol Hepatol 2004;2:309). Postmarketing surveillance has also raised concerns about cytopenias and liver function abnormalities.

- *Other biologic therapies:* A bewildering number of biologic therapies are under development for use in IBD (Gastroenterol Clin North Am 2004;33:251). These drugs are largely recombinant human proteins (cytokines, growth factors) and monoclonal antibodies. Many are in FDA phase II and III of development.

- *Other medical therapies:* In pts who do not achieve excellent control of disease with 5-ASA, steroids, or azathioprine/6-MP, other agents can be considered. **Methotrexate** is effective in 40% of steroid-dependent pts but has substantial toxicity (Nejm 1995;332:292). **Cyclosporine** has short-term efficacy (Scand J Gastroenterol 1993;28:849), but the lack of durable response and toxicity make its use minimal in clinical practice.

- *Maintenance of medical remission:* The 5-ASA agents are effective in maintaining remission in Crohn's, but the choice of agent, optimal dose, and pt populations have not yet been determined (Aliment Pharmacol Ther 1996;10:1). In practice, remission is maintained by whatever ASA preparation was used in inducing remission at a dose not lower than 2.4 gm daily. Meta-analysis shows that azathioprine and 6-MP are effective in maintenance of remission (Ann IM 1995;123:132). These agents are used to maintain remission when they are part of the initial rx that induced remission or in pts who required steroids for remission. The maintenance dose is the same as that used to induce remission. Infliximab for maintenance of remission is discussed earlier.

- *Surgical therapy:* Surgery is considered in two settings. The first is in those pts with acute complications such as obstruction, bleeding, or abscess not amenable to radiological drainage that are not responding to medical rx. The second is in pts who remain chronically ill despite medical rx. It is especially sensible to consider surgery early in medically refractory pts with a limited extent of disease. Prolonged courses of ineffective, toxic medical rx must be avoided.

- *Prevention of postoperative recurrence:* (Am J Gastro 2000; 95:1139) Endoscopic postoperative recurrence usually occurs at the neoterminal ileum, the surgically created distalmost small bowel. The mechanism for this pattern is unknown.

Endoscopic recurrence is 28% at 1 year and 77% at 3 years. Clinical recurrence rates are lower, but ultimately 30% of pts require a second resection within 10 years. Mesalamine reduces risk in most studies, but the magnitude of risk reduction is a modest 13% (GE 1997;113:1465). Surprisingly little data has been published on postoperative maintenance with azathioprine or 6-MP, though treated pts fare much better than historical controls. Steroids are ineffective. All postoperative pts should be offered maintenance rx, but the optimal dosage and agent has yet to be determined.

- *Nutrition:* Enteral feeding is effective in inducing remission in Crohn's disease but is difficult and expensive. Polymeric and elemental diets are of equal efficacy (Am J Gastro 2000; 95:735). They may be of greatest use in childhood and adolescence, when growth retardation of steroids is the greatest concern (Aliment Pharmacol Ther 1997;11:17). In pts with partially obstructive disease, a low-residue diet may reduce sx.
- *Cigarettes:* Smokers are more likely to develop Crohn's, to need surgery, to require immune-modulating drugs such as 6-MP, and to relapse than nonsmokers are (Am J Gastro 2000;95:352). Smokers should be counseled and helped to quit.
- *Perianal disease and fistulas:* (Semin Gastrointest Dis 1998;9:10) Fissures, fistula, and abscesses occur in one third of pts with Crohn's. When there is pain or fluctuance, imaging studies (eg, CT scan) and surgical drainage may be needed. In the absence of pain or fluctuance, antibiotics are the first line of rx for fistulas, though controlled data are lacking. Choices include metronidazole 250-500 mg po tid, ciprofloxacin 500 mg po bid or clarithromycin 500 mg po bid. Relapse is 70% when rx is stopped. Azathioprine/6-MP is helpful in two thirds of pts. Infliximab (5 mg/kg iv at 0, 2, and 6 weeks) is effective in closing fistulas in two thirds of pts with a median duration of response of 3 months (Nejm 1999;340:1398). This should be

tried when the less expensive measures fail and maintenance rx may be required (see "Maintenance of medical remission," earlier in this list). Surgical rx is needed to control sepsis and to treat refractory sx (Semin Gastrointest Dis 1998;9:15). Surgery should generally be avoided for treatment of skin tags, hemorrhoids, and fissures because of poor healing and risk of complications (GE 2003;125:1503).

- *Osteoporosis prevention:* Osteoporosis is common in Crohn's even when corticosteroids are not used. Most pts need calcium (1.5 gm daily) and vitamin D supplementation (800 IU daily). Prophylactic regimens to reduce steroid-induced bone loss should be instituted (GE 2003;125:937).
- *Psychosocial issues:* Psychosocial factors do not cause Crohn's but are as important to evaluate and treat as other sx of the disease. Assessing the psychosocial factors will improve compliance, minimize misunderstandings between pt and physician, and improve the pt's health status (Gastroenterol Clin North Am 1995;24:699).
- *Pregnancy:* Most pts whose disease is well controlled can expect nearly normal fertility and an uncomplicated pregnancy. The 5-ASA agents and steroids can be used in pregnancy. Metronidazole and ciprofloxacin should be avoided. The use of azathioprine/6-MP is controversial (Dig Dis 1999;17:201).

4.8   Ulcerative Colitis

Am J Gastro 2004;99:1371; Lancet 2002;359:331

Cause: No causative agent has been identified.

Epidem: (Gastroenterol Clin North Am 1995;24:467) The epidemiology of UC is similar to that of Crohn's. The incidence is bimodal, with peaks in the 3rd and 6th decades. In contrast to Crohn's, men with UC outnumber women with UC by 20%. Incidence is higher in urban areas, industrialized countries, and in those of higher socioeconomic status. Like Crohn's, UC is more common in northern latitudes (eg, incidence 15/100,000/yr in Norway and 2/100,000/yr in Spain), but in contrast to Crohn's, incidence has been stable over time. Smokers have half the risk of nonsmokers, and former smokers are at even greater risk than nonsmokers (GE 1994;106:807). First-degree relatives have 15 times increased risk of UC but not of Crohn's. Though at one time, UC was thought to be primarily a psychiatric disorder, there appears to be no greater frequency of psychiatric diagnosis in UC pts than in controls (Dig Dis Sci 1982;27:513).

Pathophys: (Gastroenterol Clin North Am 1995;24:475) Ulcerative colitis and Crohn's share many common epidemiologic and clinical features and the pathophysiologies must be closely related. UC results from a failure of the immune response to be appropriately down-regulated. The inappropriate immune response results in lymphokines (especially interleukins 4 and 10) that mediate mucosal inflammation in the colon. Colonic inflammation causes the diarrhea and bleeding that characterize the disease. The nature of the stimulus that initiates the immune response and the factors that perpetuate the response are unknown. Both genetic factors (BMJ 1993;306:20) and environmental factors contribute. UC, like Crohn's, is likely a group of closely related disorders that share final common pathways of inflammation. Current models cannot account adequately for the distribution of UC, the high frequency of autoantibodies in the disorder, or its extraintestinal manifestations.

Sx: Chronic bloody diarrhea is the hallmark of UC. It is usually associated with a sense of urgency with BMs, a sense of incomplete evacuation, and an uncomfortable sensation of rectal spasm (tenesmus). The distribution and severity of the colitis affects the clinical presentation. Pts with **proctitis** (disease confined to the rectum) may present with relatively formed BMs once or twice daily interspersed with multiple trips to the toilet to evacuate bloody mucus. With greater lengths of involved bowel (proctosigmoiditis, left-sided colitis, or pancolitis) the pt has more diarrhea, crampy lower abdominal pain, and is generally more ill. Weight loss and fever reflect more severe inflammation or a greater extent of disease. The **extraintestinal manifestations** of UC are less numerous than those of Crohn's. Acute arthropathy occurs in 10-15% of pts and typically involves single large joints or multiple small joints symmetrically. Other manifestations include sacroiliitis (9-11%), ankylosing spondylitis (1-3%), uveitis and episcleritis (5-15%), erythema nodosum (10-15%), pyoderma gangrenosum (1-2%), and sclerosing cholangitis (2-7%) (Gastroenterol Clin North Am 1999;28:255).

Si: Depending on the severity of illness, the pt may have fever, cachexia, and abdominal tenderness. Distension raises the possibility of toxic megacolon.

Crs: Most pts have a chronic relapsing illness. About 10% of pts will have a single unrelenting attack or a single attack with prolonged remission. Pts with systemic sx such as fever and weight loss are most likely to relapse. A pt in remission has a 20% chance of relapse of disease the following year, and those with active disease have a 70-80% chance of relapse in the following year (GE 1994;107:3). Those with proctitis develop disease outside the rectum about 12% of the time over the course of 10 years and have a low risk of colectomy (3-5%) (Scand J Gastroenterol 1977;12:727).

Cmplc:

- *Colorectal cancer:* (Curr Gastroenterol Rep 1999;1:496) The CRC risk for pts with UC is about 7-14% at 25 years. Older studies from referral centers overestimated the risk. The risk appears to rise after 8 years of disease and increases 0.5-1% per year of disease duration. A family hx of CRC or concurrent sclerosing cholangitis increases risk while 5-ASA rx and regular medical care decrease risk. Dysplasia, which can be defined as neoplasia confined to the mucosa, precedes invasive cancer. Pathologists classify dysplasia as low-grade, high-grade, or indefinite. Colonoscopic surveillance to detect dysplasia is widely performed but there are several practical problems with cancer prevention by surveillance for dysplasia. These include: (1) pathologists frequently do not agree on the determination of dysplasia, (2) not all resected colon specimens with cancer show dysplasia elsewhere in the specimen, (3) surveillance samples a tiny portion of the mucosa, (4) cancer can be seen within a year or 2 of surveillance, and (5) surveillance has never been conclusively proven to save lives. Despite these limitations, the ACG has published guidelines suggesting annual surveillance after 8-10 years of disease outside the sigmoid. The AHCPR guideline is colonoscopy q 1-2 yr after 8 years of pancolitis or 15 years of left-sided colitis (GE 2003;124:544).

The finding of dysplasia of any grade (confirmed by a second expert pathologist) is considered an indication for colectomy. An area of confusion is the management of dysplasia associated lesions or masses, or so-called DALMs. Some of these lesions are probably garden variety sporadic adenomas unrelated to colitis (Am J Gastro 1999;94:1746). Those DALMs that look like resectable discrete polyps can probably be managed by endoscopic polypectomy, bx of the surrounding mucosa, and surveillance (GE 1999;117:1295).

- *Osteoporosis:* Like pts with Crohn's, pts with UC are at increased risk (Am J Gastro 1999;94:878).
- *Toxic megacolon:* This is a condition in which the colon becomes dilated (>6 cm) in the presence of severe colitis and systemic toxicity. Morbidity and mortality are high. Management includes rx of the colitis, avoidance of narcotics and anticholinergics, colonic decompression and close observation for complications requiring surgery (Am J Gastro 2003;98:2363).

Diff Dx: The most common difficulty in diagnosis is distinguishing acute, self-limited infectious colitis from UC. An abrupt onset is the most useful piece of history suggesting an infectious cause. Stool studies should be obtained to rule out bacterial pathogens and amebiasis (p275). C. *difficile* is common in IBD pts but tends not to be so bloody. Ischemic colitis, CMV colitis, drug-induced colitis (especially gold), and radiation colitis round out the differential. Crohn's disease is usually distinguished from UC by the tendency of Crohn's to involve noncontiguous portions of bowel (skip lesions), to spare the rectum, by its histologic features, or by small bowel involvement. About 5-10% of pts cannot be cleanly classified as UC or Crohn's and their cases are called indeterminate colitis.

X-ray: Barium enema is too insensitive to be useful in UC. CT if done for other reasons may show thickened colon. Plain abdominal films are useful for the detection of toxic megacolon.

Endoscopy: Colonoscopy shows evidence of colitis beginning in the rectum and found in a continuous and circumferential pattern to the point of transition to normal mucosa. The colitis is characterized by granularity, friability, ulceration, and inability to visualize the underlying normal vasculature (loss of the vascular pattern) (Med Clin N Am 1990;74:51). Histology shows acute and chronic inflammation in the lamina propria and distortion of the normal architecture (eg, gland atrophy, branching). Histologic features help distinguish acute self-limited colitis due to infection from a first presentation of IBD (Scand J Gastroenterol 1994;29:318).

Rx: (Am J Gastro 1997;92:204; Gastroenterol Clin North Am 1999;28:297; GE 2004;126:1582)

- *Proctitis:* Proctitis is most effectively treated with mesalamine suppositories 500 mg pr bid for a period of 4-8 weeks, depending on severity and response. For a first mild episode it is reasonable to stop rx and wait for relapse. Maintenance rx is

individualized with a single suppository every 2nd or 3rd night.
Hydrocortisone suppositories or foam are alternatives. A rare
pt may require oral steroids.

- *Proctosigmoiditis:* For pts who are ambulatory and with no signs
  of toxicity, mesalamine enemas 4 gm pr qhs are effective,
  expensive, and work more rapidly than oral 5-ASA preparations. Steroid enemas are an alternative but systemic steroid
  absorption does occur. For pts who prefer oral rx, the aminosal-
  icylates **mesalamine** (Asacol 800-1600 mg po tid) or **balsalazide** (Colazal 2.25 gm po tid) are effective. Studies comparing these agents are too limited by methodologic problems
  to conclude that either agent is superior (Am J Gastro
  2002;97:2939). **Sulfasalazine** 2-4 gm daily in 2-4 divided doses
  is a less expensive alternative that is associated with many
  more side effects. These are mostly caused by the sulfapyridine
  portion of the sulfasalazine molecule that is released when the
  parent drug splits off the active 5-ASA molecule in the colon.
  If sulfasalazine is used, then folate 1 mg po qd should be given
  to treat impaired folate absorption from sulfapyridine.
  Olsalazine, (Dipentum), a 5-ASA dimer, is effective but is
  used less often because of diarrhea as a side effect.
- *Disease beyond the sigmoid:* Delivery of topical rx outside the
  sigmoid is less reliable, and oral rx is often needed. Mesalamine
  and balsalazide are common choices as previously described.
  Topical rx with a mesalamine enema can be added to oral rx
  for more rapid sx control.
- *When 5-ASA is not enough:* Pts with extensive colitis, weight
  loss, and anemia and those who are more disabled by their sx
  should be treated with prednisone from the outset. In addition,
  pts who are not as ill but have failed attempts at maximal
  5-ASA rx should receive prednisone. Prednisone is given at
  doses of 40-60 mg daily. The oral 5-ASA can generally be
  stopped at high doses of prednisone, though topical rx can still
  be helpful for sx relief. When sx improve, the prednisone is

tapered by 5 mg per week. The 5-ASA is resumed when the prednisone dose is reduced to 20 mg or so, but there is little science to guide the practice. Sometimes the taper must be slowed (eg, 2.5 mg a week) when the prednisone dose drops below 20 mg. For those with an inadequate response to oral steroids or for those who relapse with tapering and become steroid dependent, azathioprine/6-MP should be considered (see p 185). Surgery is a curative alternative that needs to be considered in this group of refractory pts. There is limited evidence that fish oil (as Max-EPA 6 caps po tid) is beneficial (Ann IM 1992;116:609).

- *Severe disease:* Intravenous steroids and hospitalization are needed in pts who have signs of systemic toxicity, those who fail to improve with oral steroids, or those who are too ill to maintain hydration and nutrition. Methylprednisolone 60-80 mg in divided doses or by continuous infusion is begun. ACTH can be used in a first attack but has little apparent advantage and adrenal hemorrhage is a risk. In these ill pts, concomitant 5-ASA or intravenous antibiotics may be used. In general, narcotics, antidiarrheals, and anticholinergics are avoided for fear of precipitating toxic megacolon. If pts fail to turn the corner in a week, then surgery needs to be considered. Cyclosporine can be given iv, but in some cases it may forestall rather than prevent colectomy. It is best used in centers with expertise in its use (Am J Gastro 1997;92:1424). Data on infliximab in severe colitis have been equivocal and new biologics are under development.

- *Surgery:* (Gastroenterol Clin North Am 1999;28:371) Surgery can be urgently required for hemorrhage, bleeding, and in pts who remain ill despite 7-10 days of maximal medical rx. Surgery is also indicated in pts who are steroid dependent or intolerant despite azathioprine/6-MP, or those who do not achieve a good quality of life on medical rx. Pts who have endured a prolonged attempt at medical rx rarely express regret after colectomy, despite the life changes. If surgery is required urgently, a subtotal colectomy (sparing the rectum) is less dangerous than a total colectomy, especially in medically high-risk pts. Completion proctectomy (with ileostomy or ileoanal anastomosis) can be achieved at a later date. For those having elective surgery, the choice is between total proctocolectomy with ileostomy versus ileal pouch-anal anastomosis. For proctocolectomy with ileostomy, 25-50% have leakage problems, 10-25% require a stoma revision, 15% will develop bowel obstruction, and 5% of men will become impotent. Ileoanal anastomosis was initially offered only to the young and fit, but it is now being offered to greater numbers of pts. Most surgeons perform the procedure in two stages. The first is abdominal colectomy, rectal mucosectomy (leaving the rectal muscular cuff and anal sphincter), creation of an ileal pouch as a fecal reservoir, ileal-anal anastomosis, and temporary diverting ileostomy. The ileostomy reduces dehiscence and pelvic infection and requires closure in a second operation 8 weeks later. Some surgeons skip the diverting ileostomy in low-risk pts. The functional results are good. The chief morbidity is bowel obstruction and infection. The failure rate requiring permanent ileostomy is 5-10%. Pts can expect an average of 6 BMs daily, including a nocturnal one. The major late complication is pouchitis (15%), an inflammatory condition of the ileal pouch of unknown cause, which responds to antibiotics (Gastroenterol Clin North Am 2001;30:223).

- *Survey for colorectal cancer:* As discussed in "Cmplc."
- *Osteoporosis prevention:* Osteoporosis is common in IBD even when corticosteroids are not used. Most pts need calcium (1.5 gm daily) and vitamin D supplementation (800 IU daily). Prophylactic regimens to reduce steroid-induced bone loss should be instituted (GE 2003;125:937).

4.9 Collagenous Colitis

Mayo Clin Proc 2003;78:614; Gastroenterol Clin North Am
1999;28:479

Cause: The cause is unknown, though a link to NSAIDs has been hypothesized (Gut 1992;33:683).

Epidem: Limited data available suggest an incidence of 1.8/100,000/yr. There is a 9:1 predominance in women, and a peak incidence in the 8th decade (Gut 1995;37:394).

Pathophys: The pathophysiology of the disorder is poorly understood (Dig Dis Sci 1991;36:705). Collagenous colitis is considered one of the two subtypes of **microscopic colitis.** Some have hypothesized an autoimmune etiology since there is a strong association of collagenous colitis with autoimmune disorders (like thyroiditis, Sjögren's, and rheumatoid arthritis). The collagen itself does not explain the diarrhea, which probably results from the inflammatory process. The most favored hypothesis is that the disorder is an inflammatory response to an uncommon, luminal infectious agent (Dis Colon Rectum 1996;39:573).

Sx: Chronic watery diarrhea and diffuse, crampy abdominal pain that waxes and wanes and has often been present for years prior to diagnosis.

Crs: About two thirds of pts remit with or without rx, and the remainder have a waxing and waning course. The disorder is an annoyance rather than a debilitating illness and does not have an impact on life expectancy.

Cmplc: None.

Diff Dx: The disorder should be considered in any older pt with chronic watery diarrhea. Most of these pts will be thought to have IBS until endoscopic biopsies make the diagnosis clear. The full diff dx is discussed under Chronic Diarrhea (p 26).

Lab: Fecal leukocytes are seen in 55%, but no other routine lab studies are of diagnostic help (Mayo Clin Proc 1995;70:430).

Endoscopy: At colonoscopy the mucosa is normal, or nonspecific erythema is seen. Histology is the defining feature, with features of colitis (acute and chronic inflammatory cells in lamina propria) associated with an increase in the thickness of the subepithelial collagen band (from a normal of 3 mm to an average of 15 mm) (Mayo Clin Proc 1995;70:430). The dx can usually be made at sigmoidoscopy since the vast majority of pts have involvement in the distal left colon (Mayo Clin Proc 1995;70:430).

Rx: There are few randomized trials to guide rx. The initial approach can be symptomatic. Exclusion of caffeine, lactose (p 172), and sorbitol (p 16) should be tried. Loperamide is often effective. Some pts respond to cholestyramine, metronidazole, or bismuth subsalicylate (8 tabs in 3 divided doses for 8 weeks [Gastroenterol Clin North Am 1999;28:479]). When pts remain symptomatic, 5-ASA preparations (eg, sulfasalazine 2-4 gm daily or mesalamine 2.4-4.8 gm daily in 3 divided doses) are tried. Budesonide has been effective in randomized trials (eg Gut 2003;52:248), but relapse is common and the toxicity of long-term therapy is unclear. Rarely, prednisone and surgery have been used.

4.10 Lymphocytic Colitis

This disorder has clinical features similar to collagenous colitis and a histology that is similar except for the absence of the subepithelial collagen layer. It is considered a subtype of microscopic colitis. Some have wondered if it is a precursor lesion to collagenous colitis or part of the spectrum of one illness (Am J Gastro 1995;90:1394). Lymphocytic colitis does not have the striking predominance in women seen in collagenous colitis, suggesting it may be a different disorder. The therapeutic approach is the same as for collagenous colitis.

4.11 (Diversion Colitis)

This is an inflammatory process that occurs in segments of bowel that have been diverted from the fecal stream (pts with a Hartmann's pouch or mucous fistula) (J Clin Gastroenterol 1992;15:281). Pts may present with pain or bloody mucoid discharge. Reestablishing the fecal stream cures the disorder. Fatty acid enemas can be tried in pts who are not candidates for surgery, but no benefit was seen in a small RCT (Dis Colon Rectum 1991;34:861).

4.12 Celiac Disease

Lancet 2003;362:383; Nejm 2002;346:180

Cause: Sensitivity to gluten, the protein fraction of wheat, rye, and barley.

Epidem: (BMJ 1999;319:236) The prevalence of disease used to be quoted as lower than 1/1000, but the recognition of asymptomatic or latent disease (Gut 1993;34:150) detected by serologic screening has put the prevalence in the 1/200 range. The disease can occur at any age, though childhood disease is declining. Peak incidence is in the 5th decade, with a predominance of 3:1 in women. Associated disorders include type 1 diabetes, thyrotoxicosis, IgA deficiency (2%), Sjögren's, PBC, osteoporosis, and neurologic disorders. Cigarette smoking appears to be protective (sigh!) (Gut 1996;39:60).

Pathophys: (GE 2000;119:234) Gluten, the trigger of celiac disease (aka celiac sprue, áka gluten-sensitive enteropathy) is the material that makes dough sticky and allows the making of bread. Gliadin, the alcohol-soluble fraction of gluten, contains proteins that are rich in glutamine and proline and toxic to celiac disease pts. These toxins are present in high concentrations in wheat, rye, and barley and in small concentrations in oats (which may be tolerated by some pts). The toxic proteins are absent in corn, millet, and rice. These toxic proteins resist digestion in the upper intestine (Nejm 2003;348:2573). They are deamidated by the enzyme **tissue transglutaminase,** which appears to be the autoantigen in celiac disease. The deamidated proteins ultimately bind to the HLA-DQ2 or DQ8 molecules and are recognized T cells. These activated T cells produce cytokines, which produce an immune response with hyperplasia of the mucosal crypts followed by atrophy of the small intestinal villi. The villous atrophy causes the characteristic clinical syndrome, though not all pts with abnormal mucosa develop sx. The disease begins in the proximal small intestine and the length of involvement affects the development of sx. Genetic factors are important, with a 70% concordance in monozygotic twins and strong associations with HLA-DQ2 or DQ-8 and other HLA antigens. However, genetics are not the entire explanation, and environmental factors, yet unidentified, are probably important.

Sx: The classical presentation of sprue is that of diarrhea due to malabsorption and subsequent weight loss. The diarrhea is associated with bloating, borborygmi, and relatively little pain. There has been a shift towards diagnosing pts with milder sx such as indigestion, fatigue, or iron deficiency. Associated sx may include peripheral neuropathy, ataxia, infertility, aphthous ulcerations of the mouth, sore tongue, generalized weakness, and arthritis. In severe cases, vitamin deficiency syndromes may occur. Dermatitis herpetiformis is a blistering skin disease characterized by pruritic, papulovesicular skin lesions (Nejm 1991;325:1709) that is considered a manifestation of celiac disease. About 75% of pts with this lesion have villous atrophy, and the rash responds to diet.

Si: In severe cases there is wasting, glossitis, and malnutrition. FOBT-positive stools are common (Nejm 1996;334:1163).

Crs: The vast majority of pts do well with dietary rx and become asymptomatic. Relapses are usually due to dietary exposure to gluten (often unintentional). A small group of pts do not respond to diet and are diagnosed with refractory or unclassified sprue. This is a heterogeneous group with a poor prognosis, and many are ultimately found to have T cell lymphomas (GE 2000;119:243).

Cmplc: Celiac disease is associated with lymphoma of the small intestine (RR=77), cancer of the mouth and pharynx (RR=23) and esophagus (RR=12). This risk appears to be reduced to normal after 5 years of a gluten-free diet (Gut 1989;30:333). Osteoporosis has been convincingly associated with celiac disease, and bone density should be evaluated (Gut 1994;35:150; Gut 1995;37:639).

Diff Dx: The major problem in diagnosis is failure to consider celiac disease in the differential diagnosis. A missed diagnosis is especially common in the elderly (Gut 1994;35:65). A suggestive history or a positive screening test leads to small bowel bx, which shows evidence of villous atrophy. A similar bx can be seen in tropical sprue (an infectious illness of uncertain cause [Gut 1997;40:428]), acid hypersecretion from gastrinoma, bacterial overgrowth, lymphoma, and eosinophilic gastroenteritis (Nejm 1991;325:1709). Therefore, the diagnosis is only considered certain when pts respond to a gluten-free diet.

Lab: The autoantigen in CD has been identified as **tissue transglutaminase** (tTG) (Nat Med 1997;3:797), and effective screening tests using ELISA assays are available. Susceptible individuals also develop autoantibodies to reticulin, a constituent of the extracellular matrix. These antibodies are identical to **antiendomysial** (EmA) antibodies, allowing their use as a screening test. However, EmA testing is expensive and cumbersome and is being replaced by tTG testing. IgA antiendomysial and tTG antibodies are >95% sensitive and specific but may miss cases with partial villous atrophy. Since IgA deficiency is common in celiac disease, an IgG antibody test or IgA levels are also needed. Antigliadin antibodies are helpful in partial villous atrophy and an IgG Ab is available (to detect IgA deficient pts) so this test is commonly ordered along with a tTG IgA Ab test.

Folate and iron deficiency (both absorbed in the duodenum) are common. Abnormal transaminases are common (Lancet 1998;352:26) and resolve with dietary rx. Because of the pitfalls of serologic diagnosis and the difficulty of the lifelong dietary rx, most pts go on to have small bowel biopsy for diagnostic confirmation. This may be unnecessary in symptomatic pts with a positive IgA EmA or tTG (Dig Dis Sci 1996;41:83).

X-ray: SBFT can be normal in mild disease. If disease is more advanced, there is loss or thickening of folds. In advanced cases there are featureless, dilated loops of small intestine with rapid transit of barium.

Endoscopy: Endoscopy can be normal or show reduced or absent Kerckring duodenal folds or scalloping of the folds (Nejm 1988;319:741). Bx obtained at endoscopy show the histologic abnormalities described earlier. Endoscopic findings are not sensitive (Am J Gastro 2002;97:933).

Rx: In theory, the dietary rx of celiac disease is straightforward. The pt simply avoids all products with gluten: wheat, barley, and rye. Oats are less toxic and are usually well tolerated (Nejm 1995;333:1033). Many clinicians will add oats to the diet after a period of stability on a diet without oats (though many commercial oat products are contaminated with gluten). The reality, however, is that a gluten-free diet is difficult, because modern food processing results in the addition of gluten as an additive in many foods. Consultation with a dietary expert is mandatory, and many lay organizations provide food lists and recipes. In practice, motivated pts often end up the true experts and can be helpful to those newly diagnosed. When pts do poorly, it is most often due to continued gluten ingestion. Other causes of a poor response to rx include wrong dx, lactose intolerance, pancreatic insufficiency, lymphocytic or collagenous colitis, and bacterial overgrowth

(Lancet 2003;362:383; Am J Gastro 2003;98:839). Only 50-70% pts are fully compliant with diet (Lancet 1997;349:1755). Pts should receive supplementation with folate, iron, and calcium if needed. They may not tolerate lactose well in the early stages of rx. A tTG Ab can be used to look for ongoing gluten ingestion in pts with relapsing sx. Evaluation of bone density and screening of first-degree relatives is appropriate.

4.13 Short Bowel Syndrome

GE 2003;124:1105; Gastroenterol Clin North Am 1998;27:467; GE 1997;113:1767

Cause: Extensive surgical resection of small intestine due to mesenteric vascular disease, Crohn's disease, or malignancy. Thrombotic vascular disease may be due to underlying coagulation defects.

Epidem: The epidemiology follows that of the underlying illness leading to the surgery.

Pathophys: The normal adult has about 240 cm of jejunum, 360 cm of ileum, and 160 cm of colon. Enteral nutrition and hydration cannot be generally maintained when massive resection leaves the pt with less than 70-100 cm of small bowel. After resection, there is a phase of intestinal adaptation during which hypertrophy of the mucosa increases absorptive surface area, and there is slowing of intestinal transit. A bewildering number of nutritional and hormonal factors are crucial in the adaptation process. Loss of surface area results in inadequate uptake of calories and protein (causing weight loss), poor absorption of micronutrients (especially fat-soluble vitamins), and electrolytes (especially Ca^{++}, Mg^{++}, and Zn^{++}). Bile salts and fatty acids are malabsorbed and may cause worsened diarrhea in pts with an intact colon by stimulating fluid secretion.

Sx: Diarrhea, weight loss, sx of volume depletion. Specific micronu-
trient deficiencies may result in a variety of syndromes
(Gastroenterol Clin North Am 1998;27:467).

Si: Cachexia and volume depletion.

Crs: The course is generally determined by the length of small bowel
remaining. The outcome is better in young pts and in pts with
(1) proximal intestinal resections (allowing for bile salt absorption in the distal ileum), (2) an intact ileocecal valve, and (3) an
intact colon.

Cmplc: D-lactic acidosis due to fermentation of malabsorbed carbohydrates in the colon may occur (presenting as dysarthria, ataxia, or
confusion, with an elevated anion gap). Oxalate kidney stones
(due to excessive colonic absorption of oxalate, which is bound
to malabsorbed fatty acids) and gallstones may be seen.

X-ray: SBFT may be used to estimate the remaining length of
intestine.

Rx: (Scand J Gastroenterol 1997;32:289) The initial postoperative
management problem is usually massive diarrhea that requires
TPN, fluid and electrolyte replacement, and an H2RA to minimize gastric acid volume. Early use of tube feeding is indicated,
since the intestinal adaptation process requires enteral feeding.
Antimotility agents are used (eg, loperamide 16-20 mg daily).
Reduction of fat calories may be needed in those with an intact
colon to prevent bile salt-induced diarrhea, but is not needed in
those without a colon. A mix of long-chain and medium-chain
triglycerides are used as a fat source. Pts are given fat-soluble vitamin supplements (A, D, E, and K). Parenteral Mg^{++} replacement may be needed because of diarrhea from oral preparations.
Cholestyramine may be used in pts with an intact colon who
develop bile salt-induced diarrhea. With this approach, most pts
can be gradually transitioned from TPN and enteral feeding to an
oral diet.

In pts who do not improve with these measures, continuous tube feeding with a polymeric diet, nocturnal feeds, or TPN may be needed. Those who require long-term TPN are on the slippery slope of complications from infection, TPN-induced liver disease, poor vascular access, and bacterial overgrowth. Operations to create antiperistaltic segments or to increase absorptive surface area have mixed success (Brit J Surg 1994;81:486). Small bowel transplant is a high-risk option that may be needed in those with intractable TPN complications (Lancet 1996;347:1801).

4.14 Bowel Obstruction

Lancet 1999;353:1476; Adv Surg 1997;31:1

Pathophys: Most episodes of bowel obstruction occur in the small intestine, and most of those are due to adhesions. While adhesions can be inflammatory, most of them are postoperative. Nearly a third of pts undergoing laparotomy are readmitted over the following 10 years with adhesion-related complications (Lancet 1999;353:1476). Pts having colonic resections and pelvic surgery are at higher risk. Other causes of obstruction include herniae, malignancy, Crohn's, radiation, bezoars, intussusception, gallstone ileus (obstruction by a gallstone), and volvulus. In the colon, malignancy is the most common cause of obstruction.

  Obstruction results in distension of bowel loops, edema of the bowel wall, and third spacing of intravascular volume. The distended, edematous bowel is more likely to twist, creating a closed-loop obstruction. This twist occludes the arterial blood supply and causes gangrene of the bowel (strangulation).

Sx: Colicky abdominal pain is the typical presenting sx (70%), though pain may become more steady in nature as obstruction persists (Scand J Gastroenterol 1994;29:715). Anorexia and nausea are frequently seen. Vomiting is common, especially in high-grade or proximal obstructions. Diarrhea may result transiently as the downstream bowel is emptied.

Si: Abnormal sounds and distension are the best physical exam evidence of obstruction (Scand J Gastroenterol 1994;29:715). Usually bowel sounds are high pitched, but if seen late in the illness or if strangulation has occurred, bowel sounds may be diminished or absent. Distension may be absent if the obstruction is proximal. Peritoneal signs (percussion and rebound tenderness, involuntary guarding) suggest the possibility of strangulation. Inguinal and femoral hernias should be excluded by exam.

Crs: A large proportion of pts with partial obstruction resolve nonoperatively. Of those with complete obstruction 8-23% will have strangulation at surgery. Recurrence rates are high (34% at 4 years, 42% at 10 years) except if obstruction is due to hernia. Recurrence rates are lower in pts treated operatively (29% vs 53%) and mortality rates range from 2-12% (Arch Surg 1993;128:765).

Cmplc: Strangulation with subsequent perforation, and intra-abdominal sepsis.

Diff Dx: Gastroenteritis (pain, nausea, vomiting), ileus, and pseudo-obstruction (p 210).

Lab: Leukocytosis is usually mild, and wbc >15,000/mm^3 should raise the question of ischemia. Electrolyte abnormalities and azotemia should be sought and corrected.

X-ray: (AJR Am J Roentgenol 1997;168:1171) **Plain films** of the abdomen are routine in suspected bowel obstruction. Air fluid levels in dilated small bowel are diagnostic but are seen in only 50-60% of cases. About 20-30% of films are equivocal, and 10-20% are normal and misleading. The x-ray can be normal if loops are all fluid filled or if the obstruction is proximal. An upright chest film centered on the diaphragm may show free air due to perforation.

    CT scan is very helpful in diagnosing obstruction (AJR Am J Roentgenol 1994;162:255). It can be used to visualize air or fluid-filled loops without aid of oral contrast, which can be difficult to give due to vomiting. Iv contrast should be used. Sometimes the point of obstruction can be seen. If the obstruction is caused by an extrinsic process such as mass or inflammation, CT can identify it. CT signs have also been identified for evidence of strangulation that may prompt earlier surgery.

Other **radiographic studies** may be needed. An unprepped gastrograffin enema is an efficient way to evaluate suspected large bowel obstruction and may be therapeutic if the obstruction is due to fecal impaction. In the acute setting, barium studies (SBFT or enteroclysis) are of limited value but may be of use after an episode of obstruction has spontaneously resolved. Ultrasound may be of some value in determining that obstruction exists (seeing dilated loops) but usually does not reveal the cause (Radiology 1993;188:649). It may be of most value in pregnant pts.

Rx: Third space fluid losses and electrolyte abnormalities must be rapidly corrected. Pts with a specific cause of obstruction (such as mass or hernia) and those with no prior surgery that might have led to adhesions should undergo laparotomy. Prompt surgery is needed if there is evidence of compromised bowel (peritoneal signs, toxicity, evidence of perforation). In obstruction due to suspected adhesions, an attempt should be made to avoid operation. A nasogastric tube should be placed to decompress the stomach and small bowel. Longer tubes are of no proven additional value (Am J Surg 1995;170:366). Most pts who resolve without operation begin to do so within 24-48 hours, though some experts wait as long as 5 days before giving up and proceeding with laparotomy (Am J Surg 1993;165:121). Those with partial obstructions are at low risk for strangulation. Pts are monitored frequently with physical exam for signs of compromised bowel and undergo laparotomy urgently if they develop. The role of laparoscopy is not yet defined (Surg Endosc 2000;14:154). Intraperitoneal bioresorbable membranes have been used to prevent recurrent adhesions (J Am Coll Surg 1996;183:297).

4.15 Colonic Volvulus

Adv Surg 1996;29:131

Epidem: Incidence is lowest in Western nations (1-3/100,000/yr) and higher in developing nations (12/100,000/yr in Ghana). The mean age of presentation is 60-70 in the West and 40-60 in developing nations. Institutionalized pts with chronic constipation are at high risk.

Pathophys: A volvulus is an axial twist of part of the gi tract around the mesentery, resulting in a complete or partial obstruction. Most volvulus occur in the sigmoid or the cecum. A redundant sigmoid colon contributes to sigmoid volvulus. A cecal mesentery that is not well attached to the posterior abdominal wall predisposes to cecal volvulus. Volvulus in other segments of colon is rare.

Sx: The presentation is that of bowel obstruction with distension, pain, and constipation. Since the condition may spontaneously revert, pts may have a hx of prior similar episodes.

Si: Distension is striking and is often asymmetric. Peritoneal signs are absent unless ischemia has complicated the volvulus.

Crs: Mortality is high in Western countries (14%) (where volvulus occurs in the medically unfit) and is higher in those needing emergency operations (25%) (Dis Colon Rectum 2000;43:414).

Cmplc: Intestinal gangrene from loss of vascular supply carries a 50% mortality (Dis Colon Rectum 1982;25:494).

Diff Dx: The differential includes mechanical obstruction from malignancy or diverticular disease and pseudo-obstruction (J Am Coll Surg 1996;183:297).

X-ray: Plain films are diagnostic in 80% of sigmoid volvulus, with findings of a distended sigmoid, two air fluid levels, and a bird beak deformity. Cecal volvulus can be more difficult to identify. Contrast studies can identify the bird beak deformity and may be therapeutic by decompressing the volvulus.

Rx: In sigmoid volvulus without clinical evidence of perforation or ischemia, sigmoidoscopy is the initial therapeutic approach. As the scope passes by the twist, there is a large and sometimes spectacular rush of gas as decompression occurs. The mucosa is then inspected for evidence of ischemia. A decompression tube is left behind, which may help splint the bowel in place. Surgery is indicated in fit pts because the risk of recurrence is high. Operations that tack bowel down (sigmoidopexy, suturing the sigmoid serosa to the posterior abdominal wall) are associated with higher recurrence rates (30-80%) than those that involve a bowel resection (Dis Colon Rectum 2000;43:414). However, resection carries greater operative risk. Extraperitonealization of the sigmoid without resection has been described as an alternative, with acceptable mortality and low recurrence rate (Dis Colon Rectum 1998;41:381). Cecal volvulus usually requires surgical rx.

4.16 Acute Colonic Pseudo-Obstruction

Gastro Endosc 2002;56:789; Annu Rev Med 1999;50:37

Epidem: This disorder (aka **Ogilvie's syndrome**) has been associated with a long list of conditions, notably orthopedic surgery, narcotics, anticholinergics, and chemotherapy. Many neurologic, renal, cardiac, obstetrical, and lung disorders have been described in association with this disorder. Malignancy, metabolic, and endocrine disorders may be present.

Pathophys: In pseudo-obstruction, the radiographs suggest mechanical obstruction, but no mechanical obstruction is present. The pathogenesis of acute colonic pseudo-obstruction is unknown. It is thought to represent an imbalance of sympathetic and parasympathetic stimulation.

Sx: The usual presentation is progressive abdominal distension that occurs over days in a hospitalized pt. Pain, nausea, and vomiting are variable features.

Si: Tympany to percussion and visible distension. Bowel sounds are present and may be high pitched.

Crs: The course is largely dependent on the underlying illness.

Cmplc: Perforation rates of up to 3% have been reported, and perforation is associated with a 50% mortality.

Diff Dx: The major differential point is that of mechanical obstruction. In pts with a typical clinical background, conservative measures can be employed without further evaluation. In those pts who fail to improve within 24 hours, endoscopy or unprepped, water-soluble contrast enema should be obtained to rule out mechanical obstruction.

Lab: Electrolytes, Ca^{++}, Mg^{++}, PO_4, BUN/Cr, O_2 saturation, and a CBC are routinely obtained. Leukocytosis is a finding worrisome for perforation.

X-ray: KUB shows a distended colon. Cecal diameter should be measured, because the risk of perforation becomes higher when cecal diameter reaches 10-12 cm. KUB is repeated daily until the findings resolve. A water-soluble contrast enema should be considered in all pts prior to the use of neostigmine to rule out a mechanical obstruction (Nejm 1999;341:1622; discussion 1623).

Endoscopy: See "Rx."

Rx: (Nejm 1999;341:192) Metabolic abnormalities such as acidosis, hypokalemia, hypocalcemia, hypomagnesemia, and volume depletion should be corrected. Drugs that inhibit motility (eg, narcotics, anticholinergics) should be stopped. Frequent turning of pts (or log rolling, spending 15 minutes in each of decubitus, prone, and supine positions) can be effective. An NGT and/or a rectal tube is inserted. If the pts fail to improve or worsen in the first 24 hours and if there are no contraindications, neostigmine should be used. A dose of 2 mg iv provides decompression within minutes (Nejm 1999;341:137). It should be given with the pt supine, on the bedpan, and on a cardiac monitor because of the risk of bradycardia, which may require atropine. Abdominal pain, salivation, and vomiting may occur. For pts who relapse or fail to respond to this intervention, colonoscopic decompression with a tube placed in the right colon is usually advocated (Gastrointest Endosc 1996;44:144). Surgery is indicated for those who have clinical evidence of perforation, peritonitis, or who fail all other rx.

4.17 Chronic Intestinal Pseudo-Obstruction

Annu Rev Med 1999;50:37; Gut 1997;41:675

Epidem: Rare.

Pathophys: This disorder is defined by the radiographic picture of chronic obstruction in the absence of a mechanical obstruction. A variety of underlying diseases may result in a chronic defect in gut motility. In most pts, the disorder is secondary to diseases such as scleroderma, amyloid, or a paraneoplastic syndrome associated with malignancy. In some pts, there is a defect in enteric smooth muscle (hollow visceral myopathy), and in others there is a defect of the enteric nervous system.

Sx: The predominant sx are pain, distension, vomiting, constipation, and diarrhea. A family history may suggest one of the primary disorders.

Si: Distension or signs of an associated collagen-vascular, or neurologic disease.

Crs: The course in pts with the secondary form depends on the associated disorder. The course in those with primary gut myopathy or neuropathy is that of chronic illness, pain, and malnutrition.

Cmplc: Bacterial overgrowth, malnutrition.

Diff Dx: Mechanical obstruction and mucosal disease such as Crohn's must be excluded.

Lab: A CMP, thyroid studies, Mg^{++}, and CBC are obtained. In specialty centers, motility and transit studies may be performed. Fibrosis and other morphologic abnormalities are seen on full thickness biopsies or resected specimens.

X-ray: Plain films show dilated bowel, giving a radiographic impression of obstruction though no mechanical obstruction exists.

Rx: Promotility agents are usually ineffective. Therapy is supportive with nutrition and rx of bacterial overgrowth. Surgery is indicated in severe, symptomatic distension in order to place a decompressive tube enterostomy (Am J Gastro 1995;90:2147). When there is localized pseudo-obstruction, resection or bypass can be performed.

4.18 Radiation Proctitis and Enteritis

Am J Gastro 1996;91:1309

Cause: Radiation rx for malignancy.

Epidem: Radiation colitis usually occurs in pts undergoing radiation rx for cancer of the uterus, cervix, ovaries, and prostate. In most pts, changes are confined to the rectum. It occurs in 2-5% of such pts (Dig Dis Sci 1991;36:373).

Pathophys: Radiation colitis can be acute or chronic. Acute radiation injury occurs as a result of mucosal cell injury and can last for 3 months after rx has ended. Chronic radiation colitis results from ischemia and fibrosis due to chronic effects of radiation on blood vessels and connective tissue (Dig Dis Sci 1991;36:373).

When the blood supply is compromised, pts develop friability, bleeding, ulcers, strictures, or fistulae. The rectum is the most vulnerable because it is in a fixed position in the radiation field (while other bowel loops may move) and is often in closest proximity to the target organ.

Sx: Painful rectal spasms (tenesmus), small volume stools, and bleeding are the most common acute sx. Fistulae and bleeding are the most common chronic sx.

Si: Blood in stool.

Crs: Most pts who present with mild to moderate sx are likely to improve spontaneously within 2 years (Q J Med 1983;52:40). In surgical series about 10-15% of pts will have severe, intractable sx lasting years and requiring surgery (Am J Gastro 1996;91:1309), but this probably overestimates the extent of the problem.

Cmplc: Chronic, severe blood loss is the most important complication seen. A small group develop stenosis, fistulae, or perforation.

Diff Dx: Dx is not difficult when there is a hx of radiation and endoscopic findings of neovascularization. Malignancy, infectious or ulcerative proctitis, or solitary rectal ulcer (p 298) are infrequent considerations.

X-ray: If done, a BE might show evidence of stricture or mucosal inflammation but colonoscopy is more helpful.

Endoscopy: Colonoscopy may reveal mucosal pallor or erythema, friability, or ulceration. Bizarre looking, telangiectatic blood vessels (neovascularization) may be the only gross finding and are the source of troublesome bleeding. Rectal ulcers or stricture may occur. Histology in the chronic phase shows vascular changes of subintimal fibrosis and telangiectatic vessels.

Rx: Tenesmus and pain are difficult to treat and do not respond well to topical steroids or 5-ASAs (Am J Gastro 1990;85:1537). Sucralfate enemas seem the most effective of the topical medical therapies, but long-term, randomized data are lacking (Dig Dis Sci 1999;44:973). Hyperbaric oxygen has been used but is not readily available (Dig Dis Sci 1991;36:373). Bleeding can be treated with local endoscopic measures such as laser (Gastrointest Endosc 1993;39:641), bipolar cautery (Gastrointest Endosc 1991;37:492), argon plasma coagulation, or formalin applied topically (Jama 1994;272:1822). A small, randomized trial of misoprostol rectal suppositories given during rx showed great benefit in preventing acute and chronic sx (Am J Gastro 2000;95:1961). Surgery, usually with a colostomy, is a last resort and is frequently associated with complications.

4.19 Pneumatosis Intestinalis

This condition is defined by the presence of gas in the bowel wall. Pts with this finding and evidence of bowel obstruction or ischemia need surgery, but many pts with a variety of conditions (recent anastomoses, jejunostomy tubes, IBD, lactulose use, chemotherapy, COPD) recover without surgical intervention (Ann Surg 1990;212:160).

4.20 Typhlitis

This is an uncommon disorder of localized inflammation of the cecum and ascending colon seen in neutropenic pts undergoing chemotherapy for malignancy. Surgical intervention may be required (Curr Gastroenterol Rep 2002;4:297).

4.21 Eosinophilic Gastroenteritis

Gut 1990;31:54; South Med J 1996;89:189

This is a disorder characterized by eosinophilic infiltration of the gi tract. Involvement can be in the mucosal, muscular, or subserosal layers of the gut and can occur from esophagus to colon. Pts with subserosal involvement present with bloating and ascites. Pts with mucosal or muscular involvement may present with seemingly functional sx such as dyspepsia (Dig Dis Sci 1997;42:2327). Common at presentation are nausea, vomiting, diarrhea, weight loss, anemia, protein losing enteropathy, and intestinal obstruction or perforation (South Med J 1996;89:189). About 50% of pts report a hx of allergy. The diagnosis is suspected with gi sx and eosinophilia, but the eosinophilia may be absent in 25% (Gut 1990;31:54). In these cases, the dx is made when bx show eosinophilic infiltration, but this can be patchy and the dx missed. In some cases full thickness bx may be required. The cause is unknown. Other causes of eosinophilia should be excluded. The response to steroids is usually dramatic (Am J Gastro 1993;88:70).

4.22 Meckel's Diverticulum

Am Fam Phys 2000;61:1037; Gastroenterol Clin North Am 1994;23:21

This abnormality is a diverticulum located on the antimesenteric border within 100 cm of the ileocecal valve and is found in 1-3% of individuals. In half of the pts, the diverticulum is lined by acid-producing heterotopic gastric mucosa. When the diverticulum ulcerates, it can present as lower tract bleeding. Intussusception can occur in adults, with the diverticulum as the leading edge. The gastric mucosa-containing diverticulum may be detected by Tc-99 pertechnetate scanning but false negatives do occur and diagnosis can be difficult.

4.23 Endometriosis

Endometriosis can involve the gut and can be confused with pain of gut origin. Crampy, nonpelvic pain can be seen in extensive disease, and complaints do not always intensify prior to or during menses. The disease can mimic IBD on barium studies (Arch IM 1995;155:977). It is important to consider this common disorder in women with chronic pain complaints (Obstet Gynecol 2003;102:397).

4.24 Epiploic Appendagitis

J Emerg Med 1999;17:823

The epiploic appendages are fat-containing structures hanging off the outside of the colon. These structures can cause acute abdominal pain if they infarct. The clinical presentation can suggest appendicitis or diverticulitis but the pt is not ill. The correct diagnosis is made by CT scanning, which is characteristic with a fat density adjacent to the colon with surrounding inflammatory change. The rx is with analgesia and observation and sx generally resolve within a week.

Chapter 5

Neoplastic Intestinal Disorders

5.1 Colorectal Cancer

GE 2000;118:S115; Lancet 1999;353:391

Epidem: (Gastroenterol Clin North Am 1996;25:717) Colorectal
cancer (CRC) is the second leading cause of cancer death in the
United States. The lifetime incidence of CRC for those born in
the U.S. is roughly 6% (Jama 1989;261:580). Age-specific incidence increases abruptly at age 40 and climbs steadily thereafter.
For example, for men ages 40-44, the rate is 12/100,000/yr,
climbing to 57/100,000/yr for men ages 50-54 and to
320/100,000/yr for men ages 70-74 (Ann IM 1990;113:373).
Incidence rates have been declining in whites since the 1970s
(decreased by 1.6%) but not in blacks (increased by 36% in
African American men), perhaps due to poorer access for blacks
to colonoscopy and polypectomy (Arch Fam Med 1995; 4:849).
There is a tendency in the U.S. for African Americans and lower
socioeconomic status whites to present with later stage cancers.

There is a striking geographic variation. The disease is
common in the U.S., Scandinavia, western Europe, and
Australia, but uncommon in Asia, Africa, and South America.
Immigrants to high-incidence areas experience a marked
increased incidence, suggesting that environmental factors may
be critical in the disease.

About 75% of cancers occur in pts without well-defined risk factors (GE 1997;112:594). There are several well-recognized risk factors, including:

- *Polyposis syndromes:* Familial adenomatous polyposis (FAP) (p 246) represents about 1% of the total cases, and those with the FAP gene have a near 100% rate of cancer development. Pts with the HNPCC family history represent about 1-2% of total cases and have a lifetime risk of CRC of about 80% if they inherit an HNPCC gene (p 242). Peutz-Jeghers (p 250) and juvenile polyposis (p 252) are uncommon risk factors.
- *IBD:* Those with ulcerative colitis proximal to the splenic flexure have an increased rate of CRC after 8-10 years, and this risk is 7-14% at 25 years (p 192).
- *Family hx of CRC:* Having a single first-degree relative with CRC appears to confer a lifetime risk of 12-24%. The high-risk end of the range represents people with a first-degree relative with CRC under the age of 45 (Gastrointest Endosc Clin N Am 1993;3:715; Ann IM 1993;118:785). Having 2 first-degree relatives with CRC puts the lifetime risk at 25-35%. The period of greatest excess relative risk begins under age 45 (when rates in the general population are low) (Nejm 1994;331:1669). Therefore, screening such individuals has maximum potential benefit if begun early (eg, age 40). When only a second- or third-degree relative is affected, the risk is increased to only 30-50% above that of the general population, so the screening strategy is not altered (Gastroenterol Clin North Am 1996;25:793).
  - *Family hx of adenoma:* The relative risk for pts whose first-degree relatives have an adenoma is 1.78, and this climbs to 2.59 for siblings of pts whose adenomas were diagnosed before age 60 (Nejm 1996;334:82).
  - *Prior CRC:* The risk of a second cancer is low in the first 10 years after dx but may be as high as 6.3% at 18 years (Clin Radiol 1984;35:425).

- *Prior colon adenoma:* Pts with villous or tubulovillous adenomas >1 cm have a RR for cancer of 3.6 at a mean of 14 years of follow-up (Nejm 1992;326:658).
- *Hyperplastic colonic polyps:* Hyperplastic polyps have conventionally been regarded as harmless and nonneoplastic. However, recent lines of evidence suggest that hyperplastic polyps (especially large lesions of the right colon) may be precursors of colon cancers characterized by methylation of DNA (Clin Gastroenterol Hepatol 2004;2:1). It has not yet been determined whether pts with hyperplastic polyps should be surveyed differently than pts at average risk.
- *Other risks:* Type 2 diabetes mellitus is associated with a RR=1.43 for CRC in women (J Natl Cancer Inst 1999;91:542). Population-based cohort studies do not show a link between breast cancer and CRC, though less methodologically sound studies have suggested an association (J Clin Gastroenterol 1994;19:57). Other risks include prior ureterosigmoidostomy (RR=10) (J Urol 1990;144:1110), irradiation for gynecologic cancer, acromegaly (Clin Endocrinol [Oxf] 1990;32:65), high intake of red meat (Cancer Res 1994;54:2390), dietary fat (Nejm 1990;323:1664), and cigarette smoking (J Natl Cancer Inst 2000;92:1178).
- *Protective factors:* It has long been thought that **dietary fiber** is protective for CRC after Burkitt hypothesized that the low incidence of CRC in black Africans was related to high dietary fiber. The low risk in black Africans now appears due to low animal product consumption (Am J Gastro 1999;94:1373). The data are not striking for the protective effect of fiber. A large meta-analysis showed benefit (J Natl Cancer Inst 1990;82:650), but several cohort studies show no benefit (Gastroenterol Clin North Am 1996;25:717). Current thinking is that fruit and vegetable fiber are more important

than grain fiber. The Nurses Health Study showed a clear benefit of >15 years of **folate**-containing multivitamin use (RR=0.25) and a more modest protective effect of dietary folate (Ann IM 1998;129:517).

There is strong epidemiologic evidence that **aspirin** prevents CRC. Of 11 observational studies done, 10 have shown a protective effect (Ann IM 1998;128:713). The Cancer Prevention Study II, a prospective mortality study of more than 1 million subjects, showed a 40% risk reduction in pts who used aspirin at least every other day (Nejm 1991;325:1593). Similar risk reduction was seen in the Health Professionals Study (50,000 men) after controlling for a number of confounding variables (Ann IM 1994;121:241). Despite tantalizing epidemiologic data, the only long-term, randomized study showed no differences after 5 years of randomized aspirin use (J Natl Cancer Inst 1993;85:1220). In a 12-year follow-up of this cohort (in which subjects self-selected aspirin use or not after 5 years), CRC was seen as frequently in aspirin users as nonusers (Ann IM 1998;128:713). Recent RCTs have shown a benefit of aspirin in reducing adenoma incidence in pts with prior adenoma or cancer (Nejm 2003;348:891; Nejm 2003;348:883).

Calcium supplementation shows no consistent benefit in epidemiologic studies, but an RCT demonstrated a benefit of supplementation in preventing recurrent adenomas (Nejm 1999;340:101). **Fish oil** is rich in omega-3 fatty acids, and fish oil supplements decrease the synthesis of arachidonate. Fish oil decreases the rectal mucosa proliferation of pts with adenomas (GE 1992;103:883) and is protective in a mouse model of CRC (Nutr Cancer 1991;15:1). Pts who are more **physically active** and leaner have a slightly lower risk of CRC (J Natl Cancer Inst 1997;89:948). **Postmenopausal estrogen** rx is associated with a 20% reduction in risk (by meta-analysis [Am J Med 1999; 106:574]). CRC incidence was seen to be decreased in coronary event trials of the **HMG-CoA reductase inhibitors** pravastatin (43% reduction in incidence [Nejm 1996;335:1001]) and simvastatin (19% reduction [Arch IM 1996;156:2085]).

Pathophys:

- *The progression from adenoma to carcinoma:* The molecular mechanisms that cause the formation of adenomas and their degeneration into cancers are now quite well understood (Gut 1993;34:289). The common first step is mutation of the adenomatous polyposis coli (APC) gene. This gene (an inherited mutation of which is the defect in FAP [p 246]) appears to be critical in regulating cell proliferation and programmed cell death (apoptosis) (Curr Gastroenterol Rep 1999;1:449). Defects in the APC gene might be inherited or acquired. For example, a subtle mutation in the APC gene (the I1307K mutation) is responsible for inherited cancers in Ashkenazi Jews (Nat Genet 1997;17:79). Adenomas begin as aberrant crypt foci, and their subsequent growth from small adenoma to large adenoma is marked by a series of mutations. Many of these mutations occur in DNA mismatch repair genes (the described defects in HNPCC pts [p 242]). One described defect is the activation of an oncogene, K-ras, while the other defects are primarily loss of tumor suppressor genes. Further transformation to cancer occurs with mutation of the p53 gene, and metastatic disease arises by a series of additional mutations. This sequence does not occur uniformly, and additional mutations are sure to be identified. The time required for this transformation from adenoma to cancer by multiple mutations cannot be precisely known. In the National Cooperative Polyp Study, only 5 of 1418 pts with adenomas developed cancers in 6 years; all were early stage. Using available data on incidence and prevalence of polyps and data on the average pt age difference at dx of adenoma and cancer, an expert panel estimated that a polyp probably takes an average of 10 years to transform into a malignancy (GE 1997;112:594).

This allows ample chance to interrupt the process by endo-scopic polypectomy.

- *Cancers without adenoma:* A small proportion of CRCs appear to arise without a preexisting adenoma. In their early stages, these lesions are entirely flat or minimally elevated, often with a depressed center (Gastrointest Endosc 1995;41:135), and they appear to be capable of invading submucosa. It is difficult to estimate the proportion of cancers that come from such lesions.

  - **Synchronous cancers** (cancers diagnosed at the same time as the first cancer found) occur in 2-5% of pts, and their dx affects the extent of operation about 10% of the time (Surgery 1997;122:706). **Metachronous lesions** (lesions diagnosed later in follow-up) occur in about 2% of pts with a mean lag of 9 years (Surgery 1997;122:706). The rate of metachronous lesions is higher in pts with HNPCC and in pts who present with synchronous lesions (Dis Colon Rectum 1997;40:935).

    - *Location of cancers:* There has been an unexplained trend over time for CRC to be found proximal to the sigmoid colon (Jama 1977;238:1641).

Sx: The location and characteristics of the tumor play a large part in the presenting sx of CRC. A small number of pts will present **without sx** after a positive screening test (FOBT, flex sig, or colonoscopy). Another group will present with visible **rectal bleeding.** These are more often left-sided cancers. A hx of visible rectal bleeding should be sought on ROS in health screening visits. The yield of pursuing visible rectal bleeding is very high in a primary care practice of U.S. veterans (13% polyps, 6.5% cancer, 5% IBD). There were no features on hx or exam that identified a low-risk group, and examination of the entire colon was needed for dx (Jama 1997;277:44). A **change in bowel habits** (eg, change in stool frequency or caliber from an obstructing lesion) is just as important a sx as rectal bleeding and leads to a cancer dx in a similar proportion of pts (Am J Gastro 1993;

88:1179). Profound **iron deficiency anemia** without much change in bowels suggests a right-sided cancer and is a common presentation in an otherwise well pt. Those with more advanced disease may present with fatigue or weight loss. Infrequent presentations include complete bowel obstruction requiring urgent surgery, perforation, cancer of unknown primary, and *Streptococcus bovis* endocarditis (Am J Gastro 1995;90:1528).

Si: Usually none but may have mass in abdomen, hepatomegaly if mets, or mass on rectal exam. FOBT is often positive but is not a reliable negative test.

Crs: The prognosis is based on stage of cancer at presentation (Table 5.1). The TNM staging system is preferred, and variations of the older Dukes system are out of favor. Survival correlates with stage (GE 1997;112:594).

Table 5.1   Colon Cancer Staging

Stage	Tumor (T)	Nodes (N)	Metastases (M)	5-Year Survival
I	Tumor invades submucosa (T1) or muscularis propria (T2)	None	None	>90%
II	Tumor through muscularis propria (T3)	None	None	75%
	Tumor through or beyond serosa (T4)			
III	Any T	Positive	None	50%
IV	Any T	Any N	Distant mets	<<10%

Cmplc: Bleeding, perforation, obstruction, mass effects of distant disease.

Diff Dx: The diff dx can be very broad since the sx of CRC are varied and are common to many other gut diseases. In practice, once a symptom prompts examination of the colon by imaging or endoscopy, the endoscopic biopsies lay the question to rest. The diff dx for masses on BE or CT includes adherent stool (perhaps 50% of masses called questionable on CT are stool); stricture due to ischemia; mass effect from diverticular disease or IBD; and uncommon colonic neoplasms such as lymphoma, carcinoid, and submucosal lesions.

Lab: CBC and CMP are routine. LFTs are not a sensitive indicator of metastatic disease. CEA is a measure of tumor burden and is a possible predictor of tumor recurrence and response to rx. The yield of cures due to CEA monitoring is small compared to the cost (Arch Pathol Lab Med 1995;119:1115).

X-ray: Barium enema is capable of detecting CRC and colonic polyps but is not as sensitive as colonoscopy. A positive BE requires colonoscopy for bx or polypectomy. Sensitivity figures come from a study of 2193 consecutive CRC cases in which records were reviewed for performance of BE or colonoscopy within the 3 prior years (GE 1997;112:17). This comprehensive study, which presumably mirrors general practice in the U.S., showed a sensitivity for ACBE of 85%, single contrast BE 82%, colonoscopy by gastroenterologists 97%, and colonoscopy by nongastroenterologists 87%. Cancers found at colonoscopy were more likely to be early stage. Colonoscopy outperformed BE in all segments of bowel, and BE did no better on left than right colon. When BE misses cancers, they are usually evident in retrospect (76%) and are typically missed in the barium pool or because of overlapping loops (Gastrointest Radiol 1991;16:123). Strategies to improve the efficacy of barium enema have been proposed (AJR Am J Roentgenol 1993;160:491), but the gap between the 2 studies is unlikely to close.

    CT colonography (aka virtual colonoscopy) is a new technique in which CT scanning is used to create a 3-dimensional image similar to that seen at colonoscopy (Nejm 1999;341:1496). The exam is done with a full bowel prep and insufflation of air into the colon (not actually a virtual experience). Its role in

CRC detection has not yet been established (reviewed in GE 2004;127:970). Improvements in hardware and software have resulted in polyp detection rates similar to that of colonoscopy in some studies (eg, Nejm 2003;349:2191) but the range of reported sensitivities in recent trials is enormous (52-92%). It is not clear which pts with polyps found on CT colonography would be referred for polypectomy (or which pts would be content not to intervene given the uncertainty). While all large polyps would require intervention, polyps in the 6-9 mm range cannot likely be ignored since they contain high-grade dysplasia in 2-7% and cancer in nearly 1%. It is not yet possible to determine whether CT colonography will increase or decrease the use of colonoscopy but it may entice greater numbers of pts to be screened.

Endoscopy: Colonoscopy is indicated whenever there is a reasonable probability of colorectal neoplasia. If the colon cannot be fully examined, barium enema or CT colonography can be performed to examine the nonvisualized colon. If colonic sx persist despite a negative colonoscopy, the possibility of a missed lesion needs to be considered.

Rx:

- *Diet and chemoprevention:* It is reasonable to recommend to pts a diet rich in fruit and vegetable fiber and low in fat and animal products, since such a diet appears protective for CRC and other illnesses. A daily multivitamin with folic acid (400 mcg) is possibly beneficial and low risk. Diets rich in cereal grains are more useful for treating constipation and preventing diverticular disease but could still be advocated as means of achieving a low-fat intake and for possible beneficial effects in CRC prevention. The data for aspirin are not compelling enough to recommend to the population at large for CRC prevention given the associated risks. Assuming a 50% effectiveness for aspirin in risk reduction its use would save fewer lives at greater cost than screening colonoscopy (GE 2002;122:78).

Further study is needed to define the role of chemoprevention by use of calcium supplements, aspirin, NSAIDs, and other agents (reviewed in GE 2004;126:1423).

- *Detect and remove adenomas* (see also p 236): It is now well established that the most effective means of preventing CRC is to detect and remove adenomas. The most convincing data are from the National Cooperative Polyp Study cohort. These 1418 pts had 1 or more adenomas removed and were followed for an average of 5.9 years. When compared to 3 historical reference groups (methodologically risky but the best we have) the incidence of cancer was 76-90% lower than expected (Nejm 1993;329:1977). Case control studies of screening rigid sigmoidoscopy in a large health plan (Nejm 1992;326:653) and endoscopy with polypectomy in U.S. veterans (Ann IM 1995; 123:904) demonstrated a 50% reduction in risk in the screened portions of bowel.

- *Surgery:* All stage I-III cancers should be treated surgically for an attempt at cure. Stage IV lesions are treated surgically to palliate pain, bleeding, or obstruction. The resection involves the primary tumor and its lymphatic drainage with a 5-cm proximal margin and 2-cm distal margin of normal bowel. The extent of bowel resected is usually dictated by the vascular supply of the involved segment. Laparoscopic colectomy improves the immediate postoperative course compared to the open operation and is just as effective for long-term cancer cure as the open operation (Lancet 2004;363:1187; Nejm 2004; 350:2050). Pts who present with complete obstruction require a 2-stage operation. They initially undergo diverting loop colostomy (in which a loop of colon is brought out to the skin and an ostomy with 2 barrels is created) until the bowel can be prepped and a cancer operation done.

  Rectal cancers (Gastroenterol Clin North Am 1997; 26:103) provide special challenges to the surgeon. When the tumor is in the upper rectum and an adequate margin can be obtained, a low anterior resection with primary anastomosis is performed. Generally, all tumors outside of the reach of the examining finger can be resected this way. The circular end-to-end stapler revolutionized this operation by making the anastomosis easier to perform (Dis Colon Rectum 1999;42:1369). Pts who have a low anterior resection have a higher risk of anastomotic recurrence and are followed more intensively postoperatively. For those pts in whom a bulky tumor, local spread, or very distal location prevent an anterior approach, an abdominoperineal, or AP, resection of the rectum is performed, and a permanent sigmoid colostomy is created. This procedure is associated with significant sexual dysfunction (45%) and bladder dysfunction (30%). Sphincter-sparing surgery (in the hands of specialists) can be considered if the tumor is 3 cm above the dentate line. Coloanal anastomosis has been described. Local excision may be reasonable for tumors that are within 8 cm of the dentate line, that are mobile, that have moderately or well-differentiated histology, and that are T1 or T2 by endoscopic ultrasound.

Metastatic disease to liver or lung can be approached surgically, especially if there is a solitary lesion. Adequate performance status, good hepatic reserve, and the ability to resect all evident disease are prerequisites. Tumor-free 5-year survival is 20-30% for resection of hepatic mets, and the results are highly variable for lung mets (Gastroenterol Clin North Am 1997; 26:103).

- *Chemotherapy:* The utility of chemotherapy depends on the tumor stage and location. The goal of adjuvant rx is to treat micrometastases not identified at operation (Semin Oncol 1999;26:545). For **stage III** CRCs, the combination of 5-FU and levamisole for 48 wk reduces recurrence rate by 40%, reduces death rate by 33%, and has become the standard of care (Ann IM 1995;122:321). The combination of 5-FU and leucovorin is an effective regimen that can be given over

6-8 months with tolerable toxicity (Lancet 1995;345: 939). Some authors suggest a year of rx (GE 2000;118:S115). For **stage II** CRCs, similar regimens are of less clear benefit (GE 2000;118:S115) because of the better prognosis of this group and only pooled retrospective data show benefit (J Clin Oncol 1999;17:1349).

For **stage II and III rectal** cancers, postoperative radiation and 5-FU (Nejm 1991;324:709) or preoperative radiation (Nejm 1997;336:980) improve survival. For **stage IV** CRC 5-FU is the basis for standard regimens. Meta-analysis suggests that continuous infusion gives better tumor response rates than bolus rx, but survival is about a year in any case (J Clin Oncol 1998;16:301). Irinotecan (CPT-11) in combination with 5-FU and leucovorin may become an alternative first-line rx, though it is more toxic. A variety of new agents have been evaluated, including monoclonal antibody therapies (Nejm 2004;350:2406).

Since chemotherapy has limited benefit, investigators have turned to gene therapy for advanced disease. In gene therapy, DNA is brought into tumor cell nuclei, usually by means of a viral vector. For example, trials are being conducted using adenovirus to insert wildtype p53 genetic material into cancer cells, hoping to restore programmed cell death. Other strategies include the insertion of suicide genes that could be combined with chemotherapy (Hematol Oncol Clin North Am 1998; 12:595).

- *Endoscopic therapy for obstruction:* It is possible to treat acute obstruction with placement of expandable metal stents as a bridge to a single-stage resection or as palliation (Gastrointest Endosc 1998;47:277). Major complications are common and the value of this approach needs additional evaluation.
- *The malignant polyp:* See p 241.
- *Post-rx follow-up:* About 50% of pts will have a recurrence of CRC after rx and most of these will happen within 3 years of surgery. Intensive programs of postoperative surveillance with

monitoring of CBC, CMP, CEA, CXR, FOBT, frequent endoscopy, and abdominal CT scanning have been used in various combinations with disappointing results. Using an evidence-based approach, the American Society of Clinical Oncology suggests very limited surveillance (J Clin Oncol 1999;17:1312). A preoperative or perioperative **colonoscopy** should be done to clear the colon of synchronous lesions and be repeated every 3-5 years thereafter. ACS guidelines suggest colonoscopy within 1 year after cancer resection (CA Cancer J Clin 2003;53:27). Pts with stage II or III rectal cancer *who do not receive radiation* may benefit from periodic sigmoidoscopy to look for anastomotic recurrence (eg, q 6 month × 2 yr). If resection of liver metastases would be clinically indicated, then postoperative CEA should be done q 2-3 months for ≥2 yr. Pts with elevations are evaluated fully for recurrence. About 30% of CRC does not produce CEA, and up to 44% of pts with normal preoperative CEA have elevations with recurrence. The recommendation for CEA testing is based on inconsistent evidence and was not supported in 2 other analyses (Can J Surg 1997;40:90; Lancet 2000;355:395).

Screening for colorectal cancer: (GE 2003;124:544; Am J Gastro 2000;95:868; GE 1997;112:594)

The case for screening average risk pts: CRC is a disease ideally suited to screening. As detailed earlier, CRC is the second leading cause of cancer death in the U.S., with a lifetime risk of 6%. CRC has a long asymptomatic phase and progression from adenoma to cancer occurs over a decade. During this time, precancerous polyps and early stage cancers can be identified and removed. Screening for CRC is a good investment. When measured in dollars per year of life saved, CRC screening (costing $15,000-25,000/yr saved) does well against breast cancer screening ($30,000-35,000), dual airbags in cars ($120,000) and smoke detectors in new homes ($210,000) (Am J Med 1999; 106:7S).

There are four major sets of recommendations: A conservative evidence-based approach is from the **U.S. Preventive Services Task Force.** The task force endorses screening for average risk pts older than age 50 but does not reach conclusions regarding the optimal approach (Ann IM 2002;137:129).

The most comprehensive document on screening was prepared by the **U.S. Agency for Healthcare Policy and Research (AHCPR)** (first published in GE 1997;112:594 and updated in GE 2003;124:544). This is the document that should be read most carefully for a comprehensive review of the data. A limitation of the guidelines in the document is that the panel offered a menu of choices without stating which choice was preferred. Choices for average risk pts included annual FOBT, flex sig q 5 yr, flex sig q 5 yr plus annual FOBT, ACBE q 5 yr and colonoscopy q 10 yr. For those with a first-degree relative with CRC or an adenoma, the panel suggested the same screening as for average risk pts, but beginning 10 yr earlier. The panel concluded that CT colonography and tests for altered DNA in stool were not yet ready for use outside research studies.

The **American Cancer Society** guidelines are similar except they endorse q 5-10 yr colonoscopy for those with a first-degree relative with CRC or an adenoma under age 60 (CA Cancer J Clin 2003;53:27).

The **American College of Gastroenterology (ACG),** for better or worse, has made more specific recommendations on the choice of CRC screening from the AHCPR menu of choices (Am J Gastro 2000;95:868). These guidelines make colonoscopy the screening test of choice. Since these groups reached different conclusions with the same data, it is valuable to understand the background regarding choices of screening tests:

- *Screening colonoscopy:* The effectiveness of colonoscopy as screening has not been established in RCTs or case control studies. Two lines of evidence support the use of colonoscopy. The first is a case control study that demonstrates that sigmoidoscopy with polypectomy decreases the risk of death from distal bowel cancer by 60% (Nejm 1992;326:653). The second line of evidence comes from the National Cooperative Polyp Study, in which pts who had their colons cleared of adenomas by colonoscopy had a 76-90% reduction in CRC incidence compared to other reference groups (Nejm 1993;329:1977). It is clear that removing adenomas prevents cancers and that colonoscopy is the most effective way to detect and remove adenomas.

The disadvantages of colonoscopy are the cost and the risk of perforation and/or bleeding from polypectomy. It is likely that there are not enough trained providers and units throughout the country to screen all those pts who would be eligible for screening colonoscopy but a relatively low acceptance rate has made this less of an issue.

The optimal interval for screening colonoscopy is unknown. In pts with a negative initial colonoscopy, the chances of finding a cancer or pathologically advanced adenoma at 5 yr were 0% and 1%, respectively (GE 1996; 111:1178). Based on rough estimates of the time to develop from adenoma to cancer, colonoscopy every 10 yr has been proposed (GE 1997;112:594).

• *Screening sigmoidoscopy:* Sigmoidoscopy is effective when combined with polypectomy for reducing mortality (Nejm 1992;326:653; J Natl Cancer Inst 1992;84:1572). The major limitation of sigmoidoscopy is that it leaves much of the colon unexamined. Two important studies of screening colonoscopy demonstrate that more than half of the pathologically advanced adenomas were found in pts with no adenomas distal to the splenic flexure (Nejm 2000;343:169; Nejm 2000; 343:162). Sigmoidoscopy for CRC can be likened to screening for breast cancer by mammography of one breast (Nejm 2000; 343:207). Pts screened with sigmoidoscopy will die from preventable CRC. The advantages of sigmoidoscopy are: (1) lower cost, (2) it can be performed by primary care physicians, and (3) it does not require sedation. The optimal interval for sigmoidoscopy has not been determined but the protective effect may be as long as 10 yr (Nejm 1992;326:653).

- *FOBT:* For the evidence-based purist, FOBT has the advantage of having been shown effective in 5 RCTs (Am J Med 1999;106:7S). Pts who undergo annual screening with rehydrated FOBT cards (which increases sensitivity and reduces specificity) and have colonoscopy for a positive test have a 33% reduction in mortality over 13 yr of follow-up (Nejm 1993;328:1365). Biennial screening is less effective but reduces mortality by 21% (J Natl Cancer Inst 1999;91:434). Accurate FOBT requires avoidance of raw meats and avoidance of a variety of foods and medicines (Ann IM 1997; 126:811). Immunochemical tests obviate the need for dietary restriction. The chief problem with FOBT as a screening strategy is that because of issues of compliance and lack of sensitivity only about 15% of the expected cases of CRC would be prevented in the first 10 yr of screening (Am J Gastro 2000;95:3250).

- *Screening barium enema:* There are limited data on BE in screening. In one trial in which ACBE and sigmoidoscopy were done, BE missed 26% of rectosigmoid adenomas >1 cm and 25% of cancers (Endoscopy 1995;27:159). It is difficult to make the argument that BE is a sensible screening tool (Am J Gastro 2000;95:868), though ACS and AHCPR guidelines endorse it.

Recommendations for average risk pts: Recognizing that there are limited data on which to base recommendations, the current ACG guidelines (which pick from the AHCPR options) seem reasonable (Am J Gastro 2000;95:868). The screening test of choice is colonoscopy every 10 yr beginning at age 50. The interval of 10 yr is on shaky ground and may change as more data become available. Those who have periodic colonoscopy should *not* have annual FOBT testing because most positive tests are false positives if the pt has had a recent normal colonoscopy. The alternative (where cost or available resources prohibit colonoscopy) is the combination of annual FOBT with sigmoidoscopy q 5 yr. It is, however, difficult to understand the rationale for a different choice of surveillance interval for sigmoidoscopy versus colonoscopy.

Recommendations for pts with a family hx of CRC: For pts with a first-degree relative with CRC under the age of 60 or multiple older relatives with CRC, the risk is increased 3-4 times. Colonoscopy beginning at age 40 (or 10 yr earlier than the age at which the relative was diagnosed with CRC) and done every 5 yr (3 yr for stronger histories) is suggested (Am J Gastro 2000;95:868). The risk is lower if the relative was diagnosed over age 60 (twofold risk) and the ACG guidelines suggest colonoscopy q 10 yr beginning at age 40. It is not clear why the guideline is so different (q 5 yr vs q 10 yr) for a pt whose relative was diagnosed at age 59 vs age 61. The only prospective study supports the use of a 5-yr interval of follow-up (Clin Gastroenterol Hepatol 2003;1:310).

Recommendations for pts with a family hx of adenomatous polyp: The AHCPR guideline suggests that a pt with a first-degree relative with an adenoma be considered in the same way as a pt with a first-degree relative with CRC. This is based on data from the National Polyp Study showing an increased risk for relatives of pts with adenomas (Nejm 1996;334:82). However, it is not evident why having a relative with a small tubular adenoma might confer a risk comparable to that of a CRC, and it is less clear how these pts should be screened. The ACG suggests individualizing the approach. A pt with a relative with pathologically advanced adenoma, especially a relative under the age of 60, could be screened in a similar way to those with a first-degree relative with CRC, but additional data are needed.

Recommendations for other high-risk groups: Specific guidelines are discussed separately for FAP (p 246), HNPCC (p 242), IBD (p 192), and for those with a personal history of adenoma (p 236) or CRC (p 230).

5.2   Adenomatous Colonic Polyps

GE 2003;124:544; Am J Gastro 2000;95:3053

Epidem: Cumulative incidence of 25% by age 50, 40% by age 70. Predominance in men. The prevalence of polyps >1 cm is 15% by 75 yr. Dietary risk factors for the incidence and recurrence of adenomas are similar to those for CRC (p 219) (Ann IM 1993; 118:91).

Pathophys: Adenomas are benign colonic neoplasms that are important because of their potential to degenerate into CRCs. The vast majority of CRCs arise from adenomas, and detection and removal of adenomas prevent CRC. The pathologist classifies adenomas as tubular, tubulovillous, or villous on the basis of histology. The endoscopist classifies adenomas by their size, location, and morphology. Polyps on a stalk are called pedunculated and are generally easier to resect completely. Polyps that are flat and broadly attached to the colonic wall are called sessile and are more difficult to remove as they become large. Pedunculated lesions are seen more often in the left colon, presumably due to the traction effect of formed stool on the developing polyp.

Size and histology determine risk for cancer development. Pts with an adenoma larger than 1 cm are 4 times as likely to develop a cancer at another site over a 14-yr period (Am J Gastro 1996;91:448). Severe dysplasia, the precursor of carcinoma, is most likely to develop in older pts with large polyps and in pts whose polyps include a large villous component. A large (>1 cm) villous adenoma in a pt over 60 yr old is 50 times more likely to harbor severe dysplasia than a small tubular adenoma (<5 mm) in a young pt (GE 1990;98:371). Adenomas do not regress but grow at a highly variable rate, with the majority staying stable in size but a minority growing at a rate of 2-4 mm/yr (Am J Gastro 1997;92:1117). Adenomas probably take an average of 10 yr to develop from small adenoma to cancer (GE 1997;112:594).

Adenomas develop from a mutated, monoclonal epithelial stem cell into cancers by a sequence of mutations in tumor suppressor genes and activation of cancer causing genes (oncogenes) (see "Colorectal Cancer," p 219). The National Polyp Study, designed to study surveillance and outcome in pts with newly discovered adenomas, provides data on outcomes after colonoscopic polypectomy. In pts with one or more adenomas found at index colonoscopy, 40% will have adenomas by 3 yr of follow-up. However, adenomas with advanced pathological features (>1 cm, severe dysplasia, or cancer) were found in only 3% of pts at 3 yr and only 0.5% were malignant. The rate of advanced adenoma was the same for pts who had 2 colonoscopies (at 1 and 3 yr after index exam) or a single colonoscopy at 3 yr (Nejm 1993;328:901). When these pts were evaluated at a mean of 5.9 yr, there was a 75-90% reduced rate of cancer compared to that in untreated reference groups (Nejm 1993;329:1977). It is not clear if pts with small tubular adenomas removed at endoscopy have a high risk of CRC in follow-up. In 776 pts with small tubular adenomas (single or multiple) removed at rigid sigmoidoscopy and followed up at a mean of 14 yr, rectal cancer developed in only 4 of 776 pts (Nejm 1992;326:658). However, in the National Cooperative Polyp Study, it was removal of *all* adenomas that resulted in the dramatic decrease in cancer incidence. Given the magnitude of the risk reduction seen in that study, it seems prudent to continue to survey pts with tubular adenomas unless more convincing evidence of its low yield becomes available. Large sessile polyps (>3 cm) frequently recur (25% in one series), and recurrence may occur after a negative colonoscopic inspection. Carcinoma is common in recurrences

(17%), and the risk of metachronous cancer is substantial (4%) (Gastrointest Endosc 1992;38:303).

Sx: Usually none. Large polyps may bleed. Distal polyps may prolapse out of rectum.

Si: FOBT is positive in a minority of adenomas.

Crs: Very few adenomas become cancers, with an estimated annual transformation to malignancy of 2.5 malignancies per 1000 polyps per yr. It probably takes on average 10 yr for a sporadic adenoma to become malignant if it is destined to do so. Pts with villous, tubulovillous, or adenomas >1 cm have a RR for cancer of 3.6 at a mean of 14 yr of follow-up (Nejm 1992;326:658). This is the rationale for endoscopic surveillance of pts with adenomas.

Cmplc: CRC, bleeding.

Diff Dx: Adenomas (about half of colon polyps) must be distinguished pathologically from other polyps. These include hyperplastic polyps (perhaps 30% of all polyps) which are usually <0.5 cm and frequently in the distal colon. Redundant mucosa or tags are polypoid-appearing but have normal colonic mucosa histologically. Lipomas, juvenile polyps, inflammatory polyps, pseudopolyps from IBD, submucosal lipoma, carcinoids, neurofibromas, and Peutz-Jeghers polyps round out the differential. Some polyps that look grossly like benign adenomas turn out to be carcinomas (see "the Malignant Polyp," p 241).

Lab: Adenomas are classified according to their histology. Most adenomas are tubular, with glands composed of multiple branching structures. A minority are villous adenomas (about 10%), with long fingerlike glands from the polyp surface projecting into the bowel lumen. These have the greatest risk of subsequent cancer. Some polyps (about 20-30%) contain a mix of tubular and villous elements and are called tubulovillous adenomas. The pathologist will usually describe the degree of dysplasia in the polyp. Severe dysplasia is the equivalent of carcinoma in situ, but as long as all the dysplasia is above the muscularis mucosa, invasive cancer cannot develop. The size of polyps is best estimated when polyps are in the colon rather than after fixation.

X-ray: Double contrast barium enema is 50-80% sensitive for polyps <1 cm, and 70-90% sensitive for polyps >1 cm. All positive BEs lead to colonoscopy for polypectomy, and false-positive BEs (perhaps 5%) also lead to colonoscopy. Barium enema is not the appropriate test to detect polyps unless colonoscopy is not available or cannot be completed. CT colonography (aka virtual colonoscopy), in which CT is used to create 3-dimensional images of the colon similar in appearance to those seen at colonoscopy, is an evolving technology discussed on p 226.

Endoscopy: Colonoscopy is the test of choice for the detection and removal of adenomas. However, it still has limitations (Am J Gastro 1999;94:194). Tandem colonoscopies demonstrate that an experienced examiner will miss 15% of polyps under 10 mm but will rarely miss larger polyps (J Natl Cancer Inst 1990; 82:1769).

Polypectomy is achieved by a variety of techniques. Small polyps (<5 mm) can be removed with bx forceps. Some endoscopists prefer hot bx forceps for the removal of small polyps. A hot bx forceps has an insulated core for retrieval of a specimen, but provides cautery to the polyp base. Its chief disadvantages are the risk of incomplete removal and of cautery injury to the bowel wall, especially in the right colon where the wall is thin (Gastrointest Endosc 1988;34:32). Small polyps can also be removed by snaring them with a wire loop without cautery. Larger polyps are removed by snare cautery in which a wire loop is wrapped around the base of the polyp and cautery applied (Am J Gastro 1987;82:615). Sessile polyps greater than 1 cm in diameter are generally removed in several bites to minimize the risk of cautery injury. Large polyps are easier and safer to resect after injection of a cushion of saline under the polyp. This creates a thermal barrier of colonic mucosa swollen with saline to protect the muscular wall from electric current injury (Am J Gastro 1994;89:305). Complications of endoscopic polypectomy include perforation and bleeding. Bleeding is more likely to occur with large polyps. Bleeding can usually be controlled endoscopically but may require surgery. Thermal injury can also create the **postpolypectomy syndrome,** in which pts develop pain and localized peritonitis due to a microperforation or serosal burn. Free perforations require surgery, but most pts with postpolypectomy syndrome recover within days with antibiotics (Gastrointest Endosc Clin N Am 1996;6:343).

Rx: Current guidelines for pts with nonfamilial colonic polyps (Am J Gastro 2000;95:3053; GE 2003;124:544) are:

- *Total colonoscopy and endoscopic polypectomy:* When adenomas are detected at sigmoidoscopy, total colonoscopy is generally performed and all adenomas are resected. There is a low yield of finding an advanced adenoma or cancer upon performing full colonoscopy for a single small adenoma found on flexible sigmoidoscopy in average-risk pts (Ann IM 1998;129:273). The ACG guidelines call for the decision for full colonoscopy to be individualized. However, given the benefit of screening colonoscopy (see "Pathophys") it seems reasonable to proceed in most circumstances. Pts who have a hyperplastic polyp found at sigmoidoscopy have a risk of adenomas of the more proximal colon of 18%, though this number is similar in pts who have a sigmoidoscopy without any polyps (GE 1992; 102:317). Therefore, hyperplastic polyps on sigmoidoscopy are no more an indication for full colonoscopy than is a normal sigmoidoscopy. A pt who has had a large ($\geq$2 cm) adenoma resected should have colonoscopy in 3-6 months to ensure complete resection, and if complete resection is not achieved after 2-3 sessions, surgery is usually appropriate.

- *Surgical polypectomy:* If adenomas cannot be resected at colonoscopy, colectomy is usually warranted unless the pt is a very poor surgical risk. Laparoscopic assisted hemicolectomy may allow more speedy recovery without increased complications (Mayo Clin Proc 2000;75:344).
- *Postpolypectomy surveillance:* Full colonoscopy is performed to resect all adenomas. If there is doubt as to the completeness of resection (because of multiple adenomas, prep, or other technical factors), a follow-up exam is done usually at 1 yr. For pts with 2 or fewer tubular adenomas <1 cm in size and no family hx of CRC, the guidelines call for colonoscopy in 5 yr. For those with a family hx of CRC, with >2 adenomas, with villous histology, or with an adenoma ≥1 cm, the first follow-up exam is at 3 yr. If the follow-up exam is negative at 3 yr, the surveillance interval is subsequently increased to 5 yr. Followup should be individualized to the age and life expectancy of the pt. The American Cancer Society (ACS) suggests an exam at 3 yr for all pts with adenomas (though this can be delayed to 6 yr for a small single adenoma). Another exam is recommended at 3 yr for pts with index adenomas >1 cm or with multiple adenomas or those with villous change or high-grade dysplasia (CA Cancer J Clin 2003;53:27). All others are returned to average-risk guidelines. The evidence base for anything beyond what to do for the first 3 yr after polypectomy is extrapolation from observational studies and expert opinion. For the time being, practitioners use these guidelines as a substitute for higher quality evidence. The best evidence base for risk reduction is in the National Cooperative Polyp Study, in which colonoscopy was q 3 yr for 6 yr.
- *The malignant polyp:* Pathologically, a polyp is malignant when cancer has invaded through the muscularis mucosa into the submucosa (Hum Pathol 1998;29:15). The concern with a malignant polyp is that cancerous lymph nodes may be left in

the pt if a colectomy is not done. However, most of these pts are cured by polypectomy, provided that the polyp has 3 favorable features: (1) the polyp is completely excised and recovered and the surgical margin is not involved, (2) the cancer is not poorly differentiated, and (3) there is no evidence of lymphatic or vascular invasion. In pts with polyps with these favorable features, the risk of metastatic disease in pedunculated polyps is 0.3% (GE 1986;91:419). Since the mortality of colectomy is generally higher (0.2% for the very young, 4.4% for those over age 70, an overall average of 2%), these pts are not operated on and generally do well. The polyp site is inspected in 3 months to ensure complete excision, and then the pt returns to standard adenoma surveillance (Am J Gastro 2000;95: 3053). In sessile polyps with the favorable characteristics described above, the risk may be as high as 4%, so colectomy may be appropriate if the pt is not at undue risk. However, the data are less clear for sessile malignant polyps since not as many large sessile malignant lesions are resected and followed. Large rectal lesions are probably best left to the surgeon, who has a better chance of removing them completely and sufficiently intact, to determine if polypectomy alone is curative (Endoscopy 1993;25:469).

5.3 Hereditary Nonpolyposis Colon Cancer Syndrome

GE 2001;121:198; Jama 1997;277:915

Cause: Inherited mutation of DNA mismatch repair genes.

Epidem: Mean age of onset of cancer 44 years. No gender predilection. About 1-2% of CRC is HNPCC related (GE 2001;121:1005).

Pathophys: The working definition of **HNPCC** (the Amsterdam criteria) is that it is an inherited form of CRC which may be identified when: (1) 3 or more relatives have CRC and one is first degree to the other two, (2) the cancer involves 2 generations, and (3) one of the cases occurs before the pt is 50 yr of age (Dis Colon Rectum 1991;34:424). In addition, some pedigrees will exhibit associated inherited malignancies of endometrium, small bowel, ovary, pancreas, stomach, biliary tree, brain, and transitional cell carcinoma of ureter and renal pelvis (GE 1993;104:1535). Strict application of this definition will mean the exclusion of some pts who have the disorder (as defined by the genetic defect). Broader inclusion criteria (called the modified Bethesda criteria) have been published (GE 2001;121:198). The genetic defect might be strongly suspected when (1) a pt has 2 HNPCC cancers, or (2) when a first-degree relative has an HNPCC cancer under age 50 or an adenoma under age 40. Other reasons to consider that a pt has a genetic effect include CRC with a cribriform or signet ring histology and early onset CRC or adenoma. The pedigrees with CRC alone are often referred to as Lynch Syndrome I and those with associated extracolonic cancers as Lynch Syndrome II.

The pathogenesis of HNPCC was suspected when tumors from these pts showed widespread alteration in short, repeated DNA sequences, called microsatellite instability. This suggested that replication errors occurred in tumor development and led to the identification of mutations in several genes that normally function in DNA mismatch repair (Curr Gastroenterol Rep 1999;1:449). Mutations from 4 genes, MSH2, MLH1, PMS1, and PMS2, account for 73% of the cases of HNPCC. Many mutations have been identified, but many are unknown. These defects are inherited in an autosomal dominant fashion, though not all pts who inherit the genes develop cancer (incomplete penetrance). Pts with HNPCC do not have large numbers of adenomas, but the adenomas they have occur at a younger age, are more likely to be villous, and grow into cancers at a much faster rate than sporadic adenomas (Gut 1992;33:783). Up to 70% of cancers occur proximal to the splenic flexure.

The **Muir-Torre syndrome** (sebaceous adenomas, sebaceous carcinomas, multiple keratoacanthomas, and colonic adenomas) is a variant of HNPCC (Am J Gastro 1998;93:1572).

Sx and Si: No different than sporadic CRC (see p 219).

Crs: Risk of CRC 75% by age 65. Risk of metachronous cancer is 50% at 15 yr. Risk of endometrial cancer 40% and ovarian cancer 9% by age 70 (Jama 1997;277:915).

Cmplc: Extracolonic malignancies.

Diff Dx: In the absence of a specific diagnostic marker, the dx is usually made by use of the descriptive clinical criteria. HNPCC must be distinguished from FAP (usually easy to do on basis of number of polyps), from attenuated FAP, and from other polyposis syndromes (see Section 5.4). The reality is that most HNPCC cases go unrecognized, not because it is difficult to distinguish it from other rare polyposis syndromes, but because most clinicians are unaware of its existence.

Lab: Genetic testing is now commercially available and should be offered to those at risk (GE 2001;121:198). In commercial labs, DNA from the proband is evaluated by a variety of techniques for mutations in MSH2 and MLH1. Typically the process begins by examining the tumor of the affected relative for microsatellite instability, which is present in the tumors in more than 90% of pts with a germline mutation. If a mutation is identified in the proband, then relatives can be tested. If a relative has a positive result, he or she is at high risk (80% chance of cancer). If a relative is negative with a positive proband, he or she is at average risk. If the proband has negative or ambiguous testing, gene testing for the rest of the family is meaningless because the proband probably has a mutation that cannot be identified by the test. If an affected family member is not available for evaluation, it is reasonable to offer mutation testing but it will only be meaningful if positive. Genetic counseling concerning the positive and negative consequences of a positive or negative test is mandatory (Am J Gastro 1999;94:2344).

Endoscopy: Colonoscopy is the test of choice for suspected gene carriers. Sigmoidoscopy is inadequate, because, unlike pts with FAP, those with HNPCC have few polyps and a tendency for right-sided disease.

Rx: Recommendations for management of HNPCC pts have been made by the Cancer Genetic Consortium (a panel of experts) and have been summarized (Jama 1997;277:915). Because of the high risk of development of a second cancer at a later date (a metachronous CRC), subtotal colectomy with ileorectal anastomosis is the operation of choice for pts with CRC in an HNPCC kindred. This gives an excellent functional result, with a short segment of bowel that can be easily surveyed for new adenomas. There are insufficient data to recommend for or against prophylactic hysterectomy and oophorectomy either at the time of colectomy or otherwise. The 3-5-yr intervals typical for surveillance of adenomatous polyps are inadequate for HNPCC pts, because cancer frequently develops within 3-5 yr of colonoscopy (10% at 5 yr) (Gut 1992;33:783; Am J Gastro 1994;89:1978). CRC has been reported within 1-2 yr of surveillance exams. Based on observational study evidence, the AHCPR recommendation is for colonoscopy q 1-2 yr beginning at age 20-25 (or 10 yr younger than the earliest cancer in the pedigree, whichever comes first) (GE 2003; 124:544). Screening for endometrial cancer is more uncertain. On the basis of expert opinion, annual transvaginal ultrasound and/or endometrial aspiration beginning between ages 25 and 35 have been proposed, but the benefit is unproven and the sensitivity unknown (Jama 1997;277:915). Even in known kindreds, there is frequently failure to control cancer because of problems with physician knowledge of HNPCC guidelines and problems with pt compliance (Am J Gastro 1999;94:2344; Dis Colon Rectum 1993;36:254).

5.4 Familial Adenomatous Polyposis and Related Syndromes

Lancet 2004;363:852; Mayo Clin Proc 2000;75:57

Cause: Mutation of the adenomatous polyposis coli (APC) gene.

Epidem: Frequency of gene mutation 1:5000 to 1:25,000. Prevalence 1:24,500 to 1:43,500. Autosomal dominant inheritance results in equal incidence for men and women. Seen in all races and ethnic groups.

Pathophys: (Q J Med 1995;88:853) In this disorder the pt inherits 1 normal copy of the **APC gene** and 1 mutant copy. This mutation may be inherited from a parent in an autosomal dominant pattern, or the pt may be the first with the germ-line mutation (and does not have a positive family hx, as occurs in 30%). In 80% of pts, the mutation can be identified. In most affected subjects, a frameshift or nonsense mutation results in the production of a truncated protein that can be detected in the lab. Normal APC gene expression seems important in programmed cell death (apoptosis). Disease results when the pt's normal (or wild) APC gene mutates so that the cells have 2 defective copies, 1 germline mutation and 1 acquired (somatic) mutation. Many mutations have been described, and variations in the nature of the mutation partially account for 4 different phenotypic expressions of the APC mutation, which are classic FAP, Gardner syndrome, Turcot syndrome, and attenuated APC.

In **classic FAP,** pts develop hundreds of adenomas that are almost always detectable by age 35 and that result universally in cancer by age 50. Adenomas are rare prior to age 12. Congenital hypertrophy of retinal pigment epithelium (CHRPE) is frequently seen and was formerly used in pedigree analysis. Adenomas are seen in stomach and duodenum, especially in the periampullary area, and 5-8% will develop duodenal cancer. Hyperplastic polyps of the stomach and fundic gland cysts are common. Desmoid tumors occur in 4-15% and are benign fibrous tumors that are a major cause of morbidity through intra-abdominal mass effect on bowel and vessels. Tumors of the thyroid (papillary carcinoma, usually in women) and hepatoblastomas (age 1-6; occur in <0.5%) are associated, though not common. Adenomas may occur in the ileum after ileoanal anastomosis.

In the **Gardner syndrome,** pts show adenomatous polyposis along with multiple osteomas, epidermoid cysts, desmoid tumors, and supernumerary teeth and other dental abnormalities. Sometimes simple FAP and Gardner's coexist in the same pedigree. Pts with **Turcot syndrome** have polyposis with CNS tumors, especially glioblastomas and medulloblastomas. **Attenuated APC** is a syndrome in which fewer than 100 polyps are found, extracolonic sx are uncommon, and there is a large variation in polyp number within 1 pedigree. Some of the pts with clinical features of attenuated APC actually have biallelic mutations in a base excision repair gene called MYH (Clin Gastroenterol Hepatol 2004;2:633).

Sx: The presenting sx are typically rectal bleeding, diarrhea, obstruction, and vague abdominal pain. Pts are often asymptomatic until they present with a cancer.

Si: FOBT-positive, masses from desmoid tumors in the abdomen, CHRPE (see "Pathophys"), jaw masses, epidermoid cysts.

Crs: Polyps usually develop in the late teens to 20s. Onset of cancer before age 10 or after age 50 is uncommon. In untreated pts, cancer usually develops in the 30s, with death at a mean age of 42. The common causes of morbidity in pts who undergo proctocolectomy are upper gi malignancy, desmoids, and operative complications. The proportion of pts dying from CRC has decreased. However, CRC is still the most common cause of death (Dis Colon Rectum 1996;39:384), partially because >20% of pts have no family hx and therefore are not screened and partially because those at risk often delay surgery or screening for social reasons (Brit J Surg 1997;84:74). Duodenal cancer occurs in 5% (Brit J Surg 1998;85:742).

Cmplc: Bleeding or obstruction from cancer, mass effect from desmoids, extracolonic cancers.

Diff Dx: In its classic form, FAP is not difficult to diagnose once sigmoidoscopy is done. The attenuated form, with fewer than 100 polyps, may cause diagnostic confusion.

Lab: Genetic testing should be offered to those at risk and to those with multiple polyps. Genetic testing allows the pt at risk to determine if he or she carries the gene and to plan accordingly. It also gives relief to those who do not carry the gene. The disadvantages of gene testing are possible effects on future insurability and employment, and survivor guilt in those who prove to be negative for the gene (Am J Gastro 1999;94:2344). Testing begins by looking for the truncated protein (Nejm 1993;329:1982) produced by the mutant APC gene (so-called protein truncation testing, or PTT). If the test is positive in a relative (as it is in 80% of pedigrees), then that relative has the disease. Not all APC mutations result in a truncated protein. Therefore, if the test is negative, an affected family member needs to be tested to see if that kindred makes a truncated protein. Only if truncated protein is found in an affected member of the pedigree is truncated protein a reliable negative test. For those pedigrees that do not make a truncated protein, linkage analysis (requiring at least 2 other family members) can be done with 95% sensitivity.

Endoscopy: Dramatic findings of hundreds to thousands of adenomatous polyps in colon. EGD may show gastric fundic polyps (50%), gastric adenomas (6%), or duodenal/ampullary adenomas (33-90%).

Rx:

- *Surgery:* Surgery should be performed when the pt is in the late teens. There are 3 surgical options: (1) total proctocolectomy with Brooke ileostomy, (2) subtotal colectomy with ileorectal anastomosis, and (3) total proctocolectomy with ileoanal anastomosis (Surg Oncol Clin N Am 1996;5:675). Ileostomy is not widely chosen by young pts. Ileorectal anastomosis has the advantage of being low morbidity, with an excellent functional result and no sexual dysfunction, but it has the disadvantage of the lifelong need for surveillance and the risk of fatal rectal cancer. Ileoanal anastomosis provides elimination of the CRC risk, but the functional results (fecal soilage, stool frequency, nocturnal stooling) are not as good (Ann Surg 1999;230:648). Later conversion to ileoanal anastomosis is associated with substantial morbidity (Dis Colon Rectum 1999;42:903). Most authors prefer ileoanal anastomosis (Ann Surg 1997;226:514). If rectum is not resected, then postoperative surveillance is difficult, because distinguishing small cancers from recurrent adenomas is difficult and because of problems with pt compliance. Postsurgical rectal cancer rates vary widely from 7-32% (Gastrointest Endosc Clin N Am 1997;7:111).

- *Screening those at risk:* (Mayo Clin Proc 2000;75:57) Pts at risk should undergo genetic testing. If gene testing is positive, annual sigmoidoscopy begins at age 10 and is done until adenomas are detected with surgery done in late teens. Hepato--blastoma screening is an option until age 6. Pts should undergo annual thyroid exams. In those with equivocal genetic testing, annual sigmoidoscopy begins at age 10, decreases in frequency at 25, and continues until age 50. If the genetic test is unequivocally negative, sigmoidoscopy every few yr is still suggested by some because of the possibility of lab error.
- *Postcolectomy and EGD surveillance:* If rectal anastomosis is done, surveillance every 6 months is mandatory. If total proctocolectomy is done, the ileal pouch is examined for adenomas q 3-5 yr. EGD with forward and side viewing scopes (to detect ampullary adenomas) is done starting at age 25 and every

1-5 yr thereafter depending on the findings (Brit J Surg 1998; 85:742; Lancet 2004;363:852). Sulindac may lower the risk of adenomas if the rectum is retained (GE 2002;122:641). Celecoxib may lower the risk of duodenal adenomas (Gut 2002;50:857).

5.5 Peutz-Jeghers Syndrome

Am J Gastro 2000;95:596; Lancet 1999;353:1211

Cause: A germ-line mutation in STK11, a serine/threonine kinase, the normal function of which has not been fully characterized (Nat Genet 1998;18:38; Nature 1998;391:184). Increased susceptibility comes from the germ-line defect, and polyps develop when a somatic mutation occurs in the normal copy of the gene from the unaffected parent.

Epidem: Rare disorder with estimated mutation rate of 1/200,000. Inherited as autosomal dominant trait. No gender predilection. Usually presents clinically in the first or second decade of life.

Pathophys: The syndrome is defined by the presence of characteristic melanin pigmentation of the skin and mucous membranes that are associated with gastrointestinal polyposis. The polyps are hamartomatous (aberrant, but nonneoplastic growths of tissue appropriate to the site) and occur throughout the gut. They are most frequent in the small intestine, less frequent in the stomach and colon. The polyps cause sx by obstruction, intussusception, prolapse, or bleeding.

The association of Peutz-Jeghers with **malignancy** is well established despite the fact that the polyps are not neoplastic. Difficulty in establishing the association is partly due to the heterogeneity of clinical features in different kindreds. In one recent series, the RR for cancer of any kind was 19 for women and 6 for men, with a 20 times RR for breast and gynecologic cancers (Ann IM 1998;128:896). Cancer of the pancreas at an early age and the otherwise uncommon Sertoli tumor of the testes are associated cancers (Brit J Surg 1995;82:1311).

Sx: Crampy abdominal pain due to recurrent intussusception, rectal bleeding (80%), hematemesis (10%), and anal extrusion of polyps (Lancet 1999;353:1211).

Si: Characteristic melanin spots, described as small, brown to bluish dark freckles of a few mm in diameter, are most frequently found on the lips and buccal mucosa. They also occur on palms and soles. They may fade with age and vary widely in intensity within kindreds.

Crs: The course is not benign, with obstruction, bleeding, and excess malignancy, but the morbidity is decreasing with effective rx of more recent generations (Lancet 1999;353:1211).

Diff Dx: The combination of pigmented skin lesions and polyp histology usually leaves little doubt as to the dx.

X-ray: SBFT is valuable to identify polyps and plan appropriate surgical intervention.

Endoscopy: Endoscopy reveals polyps of several mm to several cm that are usually lobulated. Polyp histology shows a core of smooth muscle fibers from muscularis mucosa extending up into the mucosa in a branching pattern that makes the polyps appear lobulated. They are covered by normal mucosa. A pattern of pseudoinvasion occurs. In this pattern, mechanical forces drive normal mucosal elements into the submucosa, where they line mucin-filled cystic spaces (Lancet 1999;353:1211).

Rx: The goal is to remove polyps to prevent sx and to reduce the risk of malignancy. The greatest problem is with small bowel polyps outside the reach of the endoscope. All polyps >1.5 cm are removed, often with frequent laparotomies and intraoperative endoscopy. Surveillance guidelines (EGD q 2 yr, SBFT q 2 yr, surveillance for breast, gonadal, and pancreatic cancer) have been published, but their efficacy is unproven (Am J Gastro 2000; 95:596).

5.6   Juvenile Polyps and Juvenile Polyposis

Brit J Surg 1995;82:14

Cause: Thus far, 2 identified mutations have been associated with this autosomal dominant disease. Mutations in the gene that codes for a protein called PTEN (Nat Genet 1998;18:12) and mutations in the cancer suppressor gene SMAD4 (a common mutation seen in pancreatic tumors) appear to create alterations in the terrain for epithelial cell growth (Curr Gastro Rep 1999;1:449). There is an association of hereditary hemorrhagic telangiectasia and juvenile polyposis in SMAD4-positive kindreds (Lancet 2004;363:852).

Epidem: This is a very rare disorder. In polyposis registries, it is seen less commonly than FAP. Therefore, gene frequency is probably less than 1:50,000. There are no gender-based differences in prevalence.

Pathophys: A juvenile polyp is a hamartomatous (nonneoplastic) polyp characterized by dilated, cystic spaces lined by columnar epithelium with an inflammatory lamina propria. Solitary juvenile polyps are said to occur in 1% of children. This disorder should be suspected when: (1) more than 3-10 juvenile polyps are seen in the colon (Arch Dis Child 1991;66:971), (2) juvenile polyps are seen throughout the gut, or (3) a juvenile polyp is found in a pt with a family hx of juvenile polyposis. The syndrome may present in a severe form in infancy, may be limited to the colon, or may involve the stomach and intestines. Pts develop multiple polyps, which may obstruct or bleed, but the chief concern is the associated CRC risk. An 18% incidence of CRC at a mean age of 37 yr has been reported in one series. The lifetime cumulative risk of CRC is about 50%. Cancer likely arises from the development of adenomatous dysplasia in a juvenile polyp (Cancer 1991;68:889) or from synchronous adenomas. There is an increased incidence of other gi cancers, especially stomach. A family hx is present in 20-50%, and presumably most of the others represent new germ-line mutations. A large number of extracolonic manifestations have been described in case reports, and it seems likely that there is a great deal of genetic heterogeneity in the syndrome. The syndrome is autosomal dominant with variable penetrance.

Sx: Bleeding, diarrhea, or obstruction from polyps.

Si: Prolapsing rectal polyps, often FOBT positive.

Crs: Highly variable, depending on number of polyps; cancer risk as above.

Diff Dx: Once histology is available, the major differential point is sporadic vs familial polyposis.

X-ray: Polyps on BE or UGI/SBFT, but endoscopy is preferred.

Endoscopy: Colonoscopy reveals polyps of 5 mm to several cm that are red, spherical, or lobulated and often are on a stalk.

Rx: For pts with so many polyps that the colon cannot be successfully cleared, surgery is recommended. Some authors are more aggressive and suggest a surgical approach for all pts, given the 50% cumulative CRC (J Am Coll Surg 1995;181:407). Others believe colectomy is not appropriate if the colon can be cleared and the pt is compliant with surveillance (Arch Dis Child 1991;66:971). Ileorectal anastomosis is the most common approach, but some advocate ileoanal anastomosis given polyp recurrences in the rectum and the need for future surveillance (J Am Coll Surg 1995;181:407). There are little data to guide the intervals of endoscopic surveillance. One approach calls for annual colonoscopy until the pt has 2 negative exams followed by extension of the exam interval (Gastrointest Endosc 1993;39:561). These authors suggest that the upper gut should be surveyed as well, with an interval of 3-5 yr if the exam is negative. Another guideline suggests both upper and lower endoscopy on a q 1-2-yr basis to beyond age 70 in those affected (Gut 2002;51 Suppl 5:V21).

5.7 Miscellaneous Polyposis Syndromes

Nejm 1994;331:1694

Cowden's Disease: Also called the multiple hamartoma syndrome, it is characterized by facial trichilemmomas and other mucocutaneous papules, fibrocystic breast disease, goiter, thyroid cancer, and multiple hamartomatous polyps of the gi tract of varying histologies. The polyps are incidental and there is no associated gi malignancy risk.

Neurofibromatosis: Submucosal neurofibromas that may cause pain or bleeding may be seen throughout the gut (Jama 1997;278:51).

Ruvalcaba-Myhre-Smith Syndrome: Macrocephaly, pigmented penile lesions, and hamartomas of the gut (Pediatr Derm 1988;5:28).

Devon Polyposis Syndrome: Recurrent inflammatory fibroid polyps requiring surgery (Gut 1992;33:1004).

5.8 Carcinoid Tumors of the Gut

Curr Opin Oncol 2002;14:38; Nejm 1999;340:858; Lancet 1998;352:799

Epidem: The incidence is low at 0.5/100,000-2.1/100,000 (Dis Colon Rectum 1997;40:349; Cancer 1997;79:813).

Pathophys: Carcinoids arise from neuroendocrine cells and contain granules rich in hormones and biogenic amines. Serotonin metabolites and other hormones are thought to be responsible for the **carcinoid syndrome** in which there is episodic flushing, wheezing, diarrhea, and eventually right-sided valvular heart disease. Carcinoid syndrome is seen only in pts with liver mets that allow release of hormones directly into the systemic circulation without clearance by the liver. A variety of kinins, prostaglandins, gastrin, somatostatin, glucagon, and other substances can be released from the tumors. The profile of released substances varies with the anatomic site (Dis Colon Rectum 1997;40:349). Serotonin is metabolized to 5-hydroxyindoleacetic acid (5-HIAA), which can be detected in the urine as a marker of the tumor. Carcinoids may occur in several sites. They can be seen as part of the MEN-1 syndrome (Ann IM 1998;129:484). **Gastric carcinoids** are usually associated with atrophic gastritis and present as small lesions in the body or fundus found incidentally at endoscopy. They can also be seen in ZE syndrome (p 145) and sporadically. Only the sporadic lesions have a high incidence of mets and carcinoid syndrome. **Small bowel carcinoids** usually arise in the distal ileum and present with obstruction or pain. They can be multicentric and are often associated with carcinoid syndrome. **Appendiceal carcinoids** usually present as incidental findings at appendectomy. In 95% of cases they are <2 cm in size and do not metastasize. Larger lesions may metastasize and cause carcinoid syndrome. **Colonic carcinoids** usually present late as large right colonic masses (Dis Colon Rectum 1994;37:482), and the carcinoid syndrome occurs in <5%. **Rectal carcinoids** are often found incidentally at endoscopy (Dis Colon Rectum 1992; 35:717). They typically contain glucagon rather than serotonin and rarely produce the carcinoid syndrome.

Sx and Si: Sx of pain or obstruction may be seen from mass effect of the tumor or mets. Most other sx are related to the **carcinoid syndrome.** Flushing is seen in 90%. In gastric carcinoid, flushing is a prolonged purple hue largely over the face and neck. In small bowel carcinoid, flushing is pink-red and of short duration. Other manifestations include secretory diarrhea (70%), abdominal pain (40%), telangiectasia (25%), wheezing (15%), and valvular heart disease (>30%).

Crs: About 45% of pts present with metastases at original dx. The 5-yr survival regardless of site is 50% but is much higher for appendiceal and rectal carcinoid (Cancer 1997;79:813). The course of metastatic disease is highly variable, with some pts having a sx-free survival of many years.

Cmplc: Carcinoid syndrome (see "Pathophys" and "Sx and Si"). Carcinoid heart disease occurs in two thirds of pts with carcinoid syndrome (Nejm 1999;340:858). Fibrotic thickening of the endocardium causes retraction of valve leaflets in the right heart, resulting in tricuspid regurgitation or, less often, stenosis. Less often there is regurgitation/stenosis of the pulmonic or left-sided valves (Circ 1993;87:1188). The cause is unknown. Niacin deficiency (pellagra, dermatitis, diarrhea, dementia) results because the precursor tryptophan is consumed by the tumor.

Diff Dx: The dx is usually considered because of sx suggestive of the carcinoid syndrome. The differential is broad depending on the presenting sx.

Lab: A 24-hr urine test for 5-HIAA is specific for carcinoid (if level >100 mmol/24 hr), though the test requires a variety of dietary and medicine restrictions for accurate performance (Lancet 1998;352:799).

X-ray: CT scan with and without contrast is used to detect hepatic mets. Radiolabeled octreotide scanning can be used to detect metastases prior to operation by the binding of somatostatin receptors on tumor cells (Nejm 1990;323:1246). Histologically, these tumors have small cells with well-rounded nuclei. They stain with chromate and with silver. Immunohistochemical stains are diagnostic by confirming the hormone content of the tumor.

Endoscopy: This is the best test for detection of gastric and intestinal lesions within reach of the endoscope.

Rx: Appendiceal carcinoids <2 cm are treated with appendectomy. Those larger than 2 cm or with extension to the base of the appendix are treated with right hemicolectomy. Rectal carcinoids are usually treated with local excision if they are <1 cm and with resection if they are >2 cm. The approach for lesions 1-2 cm in size is individualized, because it is not clear that resection is better than local excision for this group. Small bowel lesions are treated with resection. Small gastric lesions can be excised endoscopically, and larger lesions are resected.

In the **carcinoid syndrome,** pts should avoid alcohol, spicy food, and exercise, which may precipitate attacks. Octreotide, a synthetic somatostatin analog injected bid, inhibits serotonin release and is effective in 70-90% of pts if adequate doses are used (Aliment Pharmacol Ther 1995;9:387). A longer-acting analog, lanreotide, had similar efficacy in a small study and is injected only q 10 d (Cancer 2000;88:770). Hepatic mets can be resected in selected pts with long-term sx relief (Am J Surg 1995;169:36). Hepatic artery occlusion (by embolization or surgery) may be of short-term benefit (several months) in unresectable disease. There may be a benefit to adding chemotherapy to prolong the response (Ann IM 1994;120:302). Transplant for metastatic carcinoid had a surprising 69% 5-yr survival in a recent French series (Ann Surg 1997;225:355). Chemotherapy is disappointing, and there is little experience with radiation (Nejm 1999; 340:858). Rx targeted to somatostatin receptors is being investigated (Curr Opin Oncol 2002;14:38).

Chapter 6

Infectious Intestinal Disorders

Comment: The most frequently encountered infectious causes of diarrhea are summarized in Section 6.1. For a discussion of the diff dx, see Acute Diarrhea (p 22) or Chronic Diarrhea (p26). General supportive measures are outlined in those sections. For general reviews, see Dis Mo 1999;45:268 or Am J Gastro 1993;88:1667.

6.1 *Clostridium Difficile* Colitis and Antibiotic Associated Diarrhea

Nejm 2002;346:334; Am J Gastro 1997;92:739

Cause: *Clostridium difficile*, an anaerobic, spore-forming bacillus.

Epidem: The reported disease incidence has been rising steadily, probably as a result of better detection and physician awareness. The illness is more common in the elderly, in renal pts, in surgical pts, in IBD pts (Gut 1983;24:713), and in those with malignancy. Carriage rates in Europe and the U.S. are 0-3% in healthy adult subjects and 35-65% in healthy neonates. The organism is frequently acquired in the hospital through the ingestion of spores. The spores resist digestion and become vegetative when they reach the colon. Infected pts are a disease reservoir. The organism can be recovered from many surfaces in pt care areas. It is transmitted via health care workers' hands or stethoscopes (J Antimicrob Chemother 1998;41[suppl C]:59).

Pathophys: Antibiotic-associated diarrhea is a mild, self-limited illness of unknown mechanism that is associated with many antibiotics, clears with cessation of antibiotics, and causes no structural damage to the colon. C. *difficile* causes a spectrum of illness, from diarrhea without obvious macroscopic colitis to more severe forms associated with inflammatory changes in the colonic mucosa. Before the discovery of C. *difficile*, this illness was called pseudomembranous colitis because of the endoscopic and histologic findings, and it was thought to be due to *Staphylococcus aureus*. The discovery that 10% of pts given clindamycin developed pseudomembranous colitis led to the discovery that toxins produced by C. *difficile* are the cause of the illness (BMJ 1995; 310:1375). The use of broad-spectrum antibiotics is the initiating event in the vast majority of cases of C. *difficile* colitis. Changes in the normal intestinal flora seem permissive for the proliferation of the organism. The organism is most often acquired nosocomially from the environment. When the colonized pt is exposed to broad-spectrum antibiotics, there is rapid overgrowth of the organism. Almost all antibiotics have been implicated in C. *difficile* colitis, including clindamycin, penicillins, cephalosporins, quinolones, erythromycin, tetracyclines, and sulfonamides. Disease is more likely to follow high-dose, prolonged courses of rx, especially if multiple agents are used.

C. *difficile* causes colitis by the elaboration of toxins A and B in the colon lumen. Toxin A causes an inflammatory reaction and fluid secretion. Toxin B is a powerful cytotoxin in tissue culture but not enterotoxigenic in animals (Nejm 1994;330:257). A variety of other virulence factors may be important in promoting colonization and tissue destruction (J Antimicrob Chemother 1998;41[suppl C]:13). From 5-25% of strains do not produce either toxin and do not cause diarrhea.

Sx: Pts with mild disease usually present with the sudden onset of watery diarrhea during or shortly after a course of antibiotics. However, there may be a delay of many weeks between antibiotic use and illness. Those with more severe illness may have severe diarrhea, substantial abdominal pain, and fever.

Si: In mild disease, there may be mild abdominal tenderness or FOBT-positive stool. In more severe disease, fever, signs of volume depletion, delirium, and abdominal distension may be seen. Localized peritoneal signs are common in severe illness and usually improve with appropriate rx. A small subgroup will present with fulminant colitis with toxic dilatation, diffuse peritonitis, or signs of perforation.

Crs: Relapse is frequent, occurring in 15-35% of pts (mean about 20%). Most treated ambulatory pts improve over 2-3 days with appropriate rx and 95% are fully resolved after a 10-day course (Nejm 1994;330:257). However, the disease has become more virulent in the last decade with a dramatic rise in mortality and complications in hospitalized pts (Cmaj 2004;171:468).

Cmplc: Fulminant colitis with peritonitis, gram-negative sepsis, and perforation.

Diff Dx: C. *difficile* disease needs to be distinguished from simple antibiotic-related diarrhea. In pts with mild sx, this means stopping the antibiotic and waiting. In pts with moderate illness, stool studies are done for C. *difficile*. If these are negative and suspicion is high, endoscopic studies may be indicated. In pts who acquire diarrhea in the hospital, the likely causes are C. *difficile*, drugs, or enteral feeding. The yield for other pathogens in hospital-acquired diarrhea is pathetically low, and routine stool cultures are usually wasteful.

Lab: Stool **immunoassays for toxin A and B** are the most widely used tests in the U.S. They are 90% sensitive and vary by brand of test. They are highly specific. A negative test in an affected pt is, therefore, not rare in clinical practice. Ordering a second test on a different day will increase the yield (Ann IM 1995;123:835). Variant strains of toxin can be missed by commercial assays (Ann IM 2001;135:434) and 1-2% of cases involve strains that produce only toxin B (Nejm 2002;346:334). **Culture** is the most sensitive and specific test and is usually reserved for investigating outbreaks when identification of the strain may be important. **Tissue culture for toxin B** is cumbersome and only 90% sensitive. **PCR of stool for toxin B** may have the best combination of sensitivity, specificity, and cost but is not widely available (Clin Gastroenterol Hepatol 2004;2:669). **Latex agglutination** detects a C. *difficile* metabolic enzyme, not the toxin (J Clin Microbiol 1991;29:2639). It detects nonpathogenic strains and has other cross reactivities, making its specificity inadequate. Leukocytosis is common.

X-ray: KUB is usually normal in mild disease, but as disease progresses, there may be radiographic signs of colitis such as thumbprinting (irregularity in the mucosal outline of the colon about the size of a thumbprint) or toxic dilatation. CT scan, often done in severely ill pts before the dx is appreciated, may show thickening of the colonic wall due to colitis.

Endoscopy: In mild disease there is minimal or no gross colitis. When the disease progresses, there is a pathognomonic finding of pseudomembranes at colonoscopy. They are raised, yellowish plaques with a stuck on appearance that vary from a few mm to more than a cm in diameter. In severe disease they may coalesce into large segments. They are easily stripped off by the endoscope (the origin of the term pseudomembrane) (Am J Gastro 1997; 92:739). The intervening mucosa may be nearly normal or edematous, friable, and erythematous, depending on disease severity. In perhaps 10% of pts, the pseudomembranes are confined to the proximal colon and may be missed at sigmoidoscopy (GE 1982;83:1259). These pts may be difficult to dx because they may have less diarrhea given the relatively spared left colon. Neutropenic pts will not have pseudomembranes, because they do not have enough white cells to make them (BMJ 1995; 310:1375).

Rx: Whenever possible, antibiotics should be stopped. Current ACG
guidelines suggest that since many cases will resolve spontaneously,
antibiotics rx should not be routinely given (Am J Gastro
1997;92:739). This guideline is widely ignored especially in light
of increasing virulence of the disease. Most clinicians only order
a diagnostic test in pts who are significantly affected and rx all
positives. Fluid and electrolyte replacement may be needed.
Antimotility agents should be avoided since this prolongs the contact of the mucosa with toxin and may worsen the illness.

In pts with mild to moderate disease, oral **metronidazole**
250-500 mg po tid for 7-10 d is the drug of choice. Some strains
are metronidazole-resistant, but this is uncommon. In pts with
severe disease, who often cannot take oral rx, the drug is given as
500-750 mg iv q 6-8 d depending on body weight and severity of
illness. Oral **vancomycin** is wildly expensive and should be used
when pts do not respond to metronidazole, cannot tolerate
metronidazole, are critically ill, or have a contraindication to
metronidazole use (eg, pregnancy). The usual dosage for vancomycin is 125 mg po qid for 7-10 d, but doses up to 500 mg po
qid are used in pts with severe illness. Oral vancomycin should
probably be used concomitantly with iv metronidazole in pts who
are critically ill. Vancomycin given by iv does not work because
there is inadequate excretion into the colon, where the organism
lies. Some very ill pts who fail metronidazole may have S. aureus
diarrhea and may respond to oral vancomycin (Am J Gastro
1997;92:739).

Cholestyramine or colestipol bind the toxin (and vancomycin!) but are marginal therapies compared to antibiotics.
Bacitracin is less effective than vancomycin (GE 1985;89:1038),
and a variety of other agents have been used (Aliment
Pharmacol Ther 1997;11:1003).

Pts with a substantial symptomatic **relapse** should simply
receive a second course of rx with metronidazole, since the cause
of relapse is rarely drug resistance. Relapse occurs by germination

of spores in the colon, by reinfection in the hospital setting, or due to another course of antibiotics. There is no well-defined approach to pts with multiple relapses. Some experts use a prolonged course of oral vancomycin; others use intermittent vancomycin (125 mg po q 2-7 d for 1 or 2 months, tapered with a nonscientific flourish). The hope is to kill vegetative forms newly developed from the spores that escape the antibiotic. Other forms of rx include lactobacillus preparations (ineffective by RCT [Mayo Clin Proc 2001;76:883]), oral *Saccharomyces boulardii* (Aliment Pharmacol Ther 1998;12:807; GE 1989;96:981), fecal enemas, donor feces by NGT (Clin Infect Dis 2003;36:580), and iv gamma globulin (Gut 2002;51:456).

Pts with severe disease may require **surgery** for perforation or fulminant colitis with a mortality of 25-67%. A series of retrospective reviews suggest that pts are more likely to survive if they have subtotal colectomy rather than simple diversion or lesser degrees of colectomy (Dis Colon Rectum 1998;41:1435; Postgrad Med J 1998;74:216).

Pts with diarrhea should be isolated to **prevent** spread of disease. Hand washing is essential, and the load of spores and vegetative forms is reduced by thorough cleaning of the environment and equipment. Rx of asymptomatic carriers with metronidazole or vancomycin is ineffective (Ann IM 1992;117:297).

6.2 *Campylobacter*

Gastroenterol Clin North Am 2001;30:709; Clin Lab Med 1999;19:489

Cause: Most human *Campylobacter* infections are caused by *Campylobacter jejunii*, but other species, including C. *coli* and any of 12 other subspecies, may cause human disease. The organisms are gram-negative, and are curved or spiral-shaped rods.

Epidem: *Campylobacter* is the most common of the bacterial causes of diarrhea after C. *difficile*. There is a bimodal peak of incidence (infants and young adults), but it affects all ages. Sporadic cases are usually associated with undercooked or mishandled poultry and less often with other meats, untreated water, or raw milk. Epidemics are associated with raw milk or contaminated water.

Pathophys: The ingestion of as few as 500 organisms can result in infection. The bug colonizes the distal ileum and colon, where invasion occurs and intestinal absorption is inhibited, resulting in diarrhea.

Sx: The incubation period is 1-5 d. Pts typically present with crampy pain, watery diarrhea (often mixed with blood and mucus), and fever. Headache may be especially prominent and a clue to the etiology.

Crs: The typical course is a 4-5-d illness with 1 to 2 wk for complete resolution. Of those seeking medical attention, 20% have sx for longer than a wk (Am J Gastro 1993;88:1667). The relapse rate is 10-20%.

Cmplc: There is firm serologic and culture-based evidence that *Campylobacter* infection can result in Guillain-Barré syndrome (Clin Microbiol Rev 1998;11:555; Infect Dis Clin North Am 1998;12:173). A syndrome of reactive arthritis in HLA-B27 positive pts may occur (within 1-3 wk) and resolve within 6 months (Arch IM 1983;143:215). Pancreatitis has been reported in 6% of pts sick enough to be hospitalized (Arch IM 1983; 143:215).

Lab: Stool culture is the test of choice. Since the organism is fastidious, a single culture may not be adequate (Am J Gastro 1993; 88:1667). An experienced observer may be able to pick out the organism on a Gram stain using carbol fuchsin as a counterstain, because it is a curved rod, giving a gull wing appearance. There are no other rapid methods of adequate sensitivity and specificity for commercial use.

Endoscopy: Usually endoscopy is not indicated, but if done, it shows features of a nonspecific colitis with erythema, edema, and loss of the vascular pattern in involved segments.

Rx: Typically the stool culture comes back after the pt is improving and rx at that time does not shorten the illness. Pts who are slow to recover, who have continued sx of dysentery, or who are immunocompromised should be treated with erythromycin 250 mg po qid for 5 d. In a subgroup of ill pts, rx with a quino-lone (eg, ciprofloxacin 500 mg po bid × 5 d) given on presentation before the culture results are available may shorten the illness (p 25). However, increasing quinolone resistance limits the value of this approach. In Europe and Asia, quinolone resistance ranges from 41-88% and in North America the rate has climbed to over 10% (GE 2000;118:S48). Azithromycin 500 mg daily is an alternative to erythromycin.

6.3 *Salmonella*

Dis Mo 1999;45:268; Am J Gastro 1993;88:1667; South Med J 1978;71:1540

Cause: There are more than 2200 serotypes of *Salmonella*. The species most likely to cause gastroenteritis in the U.S. are *S. typhimurium*, *S. enteritidis*, *S. heidelberg,* and *S. newport*.

Epidem: About 40,000 cases are reported annually in the U.S., repre-senting about 1-5% of the actual total. Transmission is by con-taminated water or food, chiefly poultry, eggs, dairy products, and processed meats. Vertical transmission in hen eggs has created an enormous reservoir (Gut 1994;35:726). Fecal-oral spread is easily prevented by hand washing.

Pathophys: The bacteria invades intestinal and colonic epithelium, frequently resulting in bacteremia (5-10%). Pts with sickle cell disease, HIV, and immunosuppression are more prone to bac-teremia. Infected pts most commonly develop gastroenteritis and less commonly extraintestinal infections (osteomyelitis, pneumonia, arteritis, and meningitis). Those infected with the typhoid-causing or paratyphoid-causing agents develop enteric fever (not further discussed here). Following acute infection, pts commonly excrete organism for wk to months. Pts are said to be chronic carriers if excretion lasts more than 1 yr. This occurs in 1% of pts infected with nontyphoidal *Salmonella*.

Sx: Pts most often present with a mild to moderate illness of crampy abdominal pain and diarrhea. A small subgroup will present with a more severe illness with high fever and bloody diarrhea. The pts with severe illness are more likely to be the very old, the very young, and the immunocompromised.

Si: Fever, abdominal tenderness (sometimes right sided if there is prominent ileal involvement), and blood in stool.

Crs: Usually self-limited illness of several d; prolonged stool excretion, with 1% of pts developing a carrier state (>1 yr of infection).

Cmplc: Extraintestinal infections from bacteremia as listed in Pathophys. Reactive arthritis may occur.

Lab: Stool C&S.

X-ray: KUB, if done, may show evidence of colitis with thick colonic folds and thumbprinting. CT may show evidence of colonic wall thickening.

Endoscopy: If done, shows nonspecific evidence of colitis. Biopsies show acute colitis without the distortion of crypt architecture or loss of mucous gland depletion seen in IBD (Gut 1994;35:726).

Rx: Antibiotic rx does not, in general, shorten the course of the illness in otherwise healthy pts with mild to moderate illness. Rx with antibiotics should be reserved for pts with severe sx (such as high fever, bloody diarrhea, or the need to be hospitalized), pts at the extremes of age, or pts who are immunosuppressed. Choices include Tm/S 160/800 mg po bid, ciprofloxacin 500 mg po bid, or norfloxacin 400 mg po bid for 5-7 d depending on the speed of response (Am J Gastro 1997;92:1962). In the small number of pts who develop the chronic carrier state following enterocolitis, rx with a quinolone for 28 d could be considered, but this is by analogy to studies in typhoidal strains rather than by direct evidence (GE 2000;118:S48).

6.4 *Shigella*

Gastroenterol Clin North Am 2001;30:709; Am J Gastro 1993;88:1667

Cause: There are 4 species of *Shigella* organisms—*S. dysenteriae*, *S. flexneri*, *S. boydii*, and *S. sonnei*.

Epidem: The only reservoirs for *Shigella* are humans and apes. In developed nations this is largely a pediatric disease because of person-to-person spread. In the West most infections are with *S. sonnei*, which is less virulent. In contrast, in developing nations, waterborne and foodborne spread is common, and disease is often with the more virulent *S. flexneri* or *S. dysenteriae*.

Pathophys: Small infectious doses are needed and usually resist stomach acid. Clinical illness usually begins within 12 hr as invasion of the small intestine begins. Over the next few d the colon is invaded and the pt develops lower abdominal pain and in some cases bloody diarrhea.

Sx: The most common sx is large volume diarrhea (bloody in about half of pts, the classic dysentery). Most pts develop abdominal pain that is crampy and may be severe. Fever and vomiting are common.

Si: Abdominal tenderness, fever, and blood in stool.

Crs: If untreated, the illness usually lasts 1 wk, with a range of 1-30 d. Chronic relapsing sx are rare.

Cmplc: Intestinal obstruction, toxic megacolon, perforation, pneumonia, and HUS have all been described. Reiter's syndrome (arthritis, back pain, urethritis, and conjunctivitis) is seen following 1-2% of cases, most often in HLA-B27-positive pts.

Lab: Stool C&S.

Endoscopy: If done, colonoscopic findings are those of a nonspecific colitis.

Rx: Rx with antibiotics shortens the course of the illness and prevents additional person-to-person spread. Pts with disease acquired in the U.S. should be treated with Tm/S I DS tab po bid × 5 d. Pts whose illness is acquired in foreign travel should be treated with a quinolone such as ciprofloxacin 500 mg po bid, and sensitivities should be confirmed (Am J Gastro 1997;92:1962). Antimotility agents should be avoided in the very ill because they worsen illness (Jama 1973;226:1525).

6.5 *E. Coli* O157:H7

Annu Rev Med 1999;50:355; Lancet 1998;352:1207; Ann IM 1995;123:698

Cause: *Escherichia coli* O157:H7, an organism so called because it expresses the 157th somatic (O) antigen and the 7th flagellar antigen. Other Shiga toxin-producing *E. coli* produce diarrheal illness, but their role is not well defined (GE 1993;105:1724).

Epidem: Incidence of 8/100,000/yr in Britain and North America, much higher in South America. Peaks in summer. Healthy cattle are the major reservoir, but it is found in many animals, especially ruminants. The disease is most often transmitted by food or water, but person-to-person spread can be important in some settings, such as a child daycare center. Meat becomes contaminated at slaughter, especially if it is ground in processing. Undercooked ground meat is a frequent cause. Outbreaks have been associated with fresh produce and with drinking or swimming in unchlorinated water. Implicated foods range from fresh-pressed apple cider (Jama 1993;269:2217) to deer meat jerky (Jama 1997; 277:1229), emphasizing the need to involve public health authorities in investigation of cases. The infectious dose is very low (50 organisms). Fecal shedding can last for weeks after recovery.

Pathophys: The virulence of this organism is based on its production of Shiga toxins, a virulence plasmid, and on other factors not yet characterized. The organism adheres to the brush border in the colon, and the virulence factors cause cell damage leading to bloody diarrhea. HUS is caused by adherence of Shiga toxins to renal endothelial cells. This probably triggers platelet and fibrin deposition in the renal vessels, causing hemolysis of red cells and renal failure secondary to microvascular occlusion.

Sx: The illness can present as asymptomatic carriage, nonbloody diarrhea, bloody diarrhea, or HUS leading to death. Incubation period is 1-7 d. The illness usually begins as watery diarrhea that turns bloody in 70% of pts. Vomiting is common (60%), but fever is low grade and occurs in only 30% of pts.

Si: Abdominal tenderness may be marked. High fever is uncommon. Neurologic abnormalities may develop in HUS pts.

Crs: Most pts recover within 7 d. However, 3-7% of pts develop HUS. Of these, 9% die, 3% have chronic renal failure or other major sequelae such as stroke or seizures, and 25% have mild renal sequelae (Jama 2003;290:1360).

Cmplc: HUS, which is more common in the very old, very young (younger than 5 yr old), and possibly in those who receive antimotility agents or antibiotics.

Lab: Stool C&S. The organism is presumptively identified because it does not ferment sorbitol. Sorbitol-negative colonies are then tested for the O157 antigen. Leukocytosis is common.

Endoscopy: Endoscopy (which is usually unnecessary) reveals a mucosa that appears hyperemic and congested, with edema and patchy superficial ulceration that is often seen in the right colon. There is no single feature on biospy that is diagnostic. There may be features of ischemic colitis and pseudomembranous colitis seen on bx (Ann IM 1995;123:698).

Rx: Rx is supportive. It seems prudent to monitor for the development of HUS, especially in the very old and very young. Loperamide should be avoided because it may predispose to HUS (J Pediatr 1990;116:589). It is not clear if antibiotics are harmful. A small prospective cohort study of children demonstrated an increased incidence of HUS in those children who received antibiotics (Nejm 2000;342:1930) but a meta-analysis of 9 studies showed no effect (Jama 2002;288:996). Shiga toxin binding agents are a new approach but an RCT of one such agent showed no benefit (Jama 2003;290:1337). HUS requires dialysis in 50% of cases. It is crucial that the physician notify public health authorities immediately of confirmed cases or suspected outbreaks. Prompt investigation can lead to prevention of additional cases by rapid identification of the source.

6.6 Cholera and Other *Vibrio* Diseases

Lancet 2004;363:223; Am J Med 1998;104:386; Lancet 1997; 349:1825

Cause: *Vibrio cholerae*, a curved gram-negative rod. The O1 and the newly emerged O139 strains cause epidemic disease and others cause sporadic diarrhea. *Vibrio parahemolyticus* causes a diarrheal illness.

Epidem: Cholera is endemic in Asia and Africa. It was reintroduced in epidemic form to Latin America in the 1990s. A newly emerged strain (O139) has caused epidemics in India, Bangladesh, and Southeast Asia. In developed nations, it is usually a disease of returned travelers. Epidemics arise when epidemic strains are introduced into nonimmune populations. Transmission is by water, food, and person-to-person spread. *Vibrio parahemolyticus* occurs from ingestion of undercooked seafood, is common in Japan, and has been seen in coastal areas of the United States.

Pathophys: Cholera is the prototypical enterotoxic, secretory diarrhea. The organism binds to small intestinal epithelial cells and secretes the cholera toxin. The toxin induces adenylate cyclase, increases in intracellular cAMP, which increases chloride secretion, and decreases Na absorption. This causes the massive volume loss that characterizes the disease.

Sx: Massive diarrhea, up to a L per hour.

Si: Volume depletion, stupor.

Crs: Usually resolves within 6 d if vascular collapse is avoided.

Lab: Stool culture. A clinical dx is usually made in an epidemic setting.

Rx: The cornerstone of rx for cholera is rehydration. This is done orally with the World Health Organization oral hydration rx (NaCl, KCl, sodium bicarbonate, and glucose), and with iv in severe cases. Tetracycline, doxycycline, and quinolones shorten the illness. Oral vaccines show promise but may be too expensive for most of those at risk (Lancet 2004;363:223).

6.7 *Yersinia Enterocolitica*

Clin Microbiol Rev 1997;10:257

This pathogen is an uncommon cause of illness in North America. It causes an acute enterocolitis, a pseudoappendicitis, or a terminal ileitis suggestive of Crohn's disease. It may be complicated by septicemia with metastatic infection and a variety of other clinical sequelae. The dx is made by C&S, though serology may also be of use. A wide variety of antibiotics are effective.

6.8 Enterotoxigenic, Enteropathogenic, and Enteroinvasive *E. Coli*

The strains of *E. coli* that cause diarrhea are very difficult to distinguish from other nonpathogenic *E. coli* in the clinical laboratory. Virulence of these strains is caused by genes that are encoded on plasmids. Only the O157:H7 type discussed in Section 6.5 is specifically identified in common clinical practice. The enteropathogenic strain is primarily a disease of infants and may be prolonged. The enterotoxigenic type produces a diarrhea causing enterotoxin and is the major cause of traveler's diarrhea. Antibiotic rx with Tm/S or quinolones shorten the illness (p 25). The enteroinvasive type causes illness by tissue invasion (Dis Mo 1999;45:268; Am J Gastro 1997; 92:1962).

6.9 *Plesiomonas*

This facultatively anaerobic gram-negative rod causes an illness of diarrhea, fever, and blood in stool. It appears to be an invasive infection after ingestion of uncooked shellfish or travel. Antibiotics (Tm/S or tetracycline) may improve the illness (Ann IM 1986; 105:690).

6.10 *Aeromonas*

Aeromonas, a facultatively anaerobic gram-negative rod, is found in fresh and brackish water in the U.S. and is a cause of diarrhea worldwide. Sx can be chronic in adults and acute and severe in children. The diarrhea is probably caused by an enterotoxin. Several antibiotics appear effective (Gastroenterol Clin North Am 2001; 30:709).

6.11 Giardiasis

Clin Infect Dis 1997;25:545

Cause: *Giardia lamblia*, a protozoan flagellate.

Epidem: Infection results from ingestion of cysts, which can be viable for months in cool water. Most infections come from contaminated water or less commonly by fecal–oral spread. Although the cysts are often resistant to the chlorine in drinking water, they can be effectively removed by filtration. Campers are at risk from water contaminated by animals (beaver fever). *Giardia* can be endemic in areas where water treatment is inadequate, though most residents of these regions remain asymptomatic.

Pathophys: After cysts are ingested and pass into the duodenum, they change to trophozoites, the vegetative form. Some trophozoites encyst in the ileum and are excreted in stool. Tissue invasion does not occur and no toxin has been identified. The mechanism of diarrhea is not clear, but may be related to disruption of the brush border. Since pts with hypogammaglobulinemia or IgA deficiency have more severe illness, a host antibody-mediated response seems important. Malabsorption commonly occurs. Lactose intolerance is found in 20-40% of pts and may last weeks even after infection is cleared.

Sx: The incubation period is generally 1-2 wk. Most infections remain asymptomatic. Acutely symptomatic pts present with cramping, midabdominal to upper abdominal pain, bloating, flatulence, and loose, foul smelling stool. Weight loss and anorexia are common. Fever is sometimes seen at the outset of illness. There is no blood found in stools. As infection becomes more chronic, malaise and epigastric pain may predominate and diarrhea lessens.

Si: Distension, very active bowel sounds.

Crs: If untreated, the infection lasts wk to months, though it usually clears spontaneously in healthy hosts. In multiple relapses, consider recurrent infection (have the well water tested!), hypogammaglobulinemia, HIV, or other immune deficiency states.

Lab: Stool *Giardia* antigen is the test of choice and is highly sensitive and specific. Stool O&P exams are insensitive even with multiple samples. Serologic tests are of little use because they do not distinguish remote from active infection. The string test, in which the pt swallows a capsule attached to a string that is inspected for trophozoites, is cumbersome. Empiric antibiotics seem a sensible alternative.

Rx: Metronidazole 250 mg po tid for 5-7 d is the most commonly used rx in the U.S. Tinidazole 2 gm po as a single dose is just as effective and has recently been released in the U.S. (Clin Microbiol Rev 2001;14:114). Furazolidone (100 mg po qid for 7-10 d), albendazole, and paromomycin are alternatives. Quinacrine is no longer available in the U.S. because of toxicity. Because of the frequency of lactase deficiency, pts should minimize lactose intake and be warned that the lactase deficiency may last for wk and cause an apparent relapse when pts try to reintroduce milk products.

6.12 Amebiasis

Lancet 2003;361:1025; Clin Infect Dis 1999;29:1117

Cause: *Entamoeba histolytica,* a protozoan parasite. There are several nonpathogenic species, such as *E. dispar,* which is tenfold more frequent but morphologically identical to *E. histolytica.* There are species of occasional or uncertain pathogenicity, such as *Entamoeba coli* (Lancet 1991;338:254) and *Dientamoeba fragilis* (Dig Dis Sci 1996;41:1811).

Epidem: Infection is endemic in many developing nations and uncommon in nations with well-developed sanitation systems. Each year, 40-50 million cases occur. In the U.S., it is largely a disease of returned travelers and immigrants. Hepatic abscess is 7-12 times more likely in men. Spread is fecal–oral through contaminated food and water.

Pathophys: The parasite is ingested in the cyst form and produces 8 trophozoites, which attach to intestinal mucin glycoproteins and invade host cells. After invasion of the colon, distant sites of infection can develop. The most common is hepatic abscess.

Sx: Some pts remain entirely asymptomatic carriers, especially in endemic areas. Pts with amebic colitis present with the gradual onset of abdominal pain, fever, and diarrhea that becomes bloody. The gradual onset is a hallmark, and weight loss is common. Fever is infrequent in colitis alone. Amebic abscess presents as pain and fever, sometimes with an RUQ mass.

Si: In colitis, blood in stool is common (70%). A mass can be detected in pts who develop a localized segmental mass of granulation tissue called an ameboma (Gastroenterol Clin North Am 1996;25:471).

Crs: The course is usually one of good response to rx, but pregnancy, malignancy, steroid use, malnutrition, and neonatal infection are more likely to result in a fulminant picture (Clin Infect Dis 1995; 20:1453).

Cmplc: Extraintestinal disease with abscess of liver, spleen, brain, empyema, or pericarditis; abscesses may rupture; fulminant colitis occurs in <0.5% and can require surgery with a mortality of 50%.

Diff Dx: The diff dx for amebic hepatic abscess is pyogenic liver abscess, echinococcus, and HCC.

Lab: A stool test for *E. histolytica* specific antigen (Gut 1994;335: 1018) is the test of choice because it is 87% sensitive and 90%

specific. Stool O&P exams miss more than half of infections (unless multiple samples are obtained) and cannot distinguish pathogenic from nonpathogenic species. Serology is a useful adjunct (75-90% sensitive) but does not distinguish recent from remote infection and may be negative early in the course of the illness. In hepatic abscess, alk phos is elevated in 80% of pts.

X-ray: CT or ultrasound are effective for the dx of abscess.

Endoscopy: Colonoscopy should be done if the cause of colitis is in doubt. Colonoscopy is superior to sigmoidoscopy. The mucosa looks similar to that of IBD with granularity, friability, and ulcerated mucosa. The ulcers may have sharply defined borders and undermining, and are called flask shaped. Scrapings of ulcer bases are examined for trophozoites, and bx are obtained for conventional and immunochemical staining (Gastroenterol Clin North Am 1996;25:471).

Rx: Both the trophozoites and the cysts must be killed to clear the intestinal infection. Metronidazole 750 mg po tid ×10 d kills trophozoites. Tinidazole 2 gm po × 3 d is as effective and is now available in the U.S. Cysts are treated by a course of diloxanide furoate 500 mg po tid ×10 d or iodoquinol 650 mg po tid × 20 d. Asymptomatic cyst passers may be treated without the course of metronidazole. For fulminant colitis iv metronidazole is used. Other rx is available for pregnant pts and special circumstances (GE 2000;118:S48). For hepatic abscess, initial rx is with metronidazole/diloxanide. Percutaneous drainage or surgery are not needed in most cases.

6.13 Cryptosporidiosis

Nejm 2002;346:1723; Adv Parasitol 1998;40:37

Cause: *Cryptosporidium pavum*, a ubiquitous protozoan parasite.

Epidem: This is a common infection with prevalence rates of under 2% in developed nations and as high as 30% in developing nations (Epidemiol Rev 1996;18:118). It is highly infectious. Human infections come from animals (especially cattle) most often via the water supply. Large outbreaks in cities with good water treatment underscore the difficulty of controlling this agent (Ann IM 1996;124:459). About 4% of pts with HIV infection in the U.S. develop cryptosporidiosis. Other risks include malnutrition and communal living.

Pathophys: The mechanism by which *Cryptosporidia* causes a profuse watery diarrhea has not been established. No toxin has been identified, and overt intestinal destruction is rare.

Sx: After an incubation period of about 6 d, healthy hosts develop a self-limited infection marked by watery diarrhea, anorexia, abdominal pain, and sometimes fever or cough. Some HIV-infected pts have transient illness but they are more likely to have chronic illness. A minority of immunosuppressed pts will present with a fulminant illness resembling cholera in its ferocity.

Si: Volume depletion, active bowel sounds, sometimes fever.

Crs: It is a self-limited illness of days to weeks in healthy hosts. It is a chronic illness in HIV pts and portends short survival (Q J Med 1992;85:813).

Cmplc: Respiratory infection is common and can cause severe cough and dyspnea. It can be lethal in HIV pts. In HIV pts, biliary infection can cause a sclerosing cholangitis-like picture that improves with sphincterotomy.

Lab: The modified Ziehl-Neelsen acid-fast stain is the common test of choice. Fluorescent antibody tests are now commercially available and appear more sensitive than staining techniques (Clin Lab Med 1995;15:307).

Rx: Supportive rx is the most important, since highly effective antimicrobial rx does not exist. Healthy hosts clear the infection. Hosts who appear otherwise healthy and do not improve should be tested for HIV. These otherwise healthy pts with a long illness and pts with HIV infection should be treated with paromomycin 500 mg po qid × 2 wk (GE 2000;118:S48), but rx is variably effective (Postgrad Med J 1997;73:713). For pts with HIV, antivirals are a cornerstone of rx. Loperamide or other antimotility agents should be used, and octreotide can be used as symptomatic rx with some benefit.

6.14 *Cyclospora*

Infect Dis Clin North Am 1998;12:1

Cause: *Cyclospora cayetanensis*, a coccidian protozoan related to *Cryptosporidium* and *Isospora*.

Epidem: The organism is found worldwide. Disease is acquired by the ingestion of oocysts as the result of fecal contamination of water or food. The most notable outbreak in the U.S. was associated with Guatemalan raspberries (Ann IM 1999;130:210). Both outbreak (Ann IM 1995;123:409) and sporadic cases have been associated with untreated water. Travelers returning from endemic areas are at high risk.

Pathophys: After ingestion, the organism becomes an intracellular parasite of small intestinal epithelium. Understanding beyond these preliminary observations is limited.

Sx: Pts typically present with watery, bloodless diarrhea that can occur in cycles. Fatigue, anorexia, weight loss, and bloating are common. A flu-like illness may precede the diarrhea by a wk.

Si: Weight loss may be demonstrated, but physical findings are nonspecific.

Crs: In immunocompetent individuals, the infection may last for weeks with diarrhea becoming less prominent and fatigue and anorexia persisting. In HIV-infected pts, the illness may be more prolonged and is more likely to relapse.

Lab: The modified Ziehl-Neelsen acid-fast stain is the most widely used detection method. Detection is enhanced by concentration methods, and new detection techniques are emerging (Arch Pathol Lab Med 1997;121:792).

Endoscopy: Bx, if done, may show villous atrophy and crypt hyperplasia (Ann IM 1993;119:377).

Rx: A placebo-controlled trial showed that Tm/S 1 DS tab po bid × 7 d is highly effective (Lancet 1995;345:691). Repeat doses tiw may be needed to prevent relapses in AIDS pts (GE 2000;118:S48).

6.15 *Isospora Belli* and Microsporidia

Isospora belli was described as a cause of diarrhea in soldiers in World War I (hence the name). This protozoan is now almost exclusively identified in AIDS pts (Nejm 1986;315:87). Water- or food-bearing oocysts are the presumptive mode of transmission. The organism can be found in small intestinal epithelial cells and causes villous atrophy and crypt hyperplasia. Sx are watery diarrhea with crampy pain and steatorrhea. Diagnosis is made by microscopic detection of oocysts using carbol fuchsin stain. It usually responds to Tm/S 160/800 po qid ×10 d, and regimens to prevent relapse have been described (GE 2000;118:S48).

Microsporidia can cause infection in healthy hosts but is largely a pathogen of AIDS pts. There are many species that can cause a diarrheal illness. They are small and difficult to detect in stool and tissue samples. A modified trichrome stain is used in stool specimens. Albendazole is effective rx for some species (Parasitology 1998;117:S143).

6.16 *Blastocystis Hominis*

This protozoan produces an illness of diarrhea and abdominal pain. In many pts with this parasite, a second infectious agent will be found. Its presence indicates that the pt was exposed to contaminated food or water. It is noninvasive and in most cases rx is not needed. Those with persistent sx and in whom no alternative etiology is identified can be offered metronidazole 750 mg po tid for 10 d (J Clin Gastro 1990;12:525).

6.17 *Dientamoeba Fragilis*

This protozoan causes an illness of diarrhea and abdominal pain. It is associated with pinworm infection. Rx is diiodohydroxyquin in adults and metronidazole in children (Dig Dis Sci 1996; 41:1811).

6.18 Viral Gastroenteritis

Gastroenterol Clin North Am 2001;30:779; Jama 1993;269:627; Nejm 1991;325:252

Viruses are frequent causes of diarrhea. However, the rx for all of the following illnesses is supportive, and a specific dx is rarely required except in the investigation of epidemics. **Rotavirus** is a frequent cause of dehydrating diarrhea lasting 5-7 d in young children. Illness is usually not severe after age 3, and infection is often asymptomatic. It occurs more often in the winter in temperate climates and is easily diagnosed, if desired, by stool antigen testing. **Norwalk-like viruses (caliciviruses)** cause outbreaks of diarrhea, fever, vomiting, and myalgia in children and adults. Infection frequently occurs in settings such as cruise ships, camps, and nursing homes. Outbreaks have been associated with contaminated shellfish, water, or other foods. Illness lasts a d or 2. PCR testing is available in research labs and has enhanced the understanding of these viruses as causes of epidemics. **Enteric adenoviruses** cause prolonged diarrheal illnesses in infants and young children. **Astroviruses** are less well-characterized causes of diarrhea.

6.19 Diarrhea in HIV

GE 1996;111:1724

Cause: Many causes of HIV diarrhea have been identified. These include pathogens that cause illness in healthy hosts such as *Campylobacter, Salmonella, Shigella, C. difficile, Giardia*, and *Entamoeba histolytica*. Opportunistic infections such as CMV, *Cryptosporidia, Cyclospora*, microsporidia, *Isospora*, and *Mycobacterium avium* complex cause prolonged diarrhea in HIV-infected pts. Multiple pathogens are seen in up to 29% of pts (Gut 1996;39:824).

Diff Dx: The differential needs to include the causes of diarrhea seen in pts who are not HIV infected (p 26). Diarrhea secondary to drugs is common in HIV-infected pts.

Lab: Stool should be sent for O&P × 3, culture for bacterial pathogens, *C. difficile* antigen, *Giardia* antigen, microsporidia (modified trichrome), *Isospora* (carbol fuchsin), and tests for *Cryptosporidia* (acid-fast or antigen screen). At least 3 stool samples are recommended, but the optimal number is unknown (GE 1996;111:1724).

Endoscopy: Colonoscopy will demonstrate a cause (usually CMV or *Cryptosporidia*, but also adenovirus or spirochetes) in 30% of pts with negative stool studies and low CD4 counts. Most of these findings were within reach of a sigmoidoscope in one series (Gut 1996;39:824), but the yield of colonoscopy vs sigmoidoscopy was 39% vs 22% in another large series (Gastrointest Endosc 1998; 48:354). EGD is indicated and may demonstrate the cause (*Cryptosporidia, Giardia, Mycobacterium avium*, CMV, or microsporidia) in up to 44% of pts with negative stool studies and CD4 counts <200/mL (Gut 1996;39:824). Some authors suggest that colonoscopy with biopsies of the terminal ileum is just as effective as sigmoidoscopy plus EGD, and suggest that EGD adds nothing. However, these authors had a very low yield of microsporidia on their EGD bx studies (Am J Gastro 1999;94:596). In discussing a strategy with pts, colonoscopy plus EGD has the highest diagnostic yield, and any other approach has a risk of missing treatable diagnoses.

Rx: Specific causes are treated as outlined under the specific pathogens earlier in this chapter. There is no consistently effective rx for *Cryptosporidia* (Postgrad Med J 1997;73:713) or microsporidia, but rx with potent antiretrovirals restores immunity and clears the pathogens (Lancet 1998;351:256). CMV is treated with ganciclovir or foscarnet (p 101).

6.20 Intestinal Helminths

Pts with these infections do not usually present with diarrhea but rather present with nonspecific abdominal pain and eosinophilia. Important cestodes (tapeworms) include *Diphyllobothrium latum*, *Taenia*, *Hymenolepis*, and *Dipylidium caninum* (Gastroenterologist 1993;1:265). Common nematodes include (1) *Ascaris lumbricoides*, (2) *Trichuris trichiura* (whipworm; I saw one that survived a gallon of polyethylene glycol and was swimming around a colon but got away), (3) *Necator americanus* and *Ancylostoma duodenale* (hookworms) (Nejm 2004;351:799), (4) *Enterobius vermicularis* (pinworm), (5) anisakiasis (the sushi parasites) (Am J Gastro 1986;81:1185), and (6) trichinosis (Gastroenterologist 1994;2:39). Ascarids are of special interest to the gastroenterologist because they can migrate into biliary and pancreatic ducts, causing cholangitis and acting as the nidus for stones. Once the dx is made (usually by O&P exams) effective rx is available (GE 2000;118:S48).

6.21 Bacterial Overgrowth

Curr Treat Options Gastroenterol 2004;7:19; Clin Perspect Gastro 2000;3:225

Cause: Colonization of the small intestine with a high concentration of bacteria.

Epidem: The elderly are more prone to bacterial overgrowth in the absence of other identifiable risks (Am J Gastro 1997;92:47).

Pathophys: Normally the small gut contains low concentrations of bacteria ($<10^4$ cfu/mL) that provide several useful functions, including the production of vitamin K and the breakdown of unabsorbed sugars into fatty acids absorbable in the colon. Several conditions can lead to bacterial overgrowth, including loss of gastric acidity (especially iatrogenic due to PPI rx), poor motility (eg, scleroderma, diabetic neuropathy), and anatomic abnormalities (diverticula, blind loops, fistulas, strictures). Pts are usually colonized by multiple genera of oral or colonic bacteria rather than a single species (Am J Gastro 1999;94:1327). Bacteria deconjugate bile acids in the small intestine, preventing the formation of micelles (mixtures of conjugated bile salts and dietary lipids) and thus reducing the absorption of dietary fat. Deconjugated bile salts are also toxic to enterocytes, resulting in malabsorption of carbohydrates and proteins. Bacteria degrade proteins. Vitamin absorption is reduced and B_{12} levels may fall due to consumption of B_{12} by bacteria and the binding of B_{12} absorption receptors in the ileum by bacterial B_{12} metabolites.

Sx: Chronic diarrhea associated with bloating and crampy abdominal pain are the typical sx. Pts often note borborygmi and foul flatus. Weight loss is common. In the elderly, the sx may be nonspecific (anorexia, nausea) (Am J Gastro 1997;92:47).

Si: There are no specific findings on exam, though pts may have the findings of the diseases (such as scleroderma) that predispose to bacterial overgrowth.

Crs: Since the predisposing conditions are usually chronic, multiple relapses are common.

Cmplc: Pts may develop complications of malnutrition or specific vitamin deficiency syndromes (night blindness with vitamin A, neuropathy and anemia with B_{12} deficiency).

Diff Dx: The broad differential is that of chronic diarrhea (p 26).

Lab: In pts with a predisposing condition and a good clinical story, empiric rx rather than lab diagnosis is reasonable. The gold standard for laboratory diagnosis is a culture of small intestinal aspirate. This is rarely done outside the research setting because of difficulties with anaerobic cultures, the difficulty of obtaining the sample, and the potential of missing distal overgrowth. The ^{13}C-xylose breath test is the preferred method of lab diagnosis. Bacteria metabolize the labeled xylose (which healthy humans usually absorb intact) and the ^{13}C labeled CO_2 is detected in the breath. The test is >90% sensitive and specific, but expensive. Hydrogen breath tests lack sensitivity and specificity (Am J Gastro 1996;91:1795).

X-ray: SBFT may show evidence of predisposing conditions such as small bowel diverticula, strictures, or Crohn's.

Rx: If possible, the underlying predisposing condition should be treated. Usually, this is not possible. There are very limited data on antibiotic choice or duration of rx. Antibiotics are typically given in 7-10 courses. In pts with frequent relapses, antibiotic courses are given 1 wk a month using a rotating schedule. Norfloxacin (800 mg daily in divided doses) and amoxicillin-clavulanate (500/125 one tab po tid) have been shown effective in a small crossover randomized trial (GE 1999;117:794). On the basis of clinical experience rather than trials, other common choices include tetracycline 250 mg po qid, doxycycline 100 mg po bid, cephalexin 250 mg po qid, or ciprofloxacin 500 mg po bid. Metronidazole is sometimes used as a single agent but is more often combined with an agent active against aerobes.

6.22 Food Poisoning

Postgrad Med 1998;103:125; Feldman M, Scharschmidt B, Sleisenger M, eds. Sleisenger & Fordtran's gastrointestinal and liver disease. 6th ed. Philadelphia: WB Saunders, 1998:1624-1627.

Foodborne illness can be from infection or preformed toxins. Infectious causes have been discussed earlier. The most common causes of foodborne toxic illness are:

Staphylococcus aureus: Preformed enterotoxin from this organism is the most common cause of toxin-borne food poisoning. It causes an acute onset illness of nausea and vomiting with a short incubation (1-6 hr) and a duration of illness of 24 hr. Fever, cramps, and diarrhea are less prominent. The organism is transmitted from food handler to food (especially foods with high salt or sugar concentrations), where toxin is formed as the organism grows in the warm food.

Clostridium perfringens: This organism produces a toxin as it grows in bulk-cooked meat or poultry that is inadequately cooled. It causes an illness of watery diarrhea and crampy pain with an incubation of 8-24 hr and duration of 24-36 hr.

Bacillus cereus: This produces an illness of cramps, diarrhea, and vomiting. Incubation is 6-14 hr with a duration of 20-36 hr. Fever is not common. It is associated with foods kept warm for prolonged periods. A variant illness of primarily vomiting has been described.

Miscellaneous: Rarer toxic foodborne illnesses include mushroom poisoning, cholera, botulism, tetrodotoxin poisoning from pufferfish, ciguatera from fish, paralytic shellfish poisoning, and scromboid.

6.23 Whipple's Disease

Lancet 2003;361:239; Gastroenterol Clin North Am 1998;27:683

Cause: Rodlike bacilli were described in the first case reported by Whipple in 1907. The causative agent, *Tropheryma whippelii*, a gram-positive actinomycete, was first identified by ribosomal RNA sequencing and recently cultured (Nejm 2000;342:620).

Epidem: The disorder is very rare and typically found in white, middle-aged men.

Pathophys: Whipple's is a chronic, multisystem, relapsing illness. Person-to-person transmission has never been documented, and host factors are probably important. Decreased monocyte inter- leukin production may be important (Gastroenterol Clin North Am 1998;27:683). Almost any tissue can be infiltrated by the macrophages loaded with periodic acid-Schiff-positive (PAS- positive) material (degenerating bacilli) that characterize the disorder.

Sx: The presentations of the illness can be quite variable. Weight loss (often 20-30 pounds) and diarrhea due to malabsorption are the most common sx. A nondestructive arthritis is common and may precede other sx by years (Mayo Clin Proc 1988;63:539). Abdominal pain is often vague and has no specific features. Cough may be seen. CNS manifestations occur in 10-50% and may include headache, ataxia, weakness, seizures, and personality changes. Some pts present only with CNS disease (Scand J Infect Dis 1999;31:411). Up to 15% of pts never have GI sx (Medicine 1997;76:170). Ocular involvement may occur and present as iritis or visual loss.

Si: Peripheral lymphadenopathy, abdominal tenderness, hyperpigmen- tation, fever, wasting, and peripheral edema are common. Murmurs occur from endocarditis or pancarditis and friction rubs may be seen. FOBT-positive stool is common (Dig Dis Sci 1994; 39:1642).

Crs: Without rx the illness is slowly progressive, but with antibiotics prognosis is good. A symptomatic response is seen in days to weeks after antibiotics. Relapse is common (40%), months or years after successful rx (Gastroenterol Clin North Am 1998;27:683).

Diff Dx: The most difficult part of the diagnosis is considering such a rare illness when nonspecific sx are present. The combination of malabsorption, fever, adenopathy, and joint sx raise the suspicion. The dx is established by bx of involved tissue, usually small bowel bx at EGD. PCR of infected tissues may be useful in pts who lack small intestinal involvement (Nejm 1995;332:390).

Lab: Anemia (90%), malabsorption (elevated stool fat on 72-hr collection, abnormal d-xylose test), low serum carotene, hypoalbuminemia. PCR can be used to identify *T. whippelii* sequences in tissues when bx features are nondiagnostic.

X-ray: SBFT is usually abnormal with dilatation and mucosal thickening (Mayo Clin Proc 1988;63:539). CT may show adenopathy.

Endoscopy: EGD shows thickened, spaced-out folds with yellow or whitish plaques but may be grossly normal (Medicine 1997; 76:170). The typical bx shows dilated lymphatics, infiltration of the lamina propria with macrophages that stain strongly PAS-positive and contain gram-positive, AFB-negative bacilli. Since involvement can be patchy, multiple specimens should be obtained (Scand J Gastroenterol 1994;29:97).

Rx: A variety of antibiotics have been used successfully. Antibiotics that do not cross the blood–brain barrier (eg, tetracycline) should not be used (Mayo Clin Proc 1988;63:539). Tm/S is considered the first-line agent (Dig Dis Sci 1994;39:1642) and is given for a period of 12 months. Oral rx should be proceeded by a 2-wk course of ceftriaxone 2 gm iv qd (Lancet 2003;361:239). Antibiotic failures may occur (GE 1994;106:782). The value of repeat bx or PCR of cerebrospinal fluid to assess eradication has not been established.

Chapter 7

Anorectal Disorders

7.1 Hemorrhoids

GE 2004;126:1463; Prim Care 1999;26:35

Epidem: The prevalence of hemorrhoids is 80-90% in U.S. adults, with equal prevalence in men and women (Dis Colon Rectum 1983;26:435). Symptomatic hemorrhoids are unusual before age 20, peak at age 45-65, and are associated with higher socioeconomic status (GE 1990;98:380). Pregnancy is a risk factor.

Pathophys: Hemorrhoids are classified as internal or external based on the anatomic location from which they originate. Two areas are important to recognize. The anal verge is the most distal portion of the anal canal. About 2-3 cm above the verge is the dentate or pectinate line, the junction of anal and rectal mucosa. Hemorrhoids are pathologic dilatations of the normal vascular beds. Hemorrhoids are internal if they originate from the vascular bed above the dentate line, and they are external if they originate below the dentate line in the bed close to the anal verge. The point of origination, not the distal extent of the hemorrhoid, defines it as internal or external. Internal hemorrhoids are covered by rectal mucosa and have no somatic sensation, while external hemorrhoids are covered by anoderm and have the somatic sensation of skin. Internal hemorrhoids are graded based on the degree of prolapse (grade I=no prolapse, grade II=spontaneous reduction, grade III=manual reduction, grade IV=cannot be reduced). The pathogenesis of hemorrhoids is not well understood, though straining is thought to be of importance in disrupting the vascular beds. Both constipation and diarrhea are conditions associated with hemorrhoids (Dis Colon Rectum 1998;41:1534).

Sx: Internal hemorrhoids cause painless bleeding or prolapse. Blood is usually bright red and is seen on toilet tissue or around stool, or it may drip into the toilet if there is prolapse. Prolapsed hemorrhoids may result in a discharge on underwear. Painful thrombosis of internal hemorrhoids is uncommon. External hemorrhoids begin as small skin tags, cause problems with hygiene, cause perianal irritation, and can acutely thrombose, causing acute, severe pain.

Si: External hemorrhoids are visible and internal hemorrhoids are not unless prolapsed. Most internal hemorrhoids are not palpable and anoscopy is mandatory to establish their presence or absence.

Crs: Sx are usually mild and intermittent. Only a minority of pts require interventions beyond topical measures or develop complications such as thrombosis or permanent prolapse.

Cmplc: Thrombosis, presenting as acute pain.

Diff Dx: The presence of hemorrhoids is easily established and the diagnostic pitfall is usually in determining if hemorrhoids are the cause of a given sx. The differential includes other causes of rectal bleeding such as fissure, polyp, cancer, and IBD, and other causes of perianal discomfort such as abscess or fistula. A fissure should be suspected if there is pain and spasm on exam. Hemorrhoids should not be accepted as a cause of rectal bleeding without further evaluation (detailed on p 38).

Lab: Usually not indicated except in substantial, chronic bleeding.

Endoscopy: Anoscopy is easy to perform and very informative. Hemorrhoids are better assessed with an anoscope than a colonoscope, though the latter is more fun to use. At anoscopy, the dentate line is identified, the distal rectal mucosa is inspected, and hemorrhoids are identified as reddish-bluish protrusions into the lumen. Anoscopy also allows for the evaluation of fissures.

Rx: A high-fiber diet to keep stools soft is usually all that is needed for sx of painless bleeding from grade I or II hemorrhoids. Some pts experience local problems with itching or burning secondary to difficult hygiene or edema associated with the hemorrhoids. This often improves with local measures such as diaper wipes, witch hazel pads, and sitz baths. Hydrocortisone creams with or without an anesthetic are popular adjunctive rx without proven efficacy.

Rubber band ligation is effective for reducible hemorrhoids. The hemorrhoid is dragged into a hollow chamber and rubber bands deployed off the chamber around the base of the hemorrhoid. Bands are placed at least 5 mm above the dentate line to avoid pain. One hemorrhoid is done at a time, with a 2-4-wk wait between treatments. About 5-10% of pts experience achy pain, some bleeding, and rarely, pelvic sepsis is seen. Injection sclerotherapy, infrared coagulation, electrocoagulation, and laser treatment have all been used successfully. Cryotherapy should be avoided because of a high complication rate. Rubber band ligation is cheap and has the highest long-term efficacy, but it has a higher incidence of postoperative pain than infrared coagulation or injection sclerotherapy (Am J Gastro 1992;87:1600). Surgical hemorrhoidectomy is done for pts with prolapse (grades III and IV), pts with concomitant external hemorrhoids, and pts in which other methods fail. Thrombosed external hemorrhoids present with a visibly swollen, often painful mass that is filled with a firm clot. Pts presenting with acute sx should be treated with prompt evacuation of the clot for pain relief.

7.2 Anal Fissure

Brit J Surg 1996;83:1335

Epidem: A common complaint in young adults, affecting men and women equally.

Pathophys: (Scand J Gastroenterol Suppl 1996;218:78) An anal fissure is a crack in the skin of the anal canal. Acute fissures are quite superficial and are usually the result of traumatic laceration from hard, dry stool. A minority of acute fissures fail to heal and become deep, with indurated edges. Chronic fissures occur in the posterior midline in 90% of affected males and 75% of affected females. Most of the remainder occur in the anterior midline. One hypothesis is that elevated resting tone of the internal anal sphincter results in poor perfusion of the skin in the posterior midline and the failure of the fissure to heal.

Sx: The typical sx are pain with or after BMs, blood on tissue or around BMs, and itch.

Si: Acute fissures are superficial lacerations and often can be seen by parting the buttocks. Chronic fissures have heaped up edges, a fibrotic looking base, and frequently have a midline skin tag at the end of the fissure. A rectal or anoscopic exam can be difficult because of associated spasm.

Crs: Most fissures are acute and heal spontaneously. A minority become chronic (sx greater than 6-8 wk) and may have cycles of healing and recurrence.

Diff Dx: Fissures can be secondary to Crohn's, syphilis, TB, HIV, leukemia, IBD, or anal cancer. Consider these diagnoses, especially if the fissure is not midline.

Endoscopy: Anal fissures are better seen with an anoscope than a colonoscope. Topical lidocaine can be helpful, but sometimes pain and spasm are too great to proceed without general anesthesia.

Rx: Most **acute fissures** are treated by making the stool softer (high-fiber diet and fiber supplements or stool softeners such as sodium ducosate 100 mg po tid) and with topical hydrocortisone preparations with an anesthetic. Witch hazel pads, diaper wipes, or sitz baths may be soothing. **Chronic fissures** are treated by methods that lower anal sphincter pressure and presumably restore blood flow to the skin of the posterior midline. Forceful anal dilatation is effective but associated with high rates of fecal incontinence. Lateral internal sphincterotomy is the most common current surgical approach. In this procedure, the internal anal sphincter is cut in a lateral position (rather than in the posterior midline). The major problem with lateral internal sphincterotomy is incontinence, with rates as high as 35% reported (Am J Surg 1996;171: 512). Modifications such as a sphincterotomy tailored to the length of the fissure may reduce that rate (Dis Colon Rectum 1997; 40:1439). Topical nitrates dilate the anal sphincter and result in healing of fissures in 40-80% of pts (reviewed in GE 2003;124: 235). Glyceryl trinitrate 0.2% is applied twice daily to the anal canal for 6 wk and is usually well tolerated though headache is a common problem. This is a much lower concentration of nitroglycerin than is used in cardiac disease, and this concentration is not commercially available in the U.S., but can be made by a good pharmacy. Botulinum toxin injected into the sphincter is more effective than placebo (Nejm 1998;338:217) but is expensive compared with nitrates. Calcium channel blockers show promise. Since medical rx is not associated with incontinence, a trial of nitrates or botulinum makes sense as first-line treatment, followed by lateral sphincterotomy if medical rx fails (Am J Gastro 2003;98:968).

7.3 Anorectal Fistula and Abscess

Anal glands are located at the dentate line in the anal canal. If these glands become obstructed and infected acutely, the pt develops an anorectal abscess. If the infection establishes a path to the perianal skin, a chronic anal fistula is created. The diagnosis is usually not difficult, and the rx is surgical (except for fistulas related to Crohn's disease). The surgical approach is dictated by the location of the abscess or fistula (Surg Clin N Am 2002;82:1139).

7.4   Fecal Incontinence

Mayo Clin Proc 2002;77:271; Dig Dis Sci 1999;44:2488

Epidem: The prevalence of incontinence of solid stool is between 0.5 and 1.5%. It is 8 times more common in women than men, and is more common in nursing home pts. Prevalence rises markedly to 17% after age 85 (Dig Dis Sci 1999;44:2488).

Pathophys: Continence is maintained by the anal sphincter (a combination of the internal and external sphincters and the puborectalis muscle) and by the 90 degree anorectal angle. The 2 major ways in which this can be disrupted are direct damage to the sphincter and pelvic floor denervation. Specific causes of incontinence include obstetrical injury to the sphincter or its innervation (the most common cause), denervation from straining at stool, pudendal nerve injury, prior anorectal surgery, fecal impaction, cancer, rectal prolapse, other sphincter trauma, and neurologic diseases. Inadequate rectal capacity or sensation can also result in incontinence.

Sx: Pts often do not volunteer a clear hx of their incontinence. High degrees of incontinence (loss of solid stool) are usually clear by hx, but more subtle incontinence (to flatus or liquid stool) may cause a complaint of too much gas, urgency, or diarrhea. Pts will know the location of every public toilet in town and be fearful of going out. The severity can be quantified by asking about use of pads and staining of underwear.

Si: The perianal skin may show soiling or irritation. The sphincter may be visibly gaping in severe cases. Voluntary and resting tone are evaluated by the examining finger. Withdrawal of the finger should elicit a closing reflex. Perianal skin sensation should be evaluated for clues to neurologic disease. A distal rectal mass can be excluded by palpation.

Crs: The course is most often one of slowly worsening degrees of incontinence.

Diff Dx: Fistulas, rectal prolapse, proctitis, and mass lesions are the major differential points.

Lab: A variety of specialized tests can be used to evaluate fecal incontinence. These include anal manometry, endosonography, electromyography (EMG), and others. These specialized tests are not readily available to most practitioners, nor are they needed to manage most pts with this common problem. However, these tests may be needed to determine the best approach for pts who do not improve with medical rx.

Endoscopy: Flexible sigmoidoscopy is indicated to exclude structural lesions and provides the opportunity to screen the distal bowel.

Rx: Most pts respond to the combination of increased fiber to add bulk to stools and the use of antidiarrheal agents. This creates bulky dry stool that is unlikely to leak out. Loperamide is well tolerated and doses of 1-2 mg daily (not prn) are usually needed. Pts are taught that any cause of loose stool (eg, acute diarrheal illnesses, lactose intolerance, excessive sorbitol, caffeine) will aggravate the incontinence. Biofeedback has its proponents and works best in highly motivated pts. Surgical repair works well (80% success) if there is a defined defect in the external anal sphincter, but most cases lack a defined defect and are due to pelvic denervation. A variety of surgical approaches are available for these refractory pts with limited success (Surg Clin N Am 2002;82:1139).

7.5   Pruritus Ani

Surg Clin N Am 1994;74:1277

Epidem: M:F ratio 4:1 for those without demonstrable cause of perianal itching.

Pathophys: The most common mechanism for perianal itch is failure to cleanse feces from the perianal area. In some pts, dietary factors, skin disease, or psychogenic factors may perpetuate itch. In some pts, chronic use of irritating substances (such as inadequately rinsed soap) may cause a dermatitis. In many self-limited cases a cause is not identifiable.

Sx: The irresistible urge to scratch.

Si: Perianal skin may show fecal soilage, deformity, erythema, cracking of thickened skin folds, and evidence of excoriation.

Crs: Episodes are usually self-limited unless a chronic predisposing condition exists.

Cmplc: None.

Diff Dx: Many cases of perianal itching have a definable, treatable cause related to perianal hygiene. The inability to keep the perianal skin clear of feces is seen in pts with poor sphincter tone, chronic diarrhea, external hemorrhoids or skin tags, prior anal surgery, prior fistulas, or perianal abscess that heals with deformity, morbid obesity, and poor personal hygiene habits. Other pts may have underlying dermatologic, dietary, drug, gynecologic, or psychogenic causes of itch. Pinworms should be considered in children.

Lab: Scotch tape test for pinworms. Skin bx or scrapings in unusual cases to look for other primary diseases such psoriasis, fungal infection, or malignancy.

Rx: In pts with evidence of fecal soilage, the underlying cause should be treated if possible. Pts should be advised to cleanse the area with diaper wipes, witch hazel pads, or warm water, but should avoid soap. Excessive rubbing while cleansing should be avoided. Topical hydrocortisone preparations may provide relief. In most idiopathic cases, sx resolve in 4-6 wk. Purported dietary causes include caffeine, chocolate, citrus and tomato products, and dietary exclusions may be tried.

7.6   Fecal Impaction

Mayo Clin Proc 1998;73:881

Epidem: The greatest risk is seen in constipated pts and in pts who are institutionalized with mental or physical impairments.

Pathophys: The initiating event is retention of a bolus of stool due to a variety of underlying causes such as painful conditions of the anus, decreased recognition of the need to evacuate (due to drugs or CNS illness), or lack of rectal sensation. The initiating bolus dries out in the rectum, and the colon delivers more until a bolus that will not pass the diameter of the anal sphincter is created.

Sx: Those with intact mentation will usually recognize the lack of bowel movements and have rectal pain. However, the presentation can be nonspecific in pts who are mentally or physically impaired, with sx such as change in performance status, nausea, bloating, or fever. Some pts will present with apparent diarrhea as stool oozes out around the bolus.

Si: Usually a hard bolus of stool may be felt but sometimes it is softer than expected or the impaction is beyond the reach of the finger. The abdomen may be distended or tender, and stool may be palpable.

Crs: May be recurrent without adequate chronic bowel regimen.

Cmplc: Stercoral ulcers (ulcers caused by local pressure necrosis of bowel by hard, dry stool). Colonic perforation is a rare complication due to full thickness pressure necrosis.

Diff Dx: The important differential consideration is mechanical obstruction due to tumor.

Lab: Leukocytosis or electrolyte abnormalities may be present in severe cases.

X-ray: Plain films demonstrate stool in the colon and rectum and air fluid levels in more severe cases. An x-ray is not a substitute for a rectal exam.

Endoscopy: A mechanical cause of impaction should be ruled out with colonoscopy if the cause is uncertain and if the pt is in an age group where CRC is a concern.

Rx: Manual disimpaction is the first step. A topical anesthetic such as lidocaine jelly may be helpful, and conscious sedation may be a kindness in some circumstances. The anal canal is gently dilated with two fingers and the bolus is broken up by the fingers. The examiner should be well garbed for the onslaught of stool. If this is not successful or if the bolus cannot be reached, a tap water or a mineral oil enema is used. If these fail, a milk and molasses enema can be tried. A gastrograffin enema can be diagnostic and is usually therapeutic when other measures fail. When there is no evidence of obstruction, oral polyethylene solutions may be given orally or per NG tube at a rate of 100 mL/hr until clear (Dig Dis Sci 1997;42:1454).

7.7   Solitary Rectal Ulcer Syndrome

Brit J Surg 1998;85:1617

Epidem: This disorder is uncommon (1 per 100,000/yr), with onset typical in the 3rd or 4th decade. There is equal prevalence in men and women.

Pathophys: The cause is unknown. It is possible that there are different causes in different groups. Rectal prolapse (either overt or occult) and paradoxical contraction of pelvic floor muscles seem important and may cause ulceration by inducing local ischemia.

Sx: Rectal bleeding, passage of mucus, sense of incomplete evacuation, and straining at stool. Rectal prolapse is common. Some pts are asymptomatic.

Si: The ulcer may be palpable and prolapse may be identified on exam.

Crs: In about half of pts, ulcers persist over 5 yr despite rx (GE 1983;84:1533).

Cmplc: Massive bleeding or stricture formation are rare complications.

Diff Dx: The major differential considerations are malignancy, IBD, and repeated trauma. The disorder is misdiagnosed 25% of the time. The incorrect diagnoses are usually IBD or neoplasia (Dis Colon Rectum 1993;36:146).

Lab: Anorectal manometry shows a variety of abnormalities, but none help with the dx or rx.

Endoscopy: Most of these lesions are found 5-10 cm from the anal verge on the anterior rectal wall. They are usually ulcers of several cm in diameter, but the appearance is variable and multiple ulcers or raised, polypoid, or circumferential lesions may be seen. Bxs show mucosal edema, variable fibrosis, and disorientation of the smooth muscle of the muscularis that extends up into the lamina propria. EUS may show lack of puborectalis relaxation.

Rx: Topical rx are usually ineffective since they do not address the underlying defect. Fiber to minimize straining can be tried. Some pts appear to have a major behavioral component with excessive straining, and biofeedback has been used with some success (Gut 1997;41:817). Surgery is an option for the very refractory pt. Rectopexy is the most common surgery, and about 50% of pts will improve. Anterior resection is disappointing (Brit J Surg 1998; 85:1246). Colostomy is a drastic alternative.

7.8 Intussusception

Ann Surg 1997;226:134; Gastroenterol Clin North Am 1994;23:21

In this process, a leading edge of bowel invaginates in the lumen of the bowel distal to it. The lesion is uncommon in adults, and most cases are associated with neoplasia at the leading edge. Most cases of intussusception in children are not associated with an anatomic abnormality. The disorder usually presents as obstruction or bleeding and is often diagnosed as a target lesion on CT or ultrasound. The rx in adults is surgical.

7.9 Proctalgia Fugax

This is a very common disorder characterized by intermittent, unpredictable attacks of a severe, spasmodic pain in the rectum that last seconds to minutes. Between attacks, pts feel entirely well and have normal bowel movements. The cause is unknown but is probably related to internal anal sphincter dysfunction. A hereditary form has been described (GE 1991;100:805). The dx is made on the basis of the characteristic story and by the exclusion of rectal pathology by sigmoidoscopy if there is any clinical doubt. Most attacks are so brief that no rx is needed. Manual pressure applied with a flat hand to the anal area may be helpful. Hot baths and passage of flatus in a knee-chest position have been used. The hereditary form responds to nifedipine but may be a different disorder (Gut 1995;36:581). The inhaled β-agonist salbutamol shortens attacks (Am J Gastro 1996; 91:686).

7.10 Cancer of the Anal Canal

This disorder represents about 1.5% of all gi tract neoplasms. It is associated with sexual transmission of the human papilloma virus. The majority of pts do not need surgery and can be cured by combination chemotherapy and radiation. See Nejm 2000;342:792 for a comprehensive review.

7.11 Hirschsprung's Disease

This disorder results from the congenital absence of ganglion cells in the anus and a variable length of distal bowel (Curr Probl Surg 1996;33:389). This results in a functional obstruction that usually presents in the first year of life as severe constipation or sepsis due to enterocolitis. A presentation in adulthood is rare, and sx in adults usually have been present since childhood (J Clin Gastro 1984; 6:205). The rx is the surgical removal of the poorly functioning aganglionic segment.

Chapter 8

Vascular Disorders of the Gut

8.1   Acute Mesenteric Ischemia

BMJ 2003;326:1372; GE 2000;118:954

Cause: This catastrophic illness most commonly results from emboli, but it can also result from arterial or venous thrombi, low-flow states, or vasculitis.

Pathophys: Sudden occlusion of a mesenteric vessel causes ischemia that progresses to infarction, usually within 24 hours. About 50% of pts have arterial occlusion, 15% have venous occlusion, and the remainder have nonocclusive disease. This latter group often develops illness after systemic hypotension, CHF, or septic shock.

Sx: Pts develop severe abdominal pain that is often out of proportion to physical exam findings. There may be associated risk factors such as recent MI, CHF, hypercoagulable states, or evidence of preexisting chronic ischemia (postprandial pain). However, many pts have no associated risk factors.

Si: Early in the course of illness the abdominal exam may be relatively benign, but as ischemia worsens, tenderness increases, bowel sounds are lost, and peritoneal findings develop.

Diff Dx: Acute abdominal pain (p 6).

Crs: Mortality rate is high and varies with etiology. Operative mortality is greatest for arterial thrombosis (77%) and nonocclusive ischemia (73%). It is lower for arterial embolism (54%) and venous thrombosis (32%) (Brit J Surg 2004;91:17).

Lab: No single serum test is helpful in making the diagnosis. CBC with differential, CMP (to look for other causes and evaluate the anion gap as a clue to metabolic acidosis), and amylase should be obtained to help in differential diagnosis.

X-ray: Plain films are used to exclude free air requiring immediate laparotomy. Doppler ultrasonography can evaluate the proximal portions of the celiac, superior mesenteric artery (SMA), and inferior mesenteric artery (IMA), but occlusions can be asymptomatic, making the test less valuable in the acute setting. CT can show abnormalities late in the course of illness caused by SMA emboli (such as gas in bowel wall, thickened bowel, or portal venous gas), but it is insensitive prior to infarction. CT is more helpful in identifying mesenteric vein occlusions. Mesenteric angiography is the diagnostic gold standard, but experts disagree on its routine use in suspected mesenteric ischemia. Proponents of angiography in suspected AMI cite the many negative results that save a laparotomy and the positives that allow for early diagnosis. Opponents cite delays in diagnosis from lack of ready availability and the time it takes to perform the test. Local expertise will play a big role. Angiography can show embolus (either partially or completely occluding) either in the major vessels or in distal branches. It may also show evidence of nonocclusive mesenteric ischemia (NOMI), in which no occlusion is seen but there is intense microvascular vasoconstriction (Am J Surg 1996;171:405).

Endoscopy: Not indicated.

Rx: Those with suspected mesenteric ischemia and no availability of angiography go to laparotomy as do those with peritoneal signs. Rx of pts with positive angiograms depends on the finding. Major emboli are treated with embolectomy and thrombus is treated with bypass (Arch Surg 1999;134:328). Infarcted segments are

resected and a second look operation may be needed to reassess
viability of the remaining bowel (Arch IM 2004;164:1054).
Minor emboli (in smaller distal vessels) can be treated with
thrombolytics, papaverine, or anticoagulation. Superior mesenteric vein thrombus without peritoneal signs can be treated with
anticoagulation. Such pts should be evaluated for a hypercoagulable state. Nonocclusive mesenteric ischemia can be treated
with intra-arterial papaverine.

8.2   Chronic Mesenteric Ischemia

BMJ 2003;326:1372; GE 2000;118:954

Cause: Vascular thrombosis from atherosclerotic disease.

Pathophys: Most pts (90%) have severe stenosis or occlusion of 2 or
3 of their mesenteric vessels. They are unable to increase gut
blood flow in response to food. A small minority have occlusions
of SMA (7%) or celiac (2%) alone.

Sx: Pts develop pain 1-3 hr after meals that persists 1-3 hr, and sx
occur with increasing frequency over weeks to months. The pain,
aka abdominal angina, creates a fear of eating and subsequent
weight loss.

Si: Cachexia and abdominal bruits may be present.

Diff Dx: The differential is that of dyspepsia (p 4). The key to making
the diagnosis is to consider it on the list of possibilities.

Crs: The 5-yr survival of those who survive revascularization is 70%.

Cmplc: Progression to infarction, malnutrition.

X-ray: Angiography is the gold standard for diagnosis. MRI angiography rivals conventional angiography in centers with special
expertise. Other tests are available (eg, mesenteric Dopplers after
meal stimulation [Am J Surg 1995;169:476] or intestinal oxygen
consumption), but they lack sensitivity and specificity (GE

2000;118:954). Asymptomatic pts over 65 yr will frequently (18%) have abnormal Doppler studies (AJR Am J Roentgenol 1993;161:985). Some clinicians use Doppler in pts with lower pretest probability as a means of avoiding a very low yield angiography.

Rx: Surgical revascularization (by endarterectomy or bypass [Ann Vasc Surg 1998;12:299]) provides about 70-90% initial success, 10% recurrence rates, and low mortality. Mesenteric angioplasty has similar initial success rates but higher recurrence rates, leading an expert panel to recommend it only in higher risk surgical pts (GE 2000;118:954). Angioplasty can be used to restore graft patency (Cardiovasc Intervent Radiol 1987;10:43).

8.3 Ischemic Colitis

BMJ 2003;326:1372; GE 2000;118:954

Cause: This illness is caused by inadequate colonic perfusion despite grossly normal mesenteric vessels. It has been associated with prior aortic or cardiac surgery; vasculitis; hypercoagulable states (GE 2001;121:561), drugs (cocaine [Am J Gastro 1994;89:1558], NSAIDs [J Clin Gastro 1993;16:31], pseudoephedrine [Am J Gastro 1999;94:2430], bcp's [J Clin Gastro 1994;19:108]), prolonged exercise (distance running), obstructing colonic lesions, and cardiopulmonary events that cause hypotension.

Epidem: More common in the elderly.

Pathophys: The most common form of the illness is transient submucosal and mucosal hemorrhage with inflammation. More rarely there can be features of chronic colitis, stricture, or progression to full-thickness gangrene. No vascular occlusion of major vessels is evident, but pts are more likely to have underlying atherosclerosis.

Sx: Pts typically experience the sudden onset of fairly severe crampy abdominal pain and bloody diarrhea. A chronic presentation with pain, bloody diarrhea, or colonic stricture is quite unusual.

Si: Tenderness and localized peritonitis may be found.

Diff Dx: The major considerations are causes of acute bloody diarrhea: infections (*E. coli* O157:H7, *Campylobacter, Shigella,* and *Salmonella*) and IBD. In some cases, diverticulitis, acute mesenteric ischemia, or obstruction are considerations.

Crs: Most pts recover completely without surgery. Academic surgical series overestimate the severity of the illness (eg, Dis Colon Rectum 1992;35:726).

Cmplc: Colonic stricture, gangrene.

Lab: CBC with diff, CMP, and amylase are usually obtained to rule out other disorders. Stool culture, stool testing for *C. difficile*, or other stool studies might be warranted.

X-ray: Plain films are useful to rule out free air and to detect thumbprinting of the colon from mucosal edema or obstruction. A CT scan often shows evidence of colitis (Radiology 1999;211:381) and is more sensitive for perforation than KUB. CT is helpful in ruling out other causes of abdominal pain. Angiography is not indicated unless the concern is acute mesenteric ischemia (in which case pts tend to have much more steady midabdominal pain rather than crampy pain with bloody diarrhea).

Endoscopy: Colonoscopy is done to establish the dx and exclude cancer and IBD. The findings are those of a segmental colitis with friability, hemorrhage, and exudate. There can be evidence of fibrosis depending on the duration of the illness. Colonoscopy is usually done after the patient has clinically improved because of the fear of perforation. Bxs are usually nonspecific but may show suggestive coagulation necrosis. The rectum is usually spared but the splenic flexure is often involved (because it is in the watershed between peripheral branches of the SMA and IMA).

Rx: Pts are kept npo, given iv fluids, and are evaluated and treated for associated cardiopulmonary conditions. Broad-spectrum antibiotics (eg, cefotetan, ampicillin-sulbactam) are given routinely on the basis of experimental studies showing benefit, but data in humans are lacking. If pts improve, diet is advanced and antibiotics are stopped. A small number of pts will deteriorate because of the development of full-thickness gangrene or will have a refractory colitis, and they are treated surgically. Stricture may require segmental resection but may improve over time without rx.

8.4 Angiodysplasias of the GI Tract

Gastrointest Endosc Clin N Am 1997;7:509; Am J Gastro 1993; 88:807

Cause: The underlying cause of angiodysplasia is unknown.

Epidem: More common in the elderly.

Pathophys: These lesions represent ectasia of submucosal veins and overlying capillaries and may occur throughout the gi tract. They are most common in the colon. They generally do not present with massive bleeding because they are low-pressure (venous) lesions. Similar lesions can be seen in hereditary hemorrhagic telangiectasia (Osler-Rendu-Weber) disease (Dig Dis 1998;16:169), Turner's syndrome, or with the CREST syndrome. Pts with von Willebrand's disease may be very difficult to treat because of a predisposition to bleeding with minor lesions (Br J Haematol 2000;108:524). In these conditions, multiple lesions are a clinical challenge. There is an association with aortic stenosis, and valve replacement may stop bleeding. In pts without these associated disorders, lesions are most often found in the cecum and ascending colon. Left-sided lesions of clinical importance are less common. Angiodysplasias may also be seen in the small intestine or stomach.

Sx: Most pts are asymptomatic. Some may present with sx secondary to chronic anemia or with acute hematochezia.

Si: Heme-positive stool. Mucocutaneous angiodysplasia are seen in hereditary hemorrhagic telangiectasia.

Diff Dx: These lesions are considered in the differential of acute or chronic gi bleeding (p 33).

Crs: A small subgroup of pts present with recurrent gross bleeding.

Cmplc: Anemia, massive hemorrhage. Perforation from endoscopic rx.

Lab: CBC is routine. Studies of coagulation may be warranted in problematic pts to look for coagulopathies.

X-ray: Substantial lesions can be seen as a late draining vein on angiography. Angiography is used much less frequently than endoscopy for dx. Angiography has a sensitivity of only 17% compared to endoscopy (Mayo Clin Proc 1988;63:993).

Endoscopy: Lesions are red, flat, or minimally raised; may have round or stellate borders; and small vessels can often be discerned. Endoscopy is the diagnostic method of choice.

Rx: A variety of endoscopic methods have been described. Bipolar electrocautery, argon plasma coagulation, and heater probe are most widely used. Pts with recurrent bleeding may be treated with estrogens (Am J Gastro 1988;83:556), but the best RCT shows no benefit of a yr of estrogen/progesterone rx (GE 2001; 121:1073).

8.5   Abdominal Aortic Aneurysm

The gastroenterologist encounters this disorder when it presents with acute abdominal pain due to dissection or as an incidental finding on physical exam or imaging studies. Elective repair is usually appropriate for healthy pts with abdominal aortic aneurysms (AAAs) in the 5-6 cm range. Pts with smaller aneurysms can be followed with periodic ultrasound, and 60% will eventually end up with elective repair (Mayo Clin Proc 2000;75:395).

Chapter 9

Pancreas

9.1 Acute Pancreatitis

Lancet 2003;361:1447; Nejm 1999;340:1412

Cause: Many causes of acute pancreatitis (AP) have been identified (Nejm 1994;330:1198; Gastroenterol Clin North Am 1999;28:571). In most regions of the world, **gallstones** are the leading cause of AP, and **alcohol** is a close second. **Idiopathic pancreatitis** (10-25% of the total) places third on the list, though many of these cases represent a failure to diagnose gallstone disease and microlithiasis (Nejm 1992;326:589). **Hypertriglyceridemia** is a relatively common cause of AP and is seen when TG levels are >1000 mg/dL. Pancreatitis occurs more often in type V hyperlipidemia and less often in types I and IV (Gastroenterol Clin North Am 1990;19:783). A bewildering number of **drugs** have been implicated in AP (Aliment Pharmacol Ther 1996;10:23; Am J Gastro 1999;94:2417). These include azathioprine/6-mercaptopurine, L-asparaginase, 5-aminosalicylic acid compounds (mesalamine, olsalazine, sulfasalazine), didanosine (an antiretroviral), valproic acid, furosemide, cimetidine, famotidine, thiazides, lisinopril, codeine (Am J Gastro 2000;95:3295), antibiotics (tetracycline, metronidazole, nitrofurantoin, erythromycin, sulfonamides, pentamadine), and NSAIDs (ibuprofen, sulindac, celecoxib) (Arch IM 2000;160:553).

Diagnostic **ERCP** is associated with a 3-9% risk of AP and rates may be higher with sphincterotomy or sphincter of Oddi manometry. **Blunt trauma** to the abdomen can cause AP by disrupting the duct. **Infections** are always listed as a cause of AP, but in adult practice they are uncommon. Mumps, coxsackievirus, CMV, *Campylobacter*, hepatitis A, and hepatitis B have all been implicated. HIV-infected pts have a high incidence of pancreatitis associated with a variety of infections and drugs. The association of **hyperparathyroidism** with AP has received more attention than it deserves and is very infrequent (0.23% of 800 consecutive pts with hyperparathyroidism in one series) (Brit J Surg 1986;73:282). Occurrence of AP following **cardiac surgery** is thought to be related to ischemia. **Emboli** and **vasculitis** are rare causes. Scorpion venom (BMJ 1970;1:666), bites of certain spiders and the Gila monster lizard, organophosphorous insecticides, and methanol are rare **toxic** causes of AP. A rare familial form **(hereditary pancreatitis)** is associated with recurrent bouts of AP leading to chronic pancreatitis and caused by mutations in the cationic trypsinogen gene (Gut 1999;45:317). Autoimmune pancreatitis can have an acute presentation. See p 322.

Other **obstructive disorders,** such as pancreatic cancer or ampullary cancer, may obstruct the duct and cause AP. In **pancreas divisum,** the dorsal and ventral ducts of the pancreas do not fuse, and the larger dorsal duct (Santorini duct) drains through the minor papilla. If the minor duct is relatively stenotic, AP may result. Sphincter of Oddi stenosis or dysfunction (p 352) may also result in AP. Choledochal cysts (p 354) and mucinous duct ectasia (p 331), an anomalous union of the pancreaticobiliary duct (Gastro Endosc 1999;50:189) are infrequent causes.

Penetrating peptic ulcer rarely presents as AP. Crohn's disease, cystic fibrosis, and hypothermia usually present with other sx. Postpartum pancreatitis appears to be largely biliary in nature (Mayo Clin Proc 2000;75:361).

Epidem: The disorder is common with an incidence of 24/100,000 per yr in the U.K. (Brit J Surg 1987;74:398). The incidence has risen over the last 40 yr for unclear reasons. The disorder is more common in men than in women.

Pathophys: (Surg Clin N Am 1999;79:699) The means by which the numerous causes of pancreatitis result in a similar clinical illness has not been determined. Biliopancreatic reflux appears to be the important initiating event in gallstone pancreatitis (Gut 1995; 36:803). There appear to be genetic predispositions to pancreatitis caused by mutations in genes that normally function to limit the destruction of the pancreas caused by activation of trypsin from trypsinogen. The shared characteristic of the many causes of AP is premature activation of proteolytic enzymes (such as trypsin from trypsinogen) and their inappropriate retention in the acinar cell. Subsequent injury to the acinar cell causes release of cytokines and activation of the complement system. Inflammatory cells are recruited into the pancreas and result in further release of inflammatory mediators (such as platelet activating factor (PAF), TNF, IL-1, and IL-6). These cause local tissue edema, cell necrosis, and the distant, systemic effects of hypotension, fever, hypoxia, leaky capillaries, and ARDS. Improved understanding of the cascade may allow for therapeutic interventions (see Rx).

Pancreatitis is classified as interstitial, edematous pancreatitis if the pancreatic tissue remains viable. It is classified as necrotizing pancreatitis (which is more severe) if pancreatic tissue becomes nonviable.

Sx: The most common sx is upper abdominal pain, which is usually epigastric and radiates to the back. Pain is generally constant and can be severe. Nausea and vomiting are common.

Si: Fever is common and does not necessarily imply infection. Hypotension and tachycardia may be associated with volume depletion. Abdominal tenderness is greatest in the epigastrium but can be present in any area of the abdomen where the inflammatory process tracks. In more severe cases, there is distention, rigidity, percussion tenderness, or loss of bowel sounds. An upper abdominal mass may be felt if the pt develops a phlegmon or pseudocyst. Bluish discoloration of the flanks (Grey Turner sign) and of the periumbilical area (Cullen sign) is rarely seen and is due to hemorrhage in severe, necrotizing disease. The lung fields can show evidence of effusions or atelectasis. The skin may show eruptive xanthomata (reddish-yellow papules of a few mm, especially on extensor surfaces) if the cause is hyperlipidemia. Tender red skin nodules from fat necrosis are rarely seen.

Crs:

- *Causes of mortality:* The course of the illness is determined by the extent of pancreatic glandular necrosis, by the degree of surrounding tissue destruction by pancreatic juice, by the systemic effects of mediators released in the inflammatory response, and by the development of infection in areas of necrosis. Early death results from multisystem failure (the first week) and late deaths are generally due to infection. About 80% of deaths are due to septic complications. In necrotizing pancreatitis (cases with sections of nonviable pancreatic tissue) 30-40% of pts develop infection in the necrosis (World J Surg 1997;21:130). Obesity is a risk for a poor outcome (Brit J Surg 1993;80:484).
- *Clinical prediction of severity:* Several methods have been described for assessing disease severity (Surg Clin N Am 1999;79:733). Three methods of assessing severity using simple clinical and laboratory tests have been described for pancreatitis. The first method is the **Ranson** criteria. In this system, poor prognostic factors are identified by assessment on admission and at 48 hr. For **alcoholic pancreatitis** these factors are: *On admission:* (1) age >55, (2) wbc >16,000/mm^3, (3) glucose >200 mg/dL, (4) LDH >350 U/L, and (5) AST >250 U/L.

Within 48 hr of admission: (1) Drop in hct >10%,
(2) increase in BUN >5 mg/dL, (3) Ca^{++} <8 mg/dL,
(4) Base deficit >4 mmol/L, (5) fluid deficit >6 L, and
(6) pO_2 <60 mm Hg.

- If fewer than 3 risk factors are present, mortality is <1%. If 3-4 factors are present, mortality is 15% and climbs with each additional risk factor. The less cumbersome **Glasgow** criteria for **gallstone pancreatitis** are applied within the first 48 hr after hospitalization. In this system, poor prognostic factors are (1) age >55, (2) wbc >15,000/mm³, (3) glucose >180 mg/dL, (4) BUN >45 mg/dL, (5) LDH >600 U/L, (6) albumin <3.3, (7) Ca^{++} <8, and (8) pO_2 <60 mm Hg. The presence of 3 or more factors indicates increased risk. The major problem with these systems is the lack of accuracy and the need to wait 48 hr to complete staging. With the Glasgow system, 30% of pts with severe pancreatitis are missed, and 40% with 3 or more criteria have a benign course (Surg Clin N Am 1999; 79:733). The third system, the **APACHE-II** score, is more complex but may be superior to other grading systems because it can be measured daily and therefore may be more accurate (Am J Gastro 1997;92:377).

- *CT prediction of severity:* CT scan can assess severity. The prognosis is excellent when CT is normal or shows pancreatic enlargement due to edema or mild peripancreatic inflammatory changes. When fluid collections are seen, the risk of infection rises to 30-50%, and mortality is 15%. CT is also used to determine if the pancreas has become necrotic. Necrotic areas do not enhance with iv contrast. In necrotizing pancreatitis, prognosis is worse, especially if the necrosis becomes infected. The degree of inflammation and necrosis can be graded on a 10-point system that correlates with outcome (Radiology 1994; 193:297). CT contrast worsened pancreatitis in an animal model, but the clinical relevance of this observation is unclear (GE 1994;106:207).

Cmplc:

- *Systemic complications:* Pulmonary complications include hypoxia, atelectasis, and pleural effusion. In more severe cases, pneumonia or ARDS develops. Renal failure and cardiovascular collapse can result from volume depletion due to bleeding or loss of fluid into the retroperitoneum. Hypocalcemia is common and is due to precipitation of calcium with fats in the process of peripancreatic fat necrosis. Hyperglycemia results from decreased insulin levels. Coagulopathy, subcutaneous nodules from metastatic fat necrosis, retinopathy, and psychosis are uncommon.

- *Pseudocyst:* A pseudocyst is a fluid-filled cavity lined by a rind of inflammatory tissue rather than the epithelium of a true cyst. Mature pseudocysts have well-developed, thick walls and form 4-6 wk after acute illness. These are to be distinguished from the thin-walled peripancreatic fluid collections seen early in the illness.

- *Infected pancreatic necrosis:* When inflamed pancreatic cells become necrotic, they are initially sterile. However, they have the potential to become infected with enteric pathogens. Infected pancreatic necrosis can be identified by CT-guided needle bx and is usually seen after the first wk (GE 1987; 93:1315).

- *Pancreatic abscess:* A pancreatic abscess is a pancreatic fluid collection that becomes infected. It is seen in about 1-4% of cases. It requires drainage but is much less dangerous than infected necrosis.

- *Unusual complications:* Pancreatic fistulas into colon, adjacent bowel necrosis, gastric varices from splenic vein thrombosis, splenic hematoma, and acute hemorrhage into pseudocysts or retroperitoneum may be seen.

Diff Dx: See "Approach to Acute Abdominal Pain" (p 6). The diagnosis of acute pancreatitis is made on the basis of the history, physical exam, and laboratory studies and is selectively confirmed by imaging studies such as CT. In mild cases presenting late in the illness, the laboratory studies may be less helpful and the imaging is more important.

The cause of pancreatitis is usually evident from the initial H&P, labs and the transabdominal ultrasound. However, in 10-25% of cases the cause is not immediately evident. About 50% of these idiopathic cases never recur but many do and require a more extensive evaluation. There is a range of expert opinions regarding the evaluation of so-called **recurrent acute pancreatitis** (compare GE 2001;120:708 to J Clin Gastro 2003;37:238). The evaluation usually begins with CT scan to look for tumor or chronic pancreatitis. If this is negative, many experts proceed to ERCP to look for chronic pancreatitis, tumors, pancreas divisum (which is then treated by dorsal duct sphincterotomy), annular pancreas, choledochocele, and anomalous union of the pancreaticobiliary duct. Some experts evaluate the sphincter of Oddi by manometry but others do not because of risk. At the ERCP bile is aspirated and examined by microscopy for cholesterol monohydrate crystals or bilirubinate granules. If these studies are negative, tests for gene defects (see "Pathophys") or testing for autoimmune pancreatitis are undertaken (with IgG4 levels). Other experts use the combination of MRCP and EUS as the initial tests and reserve ERCP for therapy because it is risky. Many experts skip biliary microscopy and recommend biliary sphincterotomy and/or cholecystectomy if ERCP/MRCP and/or EUS is negative. The approach will vary with the local expertise in the various available modalities.

Lab: **Amylase** is a sensitive predictor of AP, but false-positive elevations may be seen due to pancreatic cancer, mesenteric infarction, bowel obstruction, perforated ulcer, and renal failure. Salivary amylase causes false positives that can be easily identified by amylase fractionation. Macroamylasemia causes a high serum amylase in the absence of pancreatitis and can be detected by fractionation. **Lipase** is more specific than amylase but can be elevated in perforated ulcer, ischemia, or obstruction (though typically such elevations are less than 3 times normal). Lipase is cleared more slowly and can be helpful if pts present days after the event. All pts should have at least a daily **CBC** and **CMP** early in the course of the illness to assess renal function, electrolytes, calcium, glucose, and liver function. Elevations of AST/ALT ($<3\times$ normal) and bilirubin may suggest gallstones as the etiology. **Triglycerides** should be obtained to exclude hypertriglyceridemia as the etiology.

X-ray: Ultrasound is a more sensitive test for gallstones than CT scanning and is indicated routinely in pts with AP and no prior hx of cholecystectomy. CT scanning with fine cuts of the pancreas and large doses of iv contrast are used to stage the disease on the basis of the degree of inflammation and the degree of necrosis. CT scanning should be done in pts who have clinically severe disease or who do not appear to be improving within a few days of admission. Plain films are needed if perforation or obstruction is suspected. CT and MRCP may be indicated in the evaluation of recurrent AP (see "Diff Dx").

Endoscopy: ERCP is indicated as a therapeutic measure in severe biliary pancreatitis or cholangitis (see "Rx"). ERCP or EUS may also be indicated in recurrent AP (see "Diff Dx").

Rx:

- *Supportive measures:* Pts are kept NPO and are given analgesia and vigorous hydration with correction and monitoring of volume status and electrolytes. Ill pts are treated in the ICU. A large fluid deficit may be seen in the first few days, and a large diuresis follows when the pt recovers. A Foley catheter is important to monitor urine output in the severely ill. An NGT does not change outcome but may provide symptomatic relief if the pt is vomiting or has an ileus. IV H2RAs minimize gastric volumes and may improve sx but not outcome. Offending drugs and alcohol are stopped. Incentive spirometry is reasonable to minimize atelectasis.

- *Antibiotics:* Early studies failed to show a benefit from antibiotic rx in pancreatitis, because the studies included many pts who did not have necrotizing pancreatitis. However, in pts with necrotizing pancreatitis, selective decontamination (with oral and rectal antimicrobials) decreases morbidity and mortality (Ann Surg 1995;222:57). This approach is nursing-care intensive, and iv antibiotics are easier. Imipenem (500 mg iv q 6-8 hr, adjusted for weight and renal function) provides excellent pancreatic tissue levels. Meta-analysis of 8 trials showed a benefit of antibiotics in reducing mortality supporting routine antibiotic use in necrotizing disease (J Gastrointest Surg 1998; 2:496).
- *ERCP:* The rationale for urgent ERCP in suspected gallstone pancreatitis is to remove the impacted stone to prevent further pancreatitis and cholangitis. Initial studies demonstrated an improvement in outcome for those with severe disease who underwent sphincterotomy (Lancet 1988;2:979). Subsequent RCTs have produced conflicting results. The benefit in one large study seems to have arisen mainly from treating cholangitis (Nejm 1993;328:228). A study that excluded pts with bilirubin ≥5 mg/dL or clinical cholangitis showed no benefit from early ERCP and showed an increased frequency of respiratory complications (Nejm 1997;336:237). A meta-analysis suggests benefit from early ERCP and sphincterotomy for removal of stones (NNT 7.6 for complications and 26 for death) (Am J Gastro 1999;94:3211). Most clinicians use ERCP selectively when clinical or laboratory studies suggest biliary obstruction or cholangitis. Recurrent bouts of AP associated with pancreas divisum can be treated with endoscopic stenting or sphincterotomy of the minor duct (Gastrointest Endosc 2000;52:9).

- *Peritoneal lavage:* In severe pancreatitis, 3 d of continuous peritoneal lavage does not improve outcome (by RCT [Nejm 1985;312:399]). Longer lavage (7 d) appears to have a benefit in reducing late infection (Ann Surg 1990;211:708) but is not widely used and has not been compared to imipenem rx.

- *Nutrition:* Pts are kept NPO in the early phases of the disease. Those with severe disease may have a prolonged illness and be unable to tolerate an oral diet. In the past such pts were typically begun on TPN to prevent nutritional complications. However, meta-analysis of recent RCTs suggest that feeding with a nasoenteric tube is both safer and cheaper and shortens hospital stay (BMJ 2004;328:1407). Pancreatic stimulation by feeding is avoided by passing the feeding tube distal to the ligament of Treitz.

- *Evaluating necrosis for infection:* In pts with necrosis on CT who improve clinically, no interventions are needed to prove that necrosis has remained sterile. However, for those who develop worsening systemic illness (fever, tachycardia, respiratory failure) or who fail to improve by the second wk, CT-guided needle aspiration should be performed to determine if necrosis is infected (GE 1987;93:1315). Pts with infection on CT bx need surgical debridement, and pts with negative aspirates are treated medically.

- *Surgical debridement:* Infected pancreatic necrosis is a clear indication for surgical debridement. A variety of surgical techniques have been described (Nejm 1999;340:1412). The benefits of debridement in those pts with early or late systemic toxicity and no evidence of infected necrosis are unproven. However, many surgeons use debridement in pts who fail to improve after prolonged medical rx (J Am Coll Surg 1995; 181:279). Debridement may also be needed if a suspected pseudocyst contains organized necrosis, because simple drainage leads to infection (Am J Gastro 1994;89:1781).

- *Pseudocysts:* (Am J Gastro 1997;92:377) Asymptomatic pseudocysts do not require intervention. The previously common practice of operating on asymptomatic pseudocysts >5 cm and present for >6 wk is not supported by current data. Symptomatic pseudocysts can be decompressed by surgical, endoscopic, or radiographic means. There are no useful comparative trials that determine the optimal approach, and local expertise is usually the determining factor. Surgical methods include cyst gastrostomy (if the cyst is adjacent to the stomach), Roux-en-Y cyst jejunostomy, and distal pancreatectomy. An endoscopic cyst gastrostomy can be made if the cyst abuts the posterior stomach (Gastrointest Endosc 1989;35:1). The cyst can be drained with a pigtail catheter as long as the main duct is not obstructed (since the cyst will not resolve if the duct is not patent), but the recurrence rate is high (Surg Gynecol Obstet 1992;175:293).

- *Cholecystectomy:* Pts with gallstones as the cause of their pancreatitis should undergo cholecystectomy as soon as the pancreatitis subsides. They should not be subjected to long delays because of the risk of recurrence (Am J Surg 1990;159:361). Common duct stones should be ruled out with intraoperative cholangiography or MRCP (p 341). If stones are found intraoperatively, they can be removed laparoscopically (in selected expert hands) or postoperative ERCP and stone extraction can be done if the expertise is available (Am J Surg 1993;165:515).

- *Rx of sludge:* Sludge appears to be a cause of AP, and rx of sludge by sphincterotomy or cholecystectomy lowers recurrence rates (Nejm 1992;326:589). However, in many pts sludge may turn out to be an incidental finding. Pancreatitis recurs in up to 20% despite rx of sludge (Gastroenterol Clin North Am 1999;28:571).

- *Therapy to reduce the systemic inflammatory response:* Since inflammatory mediators cause the systemic illness seen in pancreatitis, attempts have been made to interrupt that process.

Antiproteolytic rx, glucagon, atropine, and somatostatin are ineffective (Gut 1998;42:886). A large trial of lexipafant, a PAF inhibitor, showed no efficacy (BMJ 2000;320:244).

9.2 Chronic Pancreatitis

Lancet 2003;361:1447; GE 2001;120:682; J Clin Gastro 1999;29:225

Cause: (GE 2001;120:682) A new classification system has been proposed for chronic pancreatitis (CP) based on etiologic risk factors. It is called the **TIGAR-O** system, with each letter representing the first letter of a risk factor shown in **bold italics** in this section. The most common causes are **toxic metabolic** and the most frequent toxic cause is alcohol. About 60-70% of CP pts in developed countries have a hx of more than 6 yr of >150 gm ethanol consumption daily. Other toxic causes include cigarette smoking (Pancreas 1996;12:131), hypercalcemia, hyperlipidemia (controversial), and chronic renal failure. Most of the remainder have **idiopathic** pancreatitis, which includes a late onset and early onset group as well as the poorly understood entity of tropical pancreatitis (J Clin Gastro 2002;35:61). There appear to be **genetic** predispositions to recurrent pancreatitis caused by mutations in genes that normally function to limit the destruction of the pancreas caused by activation of trypsin from trypsinogen (Lancet 2003;361:1447). These mutations include: (1) mutations in serine protease inhibitors (SPINK1 mutation), (2) mutations in the cystic fibrosis transmembrane conductance receptor (CFTR) gene that are common in pts with apparently idiopathic CP (and no clinical evidence of cystic fibrosis) (Nejm 1998; 339:653), and (3) mutations in the cationic trypsinogen gene, which are the cause of familial pancreatitis. **Autoimmune** pancreatitis is being increasingly recognized and is characterized by lymphoplasmacytic infiltration and fibrosis, enlarged pancreas with narrowing of the main duct, elevated IgG levels (especially IgG4) and steroid responsiveness (Am J Gastro 2004;99:1605).

Recurrent and severe acute pancreatitis may lead to chronic disease in select cases. A much smaller group will have **obstruction** of the duct such as can be seen with trauma, pseudocysts, ampullary tumors, and pancreas divisum (p 312). Pancreatic insufficiency may be seen in a variety of disorders without pancreatitis, most notably in cystic fibrosis (Surg Clin N Am 1999; 79:829).

Epidem: Since the disease is frequently undiagnosed, prevalence rates of chronic pancreatitis are unknown and estimates vary from 0.04 to 5.0%. The median age of onset is 45 yr in alcoholic CP. A bimodal incidence is seen in idiopathic CP, with onset in late teens and 50s (GE 1994;107:1481).

Pathophys: (Am J Gastro 2004;99:2256) With many different etiologies, it could be surmised that several different mechanisms might lead to CP. In the case of alcohol there are probably several factors that are important for disease progression since only the minority of alcoholics develop CP. Oxidative stress, direct toxic effects, genetic defects, cycles of necrosis and fibrosis, and chronic obstruction are likely important factors in many cases. Pain may be caused by tissue necrosis, pseudocysts, elevated pancreatic duct and pancreatic interstitium pressures, ischemia, or nerve damage.

Sx: Most pts with CP have a hx of alcoholism and report recurrent attacks of upper abdominal pain radiating to the back. Attacks are partially relieved by being upright. Pain can be intermittent or chronic and unrelenting. About 10-20% of pts present without pain but with diabetes, malabsorption, weight loss, or jaundice.

Si: Epigastric tenderness or mass if a pseudocyst is present.

Crs: In CP, there is generally progressive destruction of pancreatic tissue, resulting in endocrine and exocrine dysfunction. The pain of CP tends to burn out over time and is often accompanied by the development of pancreatic insufficiency. Mortality is 50% at

25 years, but much of that is due to diseases associated with alcoholism.

Cmplc: Pancreatic cancer occurs in 4% of pts after 20 yr of disease (Nejm 1993;328:1433). Diabetes and exocrine insufficiency are late features caused by destruction of more than 80-90% of the gland. Exocrine insufficiency can result in malnutrition and fat soluble vitamin deficiency (A, D, E, and K). Pseudocysts may develop and may cause pain, rupture, become infected, bleed, or compress adjacent organs (see p 321). Portal or splenic vein thrombosis rarely occurs, but the latter may result in isolated gastric varices (Dig Dis Sci 1992;37:340).

Diff Dx: The broad differential is that of dyspepsia (p 4). In those presenting with malabsorption, the differential includes the many causes of malabsorption/maldigestion (p 30). Most pts with chronic pain from pancreatitis and normal imaging studies will go without a diagnosis unless tests of pancreatic function are used (see "Lab"). Some pts with apparent chronic pancreatitis have pancreatic cancer that may be impossible to diagnose without surgery, unless ERCP reveals a long stricture that can be brushed for diagnosis.

Lab: Amylase and lipase may be modestly elevated but are frequently normal because of the glandular destruction. LFTs can be elevated due to associated alcoholism or due to bile duct obstruction (from fibrotic or edematous changes in the pancreas). A variety of impractical and insensitive tests for pancreatic function have been described. The most sensitive is collection of duodenal juice with measurement of its protein and bicarbonate content after secretin administration (the secretin-pancreozymin test). Tests that depend on pancreatic digestion of orally administered substrates or depend on the detection of chymotrypsin or trypsin in stool can also be used to detect more subtle pancreatic dysfunction. The major problem with these tests (eg, pancreolauryl test, bentiromide test) is poor predictive value in the pts for whom the test is needed (those with chronic pain and negative imaging studies). A 72-hr stool collection for fat on a 100-gm daily fat diet is the best test for determining if diarrhea is from fat malabsorption due to exocrine insufficiency. A spot Sudan stain for stool fat is a good positive but not a reliable negative test for steatorrhea.

X-ray: Pancreatic calcifications are seen on KUB in 30% of pts. CT is more sensitive for calcifications and ductal abnormalities (75-90% depending on the study and the degree of disease [GE 1994;107:1481]) but is not as good as ERCP. MRCP is evolving as an alternative to ERCP in some centers (Am J Gastro 2002;97:347).

Endoscopy: ERCP is the imaging gold standard for diagnosis. Early disease shows mild changes in the main duct and ectasia of the side branches. In more advanced disease there is beading and dilatation of the main duct and its side branches. ERCP is not perfectly sensitive. A normal ERCP can be seen in pts whose pancreatic function test is abnormal and who subsequently develop sx of chronic pancreatitis. EUS has become a sensitive tool for the detection of chronic pancreatitis in expert hands. It may be a good alternative to ERCP when CT and MRCP are nondiagnostic because EUS is less risky (Gastro Endosc 2002; 56:S76).

Rx: (GE 1998;115:765)

- *Medical rx of pain:* Episodic pain can be treated with narcotic analgesics prescribed by one physician to minimize the abuse potential. Antidepressants such as amitriptyline can be used to minimize pain perception. **Pancreatic enzymes** can be beneficial by causing a negative feedback inhibition of pancreatic secretion by denaturing CCK-releasing peptide. A total of 6 RCTs have been reported, and a meta-analysis failed to show benefit (Am J Gastro 1997;92:2032). However, the 2 positive studies used tablet preparations rather than enzyme capsules.

Pancrelipase 6 tab po ac and qhs reduces pain by 75% in pts with mild to moderate disease (GE 1984;87:44). Suppressing pancreatic function by decreasing gastric acidity or by using octreotide does not appear to help. **Nerve blocks** with corticosteroids or alcohol are widely tried in chronic pain and are variably successful.

- *Endoscopic rx of pain:* Pancreatic stenting, which presumably relieves pancreatic ductal obstruction, has been reported in an unblinded fashion to relieve pain in up to 60% of pts with CP (Gastrointest Endosc 1999;49:S77). However, stenting also causes ductal changes that may not be reversible (Gastrointest Endosc 1996;44:268). In the absence of RCTs, these potentially morbid procedures should be limited to expert centers as parts of studies. Pancreatic stones can be removed from the main duct with improvement in pain in >50% of pts, but the relevance of pancreatic stones in causing pain is far from clear (Int J Pancreatol 1996;19:93).

- *Surgical rx of pain:* (GE 1998;115:765) The procedure of choice for pts with pain unrelieved by medical measures and associated with a dilated pancreatic duct (≥6 mm) is a lateral pancreaticojejunostomy (a so-called Puestow-type operation). It is relatively low morbidity, and pain relief in 60% of pts at 2 yr might be expected. For pts with nondilated ducts, a pancreatic resection is necessary. Thoracoscopic sympathectomy may be a less morbid alternative in expert hands (J Gastrointest Surg 2002;6:845). Distal pancreatic resections frequently fail to relieve pain unless disease is confined to the tail (eg, posttraumatic ductal strictures). Pancreaticoduodenectomy (the Whipple procedure) appears to be an effective though drastic solution. Pain relief is good (85%) even though diseased tail of pancreas is left behind.

- *Malabsorption:* Clinical malabsorption occurs in advanced disease when more than 80-90% of the gland is destroyed. Malabsorption of fat (steatorrhea) and protein (azotorrhea) occurs. Sx are treated by providing about 30,000 IU of lipase and 10,000 IU of trypsin during the postprandial period. This replacement represents only about 5% of the normal digestive output. Either tablets or enteric-coated capsules can be used. Tablets are less expensive and subject to acid degradation in the stomach (eg, pancrelipase with 8000 U lipase per tablet). Enteric-coated preparations resist acid degradation, have higher lipase concentration per tablet, and may work when uncoated preparations fail. Addition of acid suppression may improve the effectiveness of tablets.

- *Rx of other complications:* Diabetes tends to be brittle, with a high risk of hypoglycemia because of the loss of glucagon due to islet cell destruction. Pseudocysts are discussed on p 321. For pancreatic ascites, the offending leak from a disrupted duct or pseudocyst is usually treated surgically. Bile duct or duodenal obstruction generally require surgery.

9.3 Pancreatic Cancer

Lancet 2004;363:1049; GE 1999;117:1464; Lancet 1997;349:485

Epidem: (Surg Oncol Clin N Am 1998;7:67) Pancreatic cancer is the 11th leading cause of cancer in the U.S. (rate 9/100,00) but the 5th leading cause of cancer death because of a grim death-to-incidence ratio of 0.99. It is slightly more common in men and blacks. The RR for smokers is at least 1.5. A diet high in fat or meat increases risk. High intake of fiber, fruits, and vegetables lowers risk. Coffee was *erroneously* described as a risk in a widely publicized study (Nejm 1981;304:630). Alcohol has no effect. Partial gastrectomy increases risk and tonsillectomy decreases risk. The risk is 4% after 20 yr of chronic pancreatitis (Nejm 1993;328:1433). There is an association with diabetes, but it is not an independent risk factor (Nejm 1994;331:81). Occupational exposure to aromatic amines (chemical workers) may be a risk. Family hx is a risk and the disease has been associated with familial pancreatitis, HNPCC (p 242), Peutz-Jeghers (p 250), familial breast cancer, and other genetic disorders.

Pathophys: The underlying defects in pancreatic cancer are acquired and inherited mutations of cancer causing genes. The genes that become defective are tumor suppressor genes (whose normal function restrains cell proliferation), oncogenes (genes that when amplified or mutated cause cell transformation), and DNA mismatch repair genes (whose normal function is to repair replication errors). Many gene defects have been described (J Am Coll Surg 1998;187:429; Am J Surg 2003;186:279).

Sx: Abdominal pain is present in 90% of pts. The pain can be vague and nondescript and may be felt in the back. Weight loss and early satiety are common. Jaundice occurs as a relatively early finding if the tumor is in the head of the pancreas and obstructs the bile duct. It can be a late finding if the tumor causes jaundice by metastases rather than obstruction. Occasionally, pts present with acute pancreatitis (3%). New onset diabetes may precede pancreatic cancer (15%). Depression may be associated.

Si: Abdominal mass, cachexia, or jaundice may be observed.

Crs: At diagnosis, the tumor is confined to the pancreas in <10% of pts. About 40% have local spread and 50% have distant spread. Most pts die within 1 yr of diagnosis, and survival for 5 yr is less than 3%.

Cmplc: Obstructive jaundice, duodenal obstruction, effects of metastatic disease.

Diff Dx: A major diagnostic pitfall is the distinction of pancreatic cancer from chronic pancreatitis, because the clinical and radiographic pictures are similar. Pancreatic adenocarcinoma must be distinguished from other, less common tumors of the pancreatic ductal epithelium (eg, cystic neoplasms of the pancreas [p 331], tumors of the islet cells [p 331], and tumors of acinar cells or nonepithelial tissues [eg, lymphoma]). These other tumors are uncommon.

Lab: CEA and CA 19-9 may be elevated. However, elevated levels provide little in the way of prognostic information and are of no value in staging.

X-ray: CT is the single most useful test, with the detection of tumors as small as 1-2 cm and detection of local spread or distant metastases. When CT predicts unresectability, the accuracy is 90%, but when it predicts a resectable lesion, the accuracy is only 50-90%. Needle bx can be accomplished by CT guidance. It is generally reserved for pts who are felt not to be operative candidates because of radiographically unresectable disease or lack of medical fitness. Angiography is used in some centers to detect vascular invasion if surgery is being considered. Newer imaging modalities are under development (Lancet 1997;349:485).

Endoscopy: ERCP allows for the detection of ductal tumors down to 1 cm in size and separates those pts with ampullary cancer and cholangiocarcinoma who may have a greater chance of resectability. At the time of ERCP, brushings and biopsies may be obtained, and obstruction can be relieved by stent placement (see "Rx"). EUS may be superior to CT for smaller lesions, lymph nodes, and vascular invasion, but is very operator dependent.

Rx:

- *Surgery:* The first step in determining the correct approach is to stage with a combination of CT scan and other modalities. Diagnostic laparoscopy is used in some centers to determine resectability since small local metastases are frequently missed on other imaging studies. It may be especially useful in tumors of the body and tail (where tiny mets are frequent) and if ascites is present. Surgery is performed if there is no radiographic evidence of vascular invasion, no local or distant spread, and if the pt is medically fit. Almost all the potentially resectable lesions are in the head since pts develop a sx (jaundice) when the tumor is still a small size. About 80-90% of lesions are found to be unresectable. A **pancreaticoduodenectomy** (Whipple operation) with or without the pylorus-sparing modification is performed. If there is no local or vascular invasion pathologically, the 5-yr survival is 50%, but these pts are few and far between. More radical surgical approaches increase morbidity but do not improve outcome. Tumors <2 cm have better survival. A **bypass** to relieve biliary or duodenal obstruction may be indicated if the pt has unresectable disease at surgery. Intraoperative chemical **splanchnicectomy** (by injection of absolute alcohol) is effective for pain control.

- *Chemotherapy and radiation:* The role of adjuvant chemoradiation in resectable pts is uncertain (Surg Oncol Clin N Am 2004;13:567). Radiation in conjunction with 5-FU is offered to pts with locally advanced disease. Gemcitabine is an option for pts with metastatic disease and poor performance status (Ann Oncol 1999;10:140). Radiation may reduce local pain. External radiation doses are limited by the radiosensitivity of the surrounding normal structures. Intraoperative implants have been tried with minimal success (J Clin Gastro 2000; 30:230).

- *Palliation of jaundice:* Obstructive jaundice can cause pruritus, malaise, cholangitis, and abdominal discomfort that is disconcerting to pts. Pts can be palliated effectively either by stenting or surgical bypass. Those with advanced disease, the elderly, and those with poor functional status are probably best palliated with stenting. Metal stents result in fewer complications due to clogging than plastic stents changed every 3 months (Gastrointest Endosc 1998;47:1). Plastic stents are cheaper and may be appropriate if life expectancy is short. Young, fit pts may benefit from a surgical approach. In surgery, a tissue diagnosis can be made and the duodenum and the biliary obstruction are bypassed and pain can be palliated with alcohol injection of the celiac plexus (CA Cancer J Clin 2000;50:241). The advantages of this approach are a lower incidence of cholangitis due to stent obstruction and the prevention of duodenal obstruction in prolonged survivors. This comes at the cost of surgical morbidity.

- *Palliation of duodenal obstruction:* Gastrojejunostomy effectively relieves duodenal obstruction. Endoscopic duodenal stenting has been described but needs further evaluation (Gastrointest Endosc 1998;47:267).

9.4 Cystic Neoplasms of Pancreas

Nejm 2004;351:1218

Mucinous Cystadenomas and Carcinomas: (40%) These lesions have large cysts with septa and peripheral calcification, and they may have a solid component. The fluid is usually rich in tumor markers and low in amylase. The benign can be separated from the malignant only under the microscope after resection. The transformation from benign to malignant is a substantial risk, so these lesions must be resected. They can be difficult to distinguish from pseudocysts.

Serous Cystadenomas: (30-40%) These lesions have multiple small cysts with larger cysts in the periphery. There is often a central stellate calcification that allows for their identification on CT scan. They have little if any malignant potential. Serous cystadenomas that have diagnostic CT features can be followed without resection (unless they are symptomatic), though malignant transformation has been reported (Am J Surg Pathol 1989;13:61).

Mucinous Duct Ectatic Neoplasms: (20-30%) These lesions are neoplastic changes of the main pancreatic duct or side branches (Am J Gastro 1992;87:300). They produce a mucus-filled cavity that communicates with the main pancreatic duct. At ERCP, globs of mucus can often be seen being spit out of a dilated ampullary orifice. These lesions can be benign or malignant. Management depends on surgical risk and potential benefits to the pt.

Papillary Cystic Neoplasms: These are the rarest of the group and are mostly solid tumors with cystic areas of hemorrhage and necrosis and often a capsule. They are most often seen in young women. They may be benign or malignant (GE 1996;110:1909).

9.5 Islet Cell Tumors

J Clin Endocrinol Metab 1995;80:2273; J Am Coll Surg 1994;178:187

Epidem: These rare tumors have a combined incidence of 1/100,000/yr.

Pathophys/Sx/Si/Diff Dx: These tumors are derived from neuroendocrine stem cells and as tumors may secrete a variety of polypeptide hormones. Many of these are part of the multiple endocrine neoplasia (MEN) type I syndrome (tumors of pancreas, parathyroid, pituitary, adrenal cortex, and thyroid) (Ann IM 1998;129:484). Several islet cell tumors are recognized:

Insulinoma: (50% of islet cell tumors) This lesion is located in the pancreas and causes fasting hypoglycemia with associated trembling, irritability, weakness, diaphoresis, and hunger (from epinephrine release) or neurologic sx such as confusion, bizarre behavior, and seizures (from the hypoglycemia directly). They are usually single benign adenomas but can be multiple, malignant, or associated with hyperplasia rather than a discrete tumor. The differential includes other causes of fasting hypoglycemia, most notably self-administration of insulin. Reviewed in Surg Oncol Clin N Am 1998;7:819.

Gastrinoma: (10-15%) See p. 145.

Vasoactive intestinal peptide (VIPoma): (10-15%) These lesions are located in the pancreas or sympathetic chain and cause watery diarrhea, hypokalemia, hypochlorhydria, and acidosis. The diarrhea is large volume and persists with fasting. They may occur as part of the MEN type I syndrome but are usually isolated lesions. Surreptitious laxative use mimics the syndrome and the broad differential of chronic diarrhea needs to be considered (p 26).

Glucagonoma: (1%) These lesions cause the 4D syndrome: diabetes, dermatitis, depression, and DVT. The pathognomonic rash is necrotic migratory erythema in which red blotches on extremities, thighs, or perineum progress to vesicopustules that desquamate and are pruritic.

Somatostatinoma: These lesions cause diabetes, diarrhea, steatorrhea, and gallbladder disease (type A). A type B lesion is associated with neurofibromatosis and can cause gi bleeding or mass effect. They tend to be large and malignant.

Pancreatic polypeptide (PPoma): These cause no sx until they present with vascular metastases. They can be associated with the MEN type I syndrome.

Nonfunctioning tumors: These tumors, with no functioning polypeptide products, present with sx similar to adenocarcinoma of the pancreas (weight loss, pain, jaundice, mass effect).

Lab: For **insulinoma,** serial glucose and insulin levels are diagnostic. C peptide levels are useful to exclude self-administration of insulin (which is probably more common than insulinoma!). Elevated hormone levels define the **VIPoma** and **somatostatinoma.** Elevated glucagon levels or skin bx are used to diagnose **glucagonoma.**

X-ray: CT scan is used to locate the tumor and assess for metastases. Arteriography in expert hands, with transhepatic portal venous sampling of hormone levels, may provide additional information (Clin Radiol 1994;49:295). Radionuclide scanning with octreotide can be used to image tumors with somatostatin receptors and can be helpful in identifying recurrences (Semin Ultrasound CT MR 1995;16:331).

Endoscopy: Use in expert hands suggests that EUS is accurate in pre-operative localization and may obviate the need for angiography, thus reducing cost (Gastrointest Endosc 1999;49:19).

Rx: Once an islet cell tumor is suspected by clinical sx and hormone levels, the rx depends on the presence of metastases and upon whether or not a localized tumor can be found. If metastases are found, chemotherapy, usually with streptozotocin and 5-FU, is offered, with response rates up to 60% (Nejm 1980;303:1189). Resection is performed if the tumor can be localized and there are no metastases. If the tumor cannot be localized, then medical rx, or in some cases subtotal pancreatectomy, are considered. Features of the MEN-I syndrome should raise the possibility of multiple lesions. Octreotide can be used to manage diarrhea in pts with unresectable disease, especially VIPoma (Dig Dis Sci 1999;44:1148).

Chapter 10
The Biliary Tree

10.1 Cholecystitis and Biliary Colic

Am Fam Phys 2000;61:1673; Clin Perspect Gastro 2000;March:87

Epidem: The risk of gallstones rises with age. The prevalence of gallstones in young women is 5-8% and rises to 35% in women over age 75. The prevalence in men rises to 20% by age 70. Risk rises later for men, presumably because pregnancy confers earlier risk on women. Obesity is a strong risk for gallstones, especially in women, and 10-25% of pts develop stones with rapid weight loss (Ann IM 1993;119:1029). In younger age groups the M:F ratio is 2:1. Estrogen replacement rx increases risk (GE 1988;94:91). Increased levels of estrogens promote biliary cholesterol supersaturation and may account for some of the observed difference. The incidence of gallstones in pregnant pts is 2%, though sludge develops in 30% and disappears postpartum in half of these pts (Ann IM 1993;119:116). Recreational physical activity reduces risk (independent of weight).

Hypertriglyceridemia increases HMG-CoA reductase activity and thereby increases risk by promoting cholesterol secretion into bile (Semin Liver Dis 1990;10:159). Certain ethnic groups (Pima Indian women of the southwestern U.S., native Chileans) have a very high incidence. Blacks have a lower risk than whites. Spinal cord injury causes gallbladder hypomotility and changes in biliary lipids that promote stone formation (GE 1987;92:966).

Pathophys: In the U.S., 85% of stones are composed of cholesterol. Pigment stones (composed largely of calcium bilirubinate) and mixed stones represent the remainder. The pathophysiology of pigment stone formation is not understood, but the physical-chemical basis of cholesterol gallstone formation has been extensively studied. There are 3 lipid species in bile: (1) cholesterol (4%), (2) phospholipids (22%, mainly as phosphatidylcholine, aka lecithin), and (3) bile salts (67%) (Semin Liver Dis 1990; 10:159). Small amounts of bilirubin (0.3%) and protein (4.5%) are also present. Cholesterol is not water soluble (it is hydrophobic). Bile salts and lecithins have polar and nonpolar surfaces and are called "amphiphiles." The polar surfaces allow the bile salts to dissolve in water. The biliary cholesterol is carried in stable particles (micelles) made up of lecithin and bile salts.

Bile is supersaturated when the capacity of the bile salts and lecithin to keep cholesterol in solution is exceeded. **Supersaturation** is the first step in stone formation and generally occurs because of excess cholesterol secretion into bile. **Nucleation** is the initial transition from liquid cholesterol crystals to solid cholesterol crystals in bile. While many people have supersaturated bile, stones precipitate in only a small number. The most important nucleating factor is gallbladder mucin, but other pronucleating and antinucleating proteins have been identified. Gallbladder **stasis** promotes stone formation by allowing stones to grow without being expelled from the gallbladder.

- *Biliary sludge:* Sludge is a mixture of gallbladder mucin and small cholesterol or calcium bilirubinate crystals from which macroscopic stones can develop (GE 1988;95:508). Sludge can be detected at ultrasound and can cause biliary sx such as colic, cholecystitis, or pancreatitis. Pts with asymptomatic sludge can be managed expectantly. Pts who have rapid weight loss, take ceftriaxone, take octreotide, are pregnant, or have undergone organ transplantation are at risk for sludge (Ann IM 1999; 130:301).

- *Consequences of stone development:* Pts with gallstones may (1) remain asymptomatic; (2) develop biliary colic from intermittent, brief cystic duct obstruction; (3) develop acute cholecystitis from prolonged cystic duct obstruction, with secondary inflammation and bacterial infection; (4) develop chronic cholecystitis from recurrent acute bouts; (5) experience migration of stones into the common bile duct and into the duodenum that may cause pain, pancreatitis, or cholangitis; (6) develop gallbladder cancer; or (7) develop gallstone ileus (bowel obstruction by a gallstone).

- *Acalculous cholecystitis:* This condition is cholecystitis in the absence of stones. It is most often seen in pts as a complication of major surgery, trauma, or burns. The precise mechanisms are unknown (J Am Coll Surg 1995;180:232).

- *Xanthogranulomatous cholecystitis:* This abnormality is found in about 1.7% of excised gallbladders. It is a destructive, fibrosing, inflammatory condition of the gallbladder characterized by the presence of lipid-laden macrophages, which possibly develop in response to extravasated bile (J Clin Pathol 1987;40:412).

Sx:

- *Biliary colic:* Most gallstones do not cause sx. The most common sx associated with gallstones is referred to as biliary colic (Postgrad Med 1991;90:119). The hallmark of biliary colic is discrete, unpredictable attacks of pain, lasting minutes to 5 hr before subsiding. The frequency of attacks is greater at night. The pt feels well between attacks. The pain is generally epigastric or RUQ (and occasionally substernal or LUQ). The pain often radiates outside the abdomen, typically to below the scapula. Nausea and vomiting may occur. Fever is uncommon without cholecystitis. Contrary to common teaching, there is no evidence that fatty food intolerance, belching, or bloating are related to the development of gallstones (Scand J Gastroenterol 2000;35:70). For sx that occur predictably or very frequently (> once weekly), a cause other than gallstones should be considered.

- *Acute cholecystitis:* In this complication, the pt begins with an attack of biliary colic that fails to resolve. The pain tends to localize to the RUQ and may be associated with vomiting. Fever may develop. An important minority of pts may have little if any pain, especially diabetics, the immunocompromised, pts with CNS disease, and pts on steroids.
- *Acute pancreatitis:* Gallstones may first present with sx of acute pancreatitis (AP) (p 335).
- *Choledocholithiasis:* These pts may present with sx of biliary colic (frequently with radiation to the scapula), jaundice, dark urine, or pancreatitis, or they may be asymptomatic.
- *Cholangitis:* Classically these pts present with Charcot's triad: fever, RUQ pain, and jaundice. All of these findings might not necessarily be present.

Si: In biliary colic, there are usually no physical findings. In cholecystitis, localized tenderness with peritoneal findings (percussion tenderness, guarding, or rebound) may develop. Many pts will demonstrate Murphy's sign, the abrupt cessation of inspiration because of worsening of the pain when examiner is palpating the RUQ. A RUQ mass may be palpable. Pts with cholangitis typically have jaundice and fever but are not universally tender in the RUQ.

Crs: (Ann IM 1993;119:606) Most gallstones remain asymptomatic. In the group of pts who initially are asymptomatic with their stones, symptoms will later develop at a rate of 1-2%/yr. The rate may be higher (4%/yr) in the first 5 yr. Once pts develop an attack of biliary colic, the chance of recurrent attacks is high, but 30% of pts will not have a second attack within 10 yr of follow-up. The rate of AP may be higher in pts with small stones (Arch IM 1997;157:1674).

Cmplc: Gallbladder cancer (p 349). A few pts will develop a stone that is impacted in the gallbladder neck and obstructs the common duct. This is referred to as Mirizzi's syndrome (Am Surg 1994;60:889). Cholecystocholedochal fistula and gallstone ileus (obstruction of the small bowel by a stone passed through a fistula) are uncommon (BMJ 2002;325:639).

Diff Dx: Depending on the presentation, the differential is that of dyspepsia (p 4), pancreatitis (p 311), or jaundice (p 47).

Lab: Labs are normal in biliary colic. LFTs, amylase, and lipase should be obtained in the evaluation of attacks of suspected biliary pain in order to look for evidence of pancreatitis or common duct stones. In the acute passage of stones, the transaminases can be very high (200-800 U/L) and may have a pattern more suggestive of hepatitis than obstruction. If the stone passes, the LFTs rapidly normalize. If obstruction persists, the alk phos and bilirubin slowly climb and transaminases stay 2-3 times normal. A leukocytosis may be seen in cholecystitis.

X-ray:

- *Biliary colic:* Ultrasound is the test of choice for pts with suspected biliary colic. A typically quoted sensitivity is 97%, with specificity at 99%. However, since many pts with negative ultrasounds never have the gold standard test (cholecystectomy), adjusted sensitivities of 90% for sensitivity and 97% for specificity have been proposed (Arch IM 1994;154:2573). CT is insensitive and not a reliable negative. In oral cholecystogram (OCG), pts swallow giant tablets of a contrast agent. The contrast agent is excreted in bile and taken up in the gallbladder. OCG is not often used because it is less sensitive than ultrasound and because it is nonspecific if nonvisualization of the gallbladder is taken as a positive.
- *Acute cholecystitis:* Ultrasound is usually the test done first to look for gallstones in this setting. Ultrasound may reveal direct evidence of cholecystitis, such as a thickened gallbladder wall

or surrounding fluid collection. Ultrasound may show evidence of dilated bile ducts from choledocholithiasis. If ultrasound is negative and acute cholecystitis is suspected, a radionuclide scan (typically called a HIDA scan no matter what isotope is used) is performed. In normal pts, the radiolabel is excreted into bile and flows into the gallbladder. If the cystic duct is obstructed (as in acute cholecystitis), the tracer is not visualized in the gallbladder and the test is positive. The sensitivity is 97% and the specificity is 90%. Since cholecystitis may occur without stones, HIDA scanning has advantages over ultrasound in the diagnosis of acalculous cholecystitis.

- *Common duct stones:* CT and US are poor tests for common duct stones. ERCP is the test of choice for pts with a strong clinical suspicion of common duct stones (jaundice, dilated duct on US, abnormal LFTs) because of the potential for endoscopic rx. If the pt is undergoing surgery, then an intraoperative cholangiogram is a cost-effective alternative. If suspicion is low MRCP is a low-risk alternative with about 90% of the sensitivity of an ERCP (Gastro Endosc 2002;56:803).

Rx:

- *Laparoscopic cholecystectomy (lap chole):* Pts with symptomatic gallstones should undergo cholecystectomy unless there is a major medical contraindication. Asymptomatic pts are better off waiting for the development of sx than having prophylactic surgery. Those with acute cholecystitis should undergo surgery promptly after resuscitation because up to 20% will have gangrene or perforation and a delayed operation results in higher complication rates (BMJ 2002;325:639). The laparoscopic approach has replaced open cholecystectomy without a randomized trial to support its use. Shortened hospital stays, reduced pain, shorter recovery time, and consumer demand have dictated that an RCT will never be done. Expected mortality of lap chole is 0.1-0.2%, and complications occur in 5%.

These rates are similar to the rates for the open operation (Ann Surg 1993;218:129). Contraindications to the laparoscopic approach include scarring or inflammation that prevents access to the RUQ, diffuse peritonitis, and coagulopathy. Not all pts can be done laparoscopically, and some pts (about 5%) must be converted to the open operation (Nejm 1991;324: 1073). Though indications for lap chole are supposedly no different than for open chole, the advent of the laparoscopic approach has increased utilization by about 11% (Surg Endosc 1996;10:746).

- *Lap chole and the common bile duct:* Access to the bile duct is not as easy with lap chole. About 8-17% of pts who undergo cholecystectomy are diagnosed with common bile duct stones (CBDS), and 1-2% will have retained stones diagnosed after surgery (J Am Coll Surg 1998;187:584). A great deal of effort has been put into methods of predicting the presence of common duct stones based on noninvasive data such as LFTs and ultrasound findings. About 90% of pts are considered low risk for CBDS because they have normal LFTs, no bile duct dilatation, and no hx of jaundice or pancreatitis. Even in this low-risk group, the incidence of stones is 5%. Pts with rising LFTs have a very high incidence of CBDS (Gastrointest Endosc 1997;45:394). In practice, the bile duct should be imaged when there is dilatation, abnormal LFTs (unless they fall rapidly to normal), pancreatitis, or a hx of jaundice. Several approaches are possible when common duct stones are suspected. Where there is a high probability of stones (jaundice, dilated ducts, cholangitis), ERCP is often performed prior to lap chole. Centers with a high degree of expertise in laparoscopic bile duct exploration or postoperative ERCP may skip preoperative ERCP in pts with a high probability of CBDS. The role of MRCP is limited because it is not therapeutic. When preoperative ERCP or MRCP is not done, common bile duct stones can be diagnosed by intraoperative cholangiography. Pts with positive

cholangiograms undergo (1) postoperative ERCP with sphincterotomy and stone extraction (Surg Endosc 1995;9:1235),
(2) laparoscopic removal of common duct stones (in the hands
of experts) (World J Surg 1998;22:1125), or (3) conversion to
an open operation. Laparoscopic methods to explore the bile
duct have fewer complications and cost less if done at expert
centers, but those outcomes are not likely in the typical community yet (Am Surg 1999;65:135). Local expertise usually
dictates the approach.

- *Complications of cholecystectomy:* The most feared complication
  of lap chole is bile duct injury. Bile duct injuries can be (1) major transections or ligations of the ducts, (2) leaks from the
  cystic duct stump, or (3) leaks from superficial branches of the
  right hepatic ducts that are exposed at surgery (Am J Surg
  1994;167:27). Leaks occur more often in the hands of inexperi-
  enced surgeons (Brit J Surg 1995;82:307). Pts with bile duct
  injuries present with pain and, to varying degrees, abdominal
  distention, ileus, and fever. LFTs may be normal or near normal
  in pts with leaks, but jaundice develops if the duct has been
  ligated. When a leak is suspected, HIDA scan usually demonstrates the leak and imaging studies may show a fluid collection. Leaks of the cystic duct stump or branches of the right
  hepatic system can be treated by placing a stent across the
  sphincter of Oddi at ERCP (Gastrointest Endosc 1993;39:416).
  As long as the stent crosses the sphincter and reduces pressure
  in the bile duct, the leak is sealed in the vast majority of cases
  (Am J Gastro 1995;90:2128). The stent is removed several
  weeks later, and closure of the leak is verified. Some experts
  prefer to do a sphincterotomy and place a nasobiliary tube. The
  nasobiliary tube usually can be removed in a few days, when
  the edema of the sphincterotomy subsides and the pt is spared
  a second procedure. No direct comparative studies are available. Major transections may require operative intervention

and are associated with a high incidence of subsequent stricture, high cost, and mortality (Ann Surg 1997;225:268). Other notable complications are bleeding and bowel injury (Nejm 1991;324:1073). Stones may be lost into the abdomen and infrequently result in infectious or mechanical complications (Surg Endosc 1999;13:848).

- *Cholecystostomy:* Pts with acute cholecystitis who are at very high risk for surgery can be treated with the placement of a cholecystostomy drainage tube or with an ultrasound-guided gallbladder puncture without a drainage tube. These interventions can be life saving (Lancet 1993;341:1132).
- *Gallstone dissolution:* In pts who are not surgical candidates, stones may dissolve with ursodeoxycholic acid (UDCA). This drug reduces cholesterol secretion into bile and allows for dissolution of cholesterol on stone surfaces. Stones must be made of cholesterol (these stones float at OCG) and must not be calcified (determined on KUB), and the cystic duct must be patent (verified with OCG). Success rates of 30-55% can be expected. There is a high recurrence rate (43% at 4 yr) (Gut 1988;29:655). Recurrence can be reduced by UDCA or aspirin.
- *Lithotripsy:* Extracorporeal shock wave lithotripsy (ESWL) can be used to shatter stones into smaller pieces that can pass or can be more easily dissolved with UDCA. Success varies with the size and number of stones (22-90%). The procedure may be complicated by biliary colic from fragments of stones (Ann IM 1990;112:126). Organic solvents instilled directly into the gallbladder may rapidly dissolve stones, but this approach is now seldom used (Gastroenterol Clin North Am 1991;20:183).
- *Prevention of stones during weight loss:* UDCA prevents stones induced by rapid weight loss (Am J Gastro 1993;88:1705).
- *Common bile duct stones postcholecystectomy:* (Am J Gastro 1997;92:1411) Pts may present postcholecystectomy with findings suggestive of common duct stones (attacks of upper

abdominal pain radiating to the back, abnormal LFTs, dilated bile ducts, pancreatitis, or cholangitis). Pts with a high probability of stones should undergo ERCP. At ERCP, the bile duct is cannulated and injected with contrast, and a sphincterotomy is made if stones are identified. This allows extraction of stones into the duodenum with use of a balloon or wire basket to capture them. Removal of stones carries a risk of short-term complications of pancreatitis, bleeding, or perforation. The bile duct can be cleared in >90% of cases. Long-term follow-up indicates that sphincterotomy is not a benign cure-all, with stone recurrence and sphincter stenosis occurring in up to 24% of pts at 15 yr (Gastrointest Endosc 1996;44:643). Balloon dilatation of the sphincter with stone extraction has similar efficacy and complications but does not create a sphincterotomy (in an RCT [Lancet 1997;349:1124]). Long-term follow-up is lacking, and the results may not be similar outside an expert center. Sublingual nitroglycerin has also been used to extract stones through a temporarily dilated sphincter (Am J Gastro 1997;92:1440). Very large stones are more difficult to remove because the sphincterotomy cannot be made large enough for the easy passage of the stone (Gut 1993;34:1718). In these cases, the stone can be grasped in a reinforced crushing basket and then fragmented into pieces that will pass through the cut sphincter (mechanical lithotripsy). Other approaches include placement of stents, use of shock wave, laser, or electrohydraulic lithotripsy, and organic solvents for dissolution (Am J Gastro 1991;86:1561).

• *Postcholecystectomy syndrome:* These pts have the same sx that brought them to cholecystectomy or they develop new sx postoperatively that are suggestive of biliary tract pain. These pts represent 3 groups. The first is the group of pts with sphincter of Oddi dysfunction (p 352). The second is the group of pts with common bile duct stones (p 343). The third is the group of pts who came to cholecystectomy for symptoms not due to gallbladder disease. These pts might have GERD, IBS, PUD, or other serious, undiagnosed pathology. A careful review of the hx guides the choice of the next diagnostic or therapeutic step. It serves little purpose to leave the pt with the nonspecific label of postcholecystectomy syndrome.

10.2 Bacterial Cholangitis

Gastroenterol Clin North Am 2003;32:1145; Am J Gastro 1998;93:2016

Cause: In most cases cholangitis is the result of infection in a biliary tree obstructed by gallstones. Ascariasis is a common cause of cholangitis in Asia.

Pathophys: Bacteria infect bile in the common duct, usually behind an obstructing stone. Pressure rises in the biliary tree, and bacteria reflux into the systemic circulation, causing sepsis. Enteric gram-negative organisms are the most common infecting organisms but anaerobes may be seen in up to 15% of pts.

Sx: RUQ pain or upper abdominal pain sometimes radiating to the back. Some pts have no pain, and the absence of pain does not rule out cholangitis. Fever or rigors are common. Nausea and vomiting may occur.

Si: Fever, at times very high. Most pts with cholangitis have jaundice. They may have relatively little upper abdominal tenderness compared to pts who present with cholecystitis. Some will have hypotension or altered mental status.

Crs: Without relief of obstruction, mortality is very high. With ERCP mortality is still as high as 10%.

Diff Dx: The diagnosis needs to be considered in any pt with fever or a sepsis picture and abnormal LFTs. Cholecystitis and pancreatitis are the 2 most common considerations, but perforated viscus, ischemic bowel, or other intra-abdominal catastrophe may give a similar picture. Pneumonia can cause pain and abnormal LFTs with sepsis. Sepsis of any cause can cause abnormal LFTs, especially if there is associated shock liver (p453).

Lab: LFTs most commonly show an obstructive picture, with elevated bilirubin and alk phos and transaminases usually below 200 U/L. Thrombocytopenia and hypoalbuminemia are risks for a poor outcome (Nejm 1992;326:1582).

X-ray: Ultrasound may show dilated ducts and occasionally stones or gas in the bile ducts. CT is usually not needed. If oral contrast is given for a CT scan it must be purged with a laxative, because the contrast interferes with ERCP. MRCP may be of use in pts with a low probability of cholangitis but in whom the possibility cannot be completely ignored (Endoscopy 1997;29:472).

Rx: Pts with suspected cholangitis are treated with a broad-spectrum antibiotic (eg, ciprofloxacin with metronidazole, ampicillin-sulbactam) and iv fluids. Ciprofloxacin achieves higher concentrations in obstructed bile ducts than many other antibiotics achieve but this may not translate into better outcomes (Gastrointest Endosc 1994;40:716). ERCP is performed after fluid resuscitation is complete and after antibiotics are begun. In most pts, sphincterotomy and stone extraction are accomplished at the initial procedure (see p 343 for stone extraction techniques). In some critically ill pts, in pts with a coagulopathy, or in pts with multiple, large stones, a nasobiliary tube should be placed as a safe and effective alternative (Am J Gastro 1998; 93:2065). The stones can be removed electively after the sepsis is medically treated and the pt is stable. If urgent surgery is done for this group of pts, mortality is 30% (vs 10% for ERCP), and the endoscopic approach is strongly preferred (based on an RCT [Nejm 1992;326:1582]).

10.3 Cholangiocarcinoma

Nejm 1999;341:1368

Epidem: The incidence is low at 1/100,000/yr. Two out of three pts are over age 65 (Ann Surg Oncol 2000;7:55). Risk factors include PSC (10% lifetime risk, p. 391), cigarette smoking, choledochal cysts, Caroli's disease (p 355), exposure to the contrast medium thorium dioxide, and chronic infection with the parasites *Opisthorchis viverrini* and *Clinorchis sinensis*. In most cases no risk factor is identified.

Pathophys: Cholangiocarcinoma most commonly involves the distal extrahepatic bile ducts or the hilum of the liver at the bifurcation of the bile ducts (Klatskin tumor). Lesions are less commonly intrahepatic or multicentric. Acute or chronic bile duct epithelial injury is probably important in malignant transformation, but the process is not well understood.

Sx: Pts typically present with sx of biliary obstruction. Jaundice is present in >90% of pts, sometimes with associated clay-colored stool, dark urine, and pruritus. Pain is not a prominent feature. Weight loss suggests advanced disease. Cholangitis is unusual.

Si: Depending on the location of the tumor, there may be a palpable mass or a palpable gallbladder.

Crs: The 5-yr survival rate is 10-45%, with a median of 12-30 months. For pts who are not operative candidates, survival is 3-6 months (Gut 1998;42:76).

Diff Dx: The differential is that of jaundice (p 47). The chief differential considerations are usually pancreatic cancer, ampullary cancer, common duct stones, and benign biliary strictures (often associated with chronic pancreatitis or prior biliary surgery).

Lab: LFTs show elevations of bilirubin and alk phos out of proportion to transaminases. The PT may be elevated due to poor vitamin K absorption, because there is no bile in gut lumen for absorption.

CA 19-9 is the most useful serum tumor marker and is elevated in more than 80% of pts (Oncology 1996;53:488).

X-ray: Ultrasound shows evidence of dilated bile ducts but often misses the lesion, especially if the lesion is in the distal bile duct. CT scan is more sensitive and may detect nodes and local invasion. MRI can be used to detect vascular encasement. Cholangiography is the gold standard. ERCP is usually the initial study done (because it is diagnostic and therapeutic), but MRCP can provide useful information if ERCP is inadequate (Nejm 1999; 341:258). PTHC can be used if drainage cannot be achieved by ERCP alone.

Endoscopy: ERCP with brushings/bx and stent placement relieves the sx associated with jaundice. In expert centers, brush or fine-needle aspiration cytology may have a diagnostic yield as high as 75% (Gut 1997;40:671), but cytology may be negative because the tumor is desmoplastic.

Rx: Surgery is the only modality that prolongs survival. The selection of pts for resection is based on characteristics of the tumor and host (Ann Oncol 1999;10:239). Many pts are unfit due to performance status, cardiopulmonary disease, or cirrhosis (Curr Probl Surg 1995;32:1). Resection is performed for intrahepatic lesions. Hilar tumors require resection with hepaticojejunostomy. Distal tumors are treated like cancers of the head of the pancreas with a pancreaticoduodenectomy (Whipple procedure). Distal lesions are more likely to be resectable (Ann Surg 1996;224:463). Liver transplant has been used for cholangiocarcinoma associated with PSC, but results have been poor and transplant earlier in the course of PSC has been proposed (Hepatology 1996;23:1105). Radiation (external beam or intraluminal) may be of very limited benefit (Gut 1996;39:852; Brit J Surg 1995;82:1522). Chemotherapy is unhelpful. Stenting palliates jaundice. Metal stents are less likely to clog and cause cholangitis, but plastic stents are cheaper. Pts with tumors >30 mm survive a mean of 3 months, and plastic is adequate. Those with smaller tumors may be better served by metal stents (Gut 1998;42:76). Photodynamic rx prolongs survival in those who fail to clear their jaundice with stenting alone (GE 2003;125:1355).

10.4 Gallbladder Cancer

Nejm 1999;341:1368

Epidem: (Am J Gastro 2000;95:1402) The mean age of dx is 65. Women are affected more than men. Rates vary widely by country. High rates are seen in Chile (13/100,000/yr), Israel, Poland, Mexico, and Bolivia. The rate in the U.S. is 2.5/100,000/yr, with rates 50% higher in whites than blacks. Important risk factors include: (1) chronic cholecystitis and gallstones (especially if >3 cm), (2) gallbladder polyps (especially solitary, sessile, echopenic lesions >10 mm), (3) anomalous junction of the pancreaticobiliary duct (where the union is outside the duodenum and there is a very long common channel and risk for gallbladder Ca may be 25% [GE 1985;89:1258]), (4) calcified gallbladder wall (porcelain gallbladder [J Clin Gastro 1989; 11:471]), (5) typhoid, (6) PSC; and (7) heavy metal exposure through occupation.

Pathophys: It is speculated that inflammation predisposes to Ca, but the mechanism is unknown.

Sx and Si: Chronic RUQ pain, fever, malaise, weight loss, or an acute bout of cholecystitis are common presentations. A few pts will have the dx made incidentally at cholecystectomy. There may be a palpable, hard mass in the RUQ.

Crs: Most pts present with advanced disease, and 5-yr survival is 5-10%. Median survival is 3 months (Am J Gastro 2000; 95:1402).

Cmplc: Biliary obstruction.

Diff Dx: The differential is usually between inflammatory and neo-plastic disease of the gallbladder once nonspecific sx have led to an imaging test. The preoperative dx is correct prior to surgery in about 50% of pts (Ann Surg 1994;219:275).

Lab: LFTs may be cholestatic if local invasion or mass effect causes obstruction.

X-ray: Mass lesions and substantial wall thickening may be evident with ultrasound. It may be impossible to distinguish inflammatory from neoplastic disease. Curable lesions are typically missed by US and CT (World J Surg 1999;23:708). CT or MRI may provide additional staging information.

Rx: Surgery is the only effective rx, but fewer than 10% of pts have resectable disease. A second resective surgery is indicated for cancers found incidentally at laparoscopic cholecystectomy unless they are stage 0 or stage 1 (Cancer 1998;83:423). Radical surgery seems of little benefit in the U.S. (Arch Surg 1990;125:237), but may show benefit in Japan (World J Surg 1991;15:337). Chemotherapy and radiation are of little value. Since the outcome for symptomatic disease is so horrible, **prophylactic cholecystectomy** is strongly recommended for porcelain gallbladder and anomalous junction of the pancreaticobiliary duct. Prophylactic cholecystectomy might be considered for pts with gallbladder polyps >1 cm, pts with gallstones >3 cm, typhoid carriers, and elderly, Native American women with gallstones (Am J Gastro 2000; 95:1402).

10.5 Ampullary Cancer

Nejm 1999;341:1368

Cancer at the ampulla of Vater is an uncommon lesion that presents with obstructive jaundice or occasionally with pancreatitis. Ampullary adenomas are precursor lesions (Gut 1991; 32:1558). Adenomas should be excised by surgery (Brit J Surg

1997;84:948) or by endoscopic snare (Gastrointest Endosc 1993; 39:127). Ampullary adenomas are more common in pts with FAP who are at risk for ampullary cancer even after colectomy. The presentation is similar to that of pancreatic cancer and the dx is generally made when ERCP is done to assess biliary obstruction and bxs are obtained. Pancreaticoduodenectomy (Whipple procedure) is done if there is no evidence of distant disease. The 5-yr survival is 40% in expert hands (Ann Surg 1998;227:821).

10.6 Gallbladder Polyps

Am J Gastro 2000;95:1402; Brit J Surg 1992;79:227

Gallbladder polyps are found in 3-6% of pts undergoing ultrasound. The most common polyp is a cholesterol polyp, a form of cholesterolosis. These lesions are generally <10 mm, do not require intervention, and if large, can be confidently identified by fine-needle aspiration (Am J Gastro 1996;91:1591). A variety of other nonneoplastic polyps have been identified. The chief concern is the possibility that a polyp will be an adenoma and develop into a carcinoma. The risk of cancer is higher if a polyp is >10 mm, solitary, sessile, echopenic on ultrasound, or associated with gallstones (Am J Gastro 2000;95:1402). The optimal management has not been determined. Some experts suggest cholecystectomy if a polyp is >10 mm and the pt is fit (Brit J Surg 1992;79:227). The alternative is serial US though the yield will be low (Gut 1996;39:860). For smaller polyps (<10 mm), serial US (q 6 months × 3 then yearly) has been suggested with cholecystectomy for polyps that enlarge (South Med J 1997;90:481). Some experts suggest that ultrasound is not needed after a stable period of 1-2 yr (Am J Surg 2004;188:186). Many clinicians ignore small polyps, especially if they are multiple and present in a pt without substantial risks for gallbladder cancer.

10.7 Sphincter of Oddi Dysfunction (Biliary Dyskinesia)

Gastro Endosc 2004;59:525; Can J Gastroenterol 2000;14:411

Epidem: The F:M ratio is 7:1 and the disorder peaks in the 40s. About 6% of pts will complain of biliary-type pain postcholecystectomy without a definable cause such as stones.

Pathophys: The sphincter of Oddi (SO) is made of muscle fibers that maintain resting tone and are a resistor to bile and pancreatic juice flow. Pts with dysfunction of the biliary portion of the sphincter experience biliary pain, often with abnormal LFTs and ductal dilatation. Those with pancreatic sphincter involvement may have recurrent pancreatitis. Pts with suspected SO dysfunction are classified on the basis of clinical findings into 3 types (Gastro Endosc 2004;59:525). **Biliary type 1** pts have biliary pain, abnormal transaminases, and a dilated bile duct on imaging studies. All these pts are thought to have SO dysfunction. **Biliary type 2** pts have pain and either a dilated bile duct or abnormal transaminases and many of these pts will have SO dysfunction if manometry is done. **Biliary type 3** pts have pain but no other abnormalities, and <10% have SO dysfunction by manometry. A similar classification (based on abnormal pancreatic enzymes and a dilated pancreatic duct) exists for pancreatic SO dysfunction. The gold standard for diagnosis is SO manometry but many experts do not use the technique because of the high frequency of pancreatitis. At manometry some pts have SO stenosis (elevated resting pressure), which may indicate a structural lesion such as fibrosis. The remaining pts have findings of an uncoordinated sphincter that is called SO dyskinesia. It is not clear if pts with intact gallbladders develop symptomatic SO dysfunction (since the gallbladder acts as a compliance reservoir to reduce pressures and therefore pain), but a response to sphincterotomy has been reported (Gastrointest Endosc 1993;39:492).

Sx: Pts usually present years after cholecystectomy with attacks of epigastric or RUQ pain sometimes associated with radiation to the back, nausea, or vomiting. The pain can be severe and last hours. In pts with involvement of the pancreatic sphincter, sx of pancreatitis may occur.

Si: Some localized tenderness may be seen in the RUQ or epigastrium, but there is no peritonitis.

Diff Dx: Common duct stones are the major consideration in type 1 pts. Intra-ampullary tumors may mimic SO dysfunction (Gastrointest Endosc 1995;42:296). The diff dx of pancreatitis needs to be considered in pts with pancreatitis as a presenting sx (p 311). The differential is broad in type 3 pts, many of whom have high levels of somatization or depression (GE 1999;116:996).

Lab: LFTs, amylase, and lipase should be obtained 3-4 hr into an attack of pain since they may be normal if done at the onset of pain.

X-ray: Biliary scintigraphy may show abnormalities such as delayed transit time from hilum to duodenum (Dig Dis Sci 1994;39: 1985). A reputedly sensitive and specific scintigraphy score has been developed (J Nucl Med 1992;33:1216). These studies may have some role in the future as a safer alternative to manometry but they have not yet been adequately validated. An abnormal ultrasound secretin test (the pancreatic duct dilates >1 mm for >20 min in response to secretin) may be an alternative to SO manometry in recurrent pancreatitis (Dig Dis Sci 1999; 44:336). MRCP is the most useful noninvasive test to exclude other structural abnormalities such as stones.

Endoscopy: MRCP or EUS is performed to look for CBDS, and to assess ductal dilatation. ERCP is generally reserved for therapeutic intent or to perform manometry (Gastro Endosc 2002; 56:803). SO manometry is performed in selected pts in some centers (see Rx). A motility catheter is placed in either the pancreatic sphincter or biliary sphincter (depending on the clinical presentation), and manometry is performed before and after injection with CCK. The risk of pancreatitis is high (8%) and even higher (29%) if the indication for the test is recurrent pancreatitis (J Gastroenterol Hepatol 1995;10:334).

Rx:

- *Biliary SO dysfunction:* If pts have SO stenosis at manometry, sphincterotomy provides sx relief (90% vs 25% in sham-treated pts in an RCT [Nejm 1989;320:82]). In contrast, those with SO motility abnormalities in the same RCT did not benefit from sphincterotomy. Nifedipine may benefit these pts (Am J Gastro 1993;88:530). All pts with type 1 dysfunction should undergo sphincterotomy, because they get good relief and manometry may be misleadingly normal (Gastrointest Endosc 1993; 39:778). Pts with type 2 dysfunction should be considered for referral to an expert center for SO manometry (which is very operator dependent) or should undergo sphincterotomy. Sphincterotomy seems more rational given the risk and limited predictive value of manometry. Type 3 pts may have pain as part of altered visceral sensitivity and are best approached with trials of anticholinergics, antidepressants, and/or calcium channel blockers. Endoscopic rx is not warranted.
- *Pancreatic SO dysfunction:* Pts with recurrent pancreatitis and SO dysfunction may benefit from biliary sphincterotomy, which is much less morbid than pancreatic sphincterotomy. However, many such pts do not benefit and go on to endoscopic pancreatic sphincterotomy often with temporary stent placement to reduce the risk of pancreatitis (Gastroenterol Clin North Am 2003;32:601).

10.8 Choledochal Cysts and Choledochocele

Lancet 1996;347:779; Ann Surg 1994;220:644

Cause: Unknown, but there may be both congenital and acquired cysts.

Epidem: In the West, 1/15,000 live births; more common in Japan.

Pathophys: There are 5 recognized types of cysts: type I (dilatation of the common bile duct), type II (bile duct diverticulum), type III (cyst of the intramural common bile duct protruding into the duodenal lumen, also called a choledochocele), type IV (multiple cysts of the intra- and/or extrahepatic bile ducts), and type V (focal dilatations of the intrahepatic bile ducts, also called Caroli's disease).

Sx: In children sx are typically pain, jaundice, and failure to thrive. Adults may have similar sx but are more likely to develop pancreatitis, bile duct stones, and gallbladder or bile duct malignancy.

Si: Usually none, but jaundice and a mass may be present.

Cmplc: Cholangiocarcinoma, pancreatitis, and bile duct stones may occur.

Diff Dx: Since these lesions are rare, they are usually not considered high on the list of causes of abdominal pain, jaundice, or pancreatitis. Once the bile duct is imaged (for whatever reason) the dx becomes evident.

Lab: Abnormal LFTs or amylase/lipase, depending on the presentation.

X-ray: MRCP is the best noninvasive test to diagnose and characterize the cysts.

Endoscopy: ERCP is reserved for pts who are thought to need endoscopic rx. Type III lesions (choledochocele) are being increasingly recognized and treated during ERCP.

Rx: Once identified, all cysts except type III should be excised with biliary bypass (Ann Surg 1994;220:644). If they are drained there is a risk of later malignancy, stones, or stricture. Type III lesions (choledochocele) can be treated with sphincterotomy (to relieve obstruction or remove stones), but the endoscopist must recognize the possibility of associated cholangiocarcinoma (Endoscopy 1995;27:233).

10.9 HIV-Related Biliary Disease

Clin Liver Dis 2004;8:213; Gastroenterol Clin North Am 1997;26:323

AIDS-related cholangitis presents with cholestatic LFTs, abdominal pain, and fever. There may be evidence of ampullary stenosis and/or radiographic findings that look like sclerosing cholangitis of the biliary tree (Am J Med 1989;86:539). The cause is unknown, though a variety of AIDS-related pathogens have been described in these pts. Rx is directed at any associated pathogen, and sphincterotomy appears effective for the pain of ampullary stenosis. Pts with HIV can develop **acalculous chole-cystitis** secondary to opportunistic infections, usually CMV, *Cryptosporidium*, or *Isospora*. The presentation is usually that of chronic RUQ pain, fever, and cholestatic LFTs due to associated biliary tree involvement. Rx is cholecystectomy though survival is short because this disorder is a late finding in AIDS (Gastro-enterol Clin North Am 1997;26:323). These disorders are becoming less frequently seen with the advent of highly active effective antiretroviral therapy (HAART).

10.10 Painful Rib Syndrome

Gut 1993;34:1006; Lancet 1980;2:632

Epidem: This condition accounts for 3-5% of gi clinic referrals in 2 series.

Pathophys: The syndrome is defined by (1) pain in the RUQ or lower chest and (2) tenderness at the costal margin that reproduces the pt's complaints. The cause of the pain is uncertain but has been attributed to abnormal mobility of the lower intercostal joints.

Sx: The pain is frequent, and often worsens with bending forward or stooping. Pts may avoid lying on the affected side. Pain is often decreased when the pt lies down or stretches. Pain may be constant or intermittent.

Si: The exam is normal except when the costal margin is palpated. Hooking the fingers under the costal margin and lifting is especially useful for reproducing the pain and convincing pts that the dx is correct.

Crs: About 70% of pts report persistent pain at a mean follow-up of 8 yr after dx. About 30% of pts had a second referral for the same pain even after a firm dx was made. For the vast majority, the pain is a nuisance and is not disabling.

Diff Dx: See "Dyspepsia," p 47.

Rx: No specific rx or testing is usually needed. In pts with refractory pain, intercostal nerve block may be helpful (Postgrad Med 1989; 86:75). Surgery to excise the offending rib has been reported (Brit J Surg 1984;71:522).

Chapter 11

Infections of the Liver

11.1 Hepatitis A

Lancet 1998;351:1643; Gastroenterologist 1996;4:107

Cause: The hep A virus, a small, nonenveloped RNA virus of the genus *Hepatovirus*. There are 4 stable human genotypes and one serotype.

Epidem: (J Infect Dis 1995;171 Suppl 1:S2) Hep A is commonly acquired before age 5 in developing nations of Africa, Asia, and Latin America, where seroprevalence is greater than 90% before adulthood. In Western nations, the seroprevalence is falling and is about 43% in the U.S. The spread is fecal–oral with secondary attack rates of about 20-50% in households. The incubation period is 15-50 days. The virus can be found in feces for about 2 weeks prior to and up to several weeks after the onset of clinical illness. Risk factors for hep A in the U.S. include (1) household or sexual contact of a pt, (2) employee or participant in daycare, (3) traveler, and (4) food (including bivalve shellfish) or water-borne outbreaks. There is no risk factor present in 45% of cases (Am Fam Phys 1996;54:107).

Pathophys: After oral ingestion, the virus is transported across the intestinal epithelium and into hepatocytes. The virus replicates within hepatocytes. Hepatocellular damage results from the host's immune response against infected cells (J Clin Lab Immunol 1993;40:47). Once jaundice occurs, viral titers fall as antibodies are produced against the virus.

Sx: A prodrome of fever, malaise, anorexia, nausea, and vomiting is usually seen in adults. The prodromal sx recede and jaundice develops. In children, the illness is usually anicteric and presents with flulike sx of pharyngitis, cough, runny nose, photophobia, and headache. Diarrhea is seen in 50% of children but is uncommon in adults.

Si: Jaundice and hepatomegaly are usually noted, but splenomegaly is less common. Spider angiomata may develop but recede after the illness. Posterior cervical nodes may be seen. A cutaneous vasculitis is rare. Impending hepatic failure may be heralded by confusion, irritability, and asterixis.

Crs: The case fatality rate is quoted at 0.35%. However, so many cases go unrecognized that this is probably an overestimate. About 70% of the fatalities occur in the 8% of pts infected after age 50. The typical course is a 3-6 month clinical illness. Jaundice usually lasts 6-8 weeks. LFTs resolve with the clinical sx. **Fulminant hepatic failure** develops in 0.14-0.35% of pts hospitalized for hep A. These pts develop worsening LFTs, markedly prolonged PT, and change in mental status. About 70-95% of them go on to develop cerebral edema, multiple organ failure, and death. **Relapsing hep A** occurs in 3-20% of all cases. These pts make an apparent clinical recovery, and weeks to months later develop recurrent illness with worsening LFTs and viral shedding. They ultimately recover (J Clin Gastro 1999;28:355). **Prolonged cholestatic hep A** is seen in 3-5% of pts. These pts have bilirubin >10 mg/dL, alk phos 3-5 times normal, and recover after an illness lasting months (Ann IM 1984;101:635).

Cmplc: Pancreatitis (Am J Gastro 1992;87:1648), renal failure (Clin Nephrol 1993;39:156), cholecystitis (Ann IM 1994;120:398), fulminant hepatic failure, Guillain-Barré syndrome (Intern Med 1994;33:799), thrombocytopenic purpura (J Clin Gastro 1993;17:166), vasculitis, and arthritis may occur.

Diff Dx: See p 42.

Lab: The diagnosis is made by demonstrating the presence of the IgM ab to hep A, which is always present during acute illness and which persists for 3-6 months. The presence of IgG ab without detectable IgM indicates prior infection and current immunity. Transaminases range from 500-5000 U/L. Bilirubin is usually less than 10 mg/dL but may go to 20 mg/dL in uncomplicated disease. A PT should be obtained as a marker of severity. Atypical lymphocytes are common.

X-ray: Ultrasound or MRCP may be indicated if obstructive jaundice is a clinical question.

Rx: In most pts the rx is on an outpatient basis with abstinence from alcohol, moderate activity, and diet as tolerated. Bed rest is unnecessary (Nejm 1969;281:1421). Enteric precautions to minimize household spread are crucial.

Two **vaccines** are commercially available in the U.S., and others are under development. They are killed, attenuated virus vaccines that induce an antibody response in almost all healthy pts within a month. Havrix or VAQTA are given to adults in a dose of 1.0 mL im, followed by a booster of 1.0 mL 6-12 months later. They are indicated for travelers to endemic areas, those who live in endemic areas (including many American states), pts with chronic liver disease (especially hepatitis C [Nejm 1998; 338:286]), pts with clotting disorders (because of concentrated blood product use), in community outbreaks, for men who have sex with men, and for illicit drug users. Other high-risk occupations might be targeted (sewage workers, daycare workers). Universal vaccination has been proposed but many practical barriers exist. A combination hep A and hep B vaccine (Twinrix) in a dose of 1.0 mL at 0, 1, and 6 months may be useful for adults needing both vaccines. The vaccine can also be used to prevent secondary spread (NNT=18 to prevent one secondary case)

(Lancet 1999;353:1136), but a direct comparison to immuno-globulin in this setting has not been done.

Prophylaxis with immunoglobulin is used for postexposure prophylaxis of household contacts and as primary prevention in infants where vaccine experience is limited. Immunoglobulin is given in a dose of 0.02 mL/kg as a single im injection as soon as the index case is recognized (Am Fam Phys 1996;54:107). It provides protection if given within 2 weeks of exposure and lasts about 4-6 weeks. Doses of 0.06 mL/kg provide protection for travelers for up to 6 months, but vaccine is preferable.

11.2 Hepatitis B

Clin Gastroenterol Hepatol 2004;2:87; Lancet 2003;362:2089; Ann IM 2000;132:723

Cause: The hep B virus, a DNA virus of the hepadnaviridae family. The virus is made up of a circular, partly double-stranded piece of DNA that is surrounded by a core called the nucleocapsid, which is then surrounded by an envelope. The envelope is antigenic (the hep B surface antigen or HBsAg) and the nucleocapsid is antigenic (the hep B core antigen or HBcAg). Immunity to HBsAg is protective and is the basis of natural and vaccine-induced immunity. The hep B e antigen (HBeAg) is derived from the core gene, which is modified and exported from liver cells. It is a marker for active replication of virus and is seen in pts with circulating hep B viral DNA.

Epidem: In endemic areas (Africa, Southeast Asia, China), 50% of the population become infected and 8% become chronic carriers. Infection is spread from mother to neonate (vertical transmission) or from child to child. In low-prevalence areas (North America, Europe), disease is spread sexually between young adults. Other risks in developed nations are iv drug use, occupational exposure, blood exposure, dialysis, or nosocomial transmis-

sion (Nejm 1992;326:721). About 20-30% of pts have no identified risk. Transmission from infected surgeons to pts has been
reported (Nejm 1997;336:178). The U.S. prevalence is 0.35% for
chronic infection and 5% for lifetime risk of infection. Hep B is
the leading cause of cirrhosis and hepatocellular carcinoma
worldwide.

Pathophys: Clinical hepatitis is the result of the host response to viral
antigens presented on the surface of hepatocytes. If the match
between the host T cell repertoire and the antigens expressed on
hepatocytes is good, immune activation results. In this case the
infected hepatocytes are cleared, the circulating infective virions
are neutralized by anti-HBs and the host clears the infection. If
the immune response is inadequate, infection persists. For the
first 2-4 weeks of adult infection, there is viral replication but no
hepatocyte destruction since the immune response has not been
developed. Levels of viral DNA are high and HBsAg is present,
but the patient is not sick and ALT is normal. When the immune
response is activated, DNA levels drop, hepatocytes are killed,
the ALT rises, and the patient becomes ill. This usually lasts a
few weeks if the patient has the typical acute hepatitis, but in
those destined for chronic hepatitis, this destructive process lasts
for yr and results in cirrhosis. When the immune response eliminates infected cells, viral replication stops, viral DNA falls
markedly (though small amounts may be found by PCR), and
HBeAg disappears. At this stage, the viral genome integrates into
the host DNA, causing expression of HBsAg on hepatocytes. Pts
diagnosed at this stage are commonly called "healthy carriers,"
though this term may be misleading because many of them may
have substantial liver disease. Finally, anti-HBs appears and the
host is protected from activation of infection or new infection.

To be considered a **healthy carrier** (recently renamed **inactive carrier**), pts should have no sx, normal ALT, no evidence of
HBeAg or hep B viral DNA and, ideally, a normal or near

normal liver bx (Hepatology 1987;7:758). These pts do not require antiviral rx but need to be monitored to determine if the disease flares (with viral replication) and to consider evaluation for HCC. The majority of such pts in the West (where disease is often acquired horizontally) do well and appear to be at minimal risk for HCC (GE 1994;106:1000; Ann IM 1993;118:191). Healthy carriers in areas endemic for neonatal transmission (Taiwan, Japan, and Alaska) have a high risk of HCC (Hepatology 1987;7:764).

Mutations occur in all regions of the genome. **Mutant viruses** have been identified with severe disease and in asymptomatic carriers. The precore mutants do not make HBeAg, and replicative infections may escape laboratory detection unless DNA levels are obtained (Gut 1993;34:1).

Sx: Most pts with acute hep B have a subclinical illness. Those with clinically detectable illness usually present with jaundice, malaise, anorexia, and fever. Those with chronic hep B are usually asymptomatic but may complain of fatigue or malaise.

Si: In acute infection, jaundice, tender hepatomegaly, and fever. There may be stigmata of chronic liver disease (p 42).

Crs: Most adult pts have an acute hepatitis that clears within 6 months. About 3-5% develop chronic hepatitis. Up to half of acutely infected adults are symptomatic. Pts are said to have chronic hepatitis if they have HBsAg detectable in the serum for more than 6 months or have HBsAg with no evidence of IgM anti-HBc. About 95% of infected neonates and 30% of children under age 6 have an asymptomatic illness that becomes chronic. Those adults with chronic hepatitis have a risk of progression to cirrhosis of 20% at 4 yr (Gut 1991;32:294). Fulminant hepatitis with coagulopathy, encephalopathy, and cerebral edema occurs in <1% of cases of acute hep B (Nejm 1993;329:1862). Any of the complications of end-stage liver disease may occur (p 429). Pts with concurrent hep C infection have aggressive liver disease, but HIV-infected pts do not have more severe liver disease than those not infected (Ann IM 1992;117:837).

Cmplc: Hep D (Delta) infection, a passenger virus that requires hep B for replication and causes severe liver disease (p 377). HCC (p 413) complicates long-standing hep B infection. It usually occurs in those with cirrhosis 25-30 yr after the onset of infection. Polyarteritis nodosa (HTN, eosinophilia, abdominal pain, rash, polyarthritis, and necrotizing vasculitis involving gut, kidneys, and CNS) is a rare but serious complication of hep B infection (Lupus 1998;7:238). Glomerulonephritis (Ann IM 1989; 111:479) and leukocytoclastic vasculitis (J Clin Gastroenterol 1995;21:42) are uncommon complications.

Diff Dx: See p 42.

Lab: **Acute infection** is diagnosed by the presence of HBsAg and IgM anti-HBc in the serum. In some very early cases, IgM anti-HBc may be absent, and it becomes positive later in the course. In those recovering from acute infection, IgM core disappears while the IgG core ab appears. HBsAg is cleared in about 24 weeks and anti-HBs appears about 8 weeks later, indicating complete recovery and future immunity. During the gap between the disappearance of HBsAg and the appearance of anti-HBs (the window), the dx is made by the presence of IgM anti-HBc. IgG antibody to the core antigen (anti-HBc) develops and usually lasts a lifetime. If IgM anti-HBc is present, the patient has likely been recently infected, because the IgM fraction usually clears within 8 months of infection. A small number of pts with a flare of chronic hep B will produce IgM anti-HBc. HBeAg is present during acute infection and clears early in the illness. In **chronic infection,** HBsAg is present in the serum for a period of greater than 6 months (by definition). The IgM anti-HBc is usually absent. The HBeAg is present and DNA levels are high when viral replication is high. The precore mutants may produce active infection but do not make the HBeAg and may escape laboratory detection unless DNA levels are checked. These pts are said to have HBeAg negative chronic hepatitis B.

Liver bx in cases of chronic hepatitis shows variable portal zone inflammation, focal hepatocyte necrosis, and ground glass hepatocytes (containing HBsAg). As the degree of injury progresses, there is more severe necroinflammatory change with eventual bridging or multiacinar fibrosis (Am J Clin Pathol 2000;113:40). Older descriptive terms such as "chronic persistent hepatitis" or "chronic active hepatitis" are no longer used. Instead, pathologists describe the degree of both inflammation and fibrosis (categorized as mild, moderate, marked, and very marked). The histologic patterns have no correlation with sx. The utility of bx is debatable, because the decision to treat is based on evidence of viral replication rather than histology. However, the bx does have value for staging the disease.

Rx: (Clin Gastroenterol Hepatol 2004;2:87)
- *Acute hep B:* There is no specific rx of acute infection. Precautions are taken against household, sexual, or other blood-borne spread (no sharing of utensils, razors, toothbrushes, or common bathing). There is no reason to restrict activity. Pts are followed for the development of complications suggesting decompensated liver disease.
- *Inactive carriers:* Monitoring with ALT q 6-12 months is recommended. If ALT rises DNA levels are obtained and the pt is further evaluated. Screening for HCC may be considered (p 413).
- *Chronic hep B without cirrhosis:* Hepatocytes with replicating virus are the target of the host-mediated immune destruction that causes fibrosis. Therefore, the goal of rx is to convert replicative infection into nonreplicative infection. Success is determined by the loss of HBeAg and measurable viral DNA in serum (seroconversion). Most successfully treated pts will continue to have HBsAg in serum, but their infection is no

longer replicative and destructive. All pts being considered for rx should have detectable HBsAg and measurable viral DNA in the serum (usually at levels $>10^5$ copies/mL). Pts with lower levels of DNA may still have significant disease and liver bx may be helpful in identifying the need to treat. DNA levels and ALT should be monitored q 6 month in those with low levels of DNA and normal ALT who are not initially treated.

The current choices of rx are interferon α-2b or the nucleoside analogs lamivudine and adefovir. **Interferon α-2b** is most effective in pts with high ALTs (>200 U/L) and low levels of viral DNA. These pts usually have active-looking hepatitis on bx. Meta-analysis indicates that about 33% of treated pts vs 12% of controls will clear HBeAg within 3-6 months of rx (Ann IM 1993;119:312). Pts who respond have a better long-term survival and fewer complications (Nejm 1996;334:1422). Typically a dose of 5 million units sc qd (or 10 million units tiw) for 16 weeks is given. Treated pts must have well-compensated liver disease since rx may cause a severe flare (BMJ 1993;306:107). Side effects can be difficult (p 374).

Lamivudine or **adefovir** should be used in pts who do not have the high ALT or low viral DNA levels that are associated with a good response to interferon. They are often preferred as first-line rx because of tolerability; this includes pts who would be candidates for interferon. Lamivudine and adefovir are easier to use and less expensive than interferon. Both are good choices for pts with normal ALT, decompensated cirrhosis, or HBeAg-negative (precore) mutants. Lamivudine is a nucleoside analog that inhibits reverse transcriptase and decreases replication. At a dose of 100 mg per day, about 17% of pts will clear HBeAg after 1 yr, and most will have histologic improvement (Nejm 1998; 339:61). Pts who fail to convert should continue rx because 10% will likely seroconvert in the next yr (GE 2000;119:172). Lamivudine-resistant mutants (called YMDD mutants) emerge in up to a third of pts after 1 yr of rx and cause a flare of hepatitis

(Hepatology 1999;30:567). Pts should be monitored at least every six months for a rise in DNA level and ALT that might indicate the emergence of a mutant strain and a need to change rx. Lamivudine is well tolerated, with side effects of nausea, anorexia, anemia, leukopenia, and neuropathy. Pts who become HBeAg and DNA negative can stop rx after an additional 6 months. Those who lose HBeAg but have stable detectable levels of DNA might also stop rx after 6 additional months but are at greater risk of reactivation.

Adefovir has similar efficacy to lamivudine but the development of resistant mutants is uncommon. In a dose of 10 mg daily, side effects are similar to those of placebo. Weakness, abdominal pain, and headache are the most common side effects. Renal toxicity has been seen at higher doses. Adefovir is the drug of choice for lamivudine resistance (GE 2004;126:81). Duration of therapy is determined as described for lamivudine. Combination rx and use of other nucleosides are under investigation.

Pts with chronic hep B should receive **hep A vaccine** (p 361).

- *Rx of cirrhotics:* Both compensated and decompensated cirrhotics should be treated with lamivudine or adefovir. Adefovir is probably the better choice because cirrhotics may not withstand a flare of disease due to the emergence of lamivudine resistant mutants.
- *Screening for hepatocellular carcinoma:* See p 413.
- *Passive immunization:* Serum containing high titers of anti-HBs can be used to create an enriched IgG preparation called HBIG. It is used for postexposure prophylaxis (usually with vaccine) for newborns of infected mothers, those with exposure to HBsAg-positive blood or body fluids, and those infected pts receiving a transplant.
- *Vaccination:* (Nejm 2004;351:2832) Vaccines are prepared with yeast by recombinant techniques. A series of 3 im injections

produces immunity in >90% of young adults. It is less effective in the elderly, in pts on hemodialysis, and in the immunocompromised. Combination of vaccine with HBIG is 79-98% effective in preventing chronic infection in newborns of HBeAg-positive women (Clin Microbiol Rev 1999;12:351). Though levels of anti-HBs become very low in most pts over yr, protection against clinically apparent acute infection or chronic infection persists. Booster doses are not recommended (except in dialysis pts [Am J Kidney Dis 1998;32:1041]). Vaccine in the U.S. is currently suggested for (1) all high-risk adults, (2) infants (to prevent childhood acquisition), and (3) adolescents who were not vaccinated as children so that they can be immune before they reach the age of high-risk sexual and drug using behavior. Two recombinant vaccines are available. The recommended adult doses are Engerix-B 20 mg or Recombivax 10 mg in 3 im doses at months 0, months 1-2, and months 6-12. A combination hep A and hep B vaccine (Twinrix) in a dose of 1.0 mL at 0, 1, and 6 months may be useful for adults needing both vaccines. Postvaccine testing for anti-HBs is needed only for high-risk groups (such as health care workers, dialysis pts, men who have sex with men).

- *Transplantation:* (Ann IM 1997;126:805) Pts undergoing liver transplant for hep B have diminished survival (73% at 1 yr, 44% at 5 yr) compared to those who undergo liver transplant for other indications. They also have a high incidence of recurrent infection (90%), especially if they have markers of active replication (HBeAg and viral DNA) at the time of transplant. Pts with fulminant hep B and those who are negative for markers of viral replication do well and are good candidates for transplant. The combination of lamivudine and HBIG appears to be the most promising for prevention of recurrence (Hepatology 1998;28:585).

11.3 Hepatitis C

Jama 2003;289:2413; Lancet 2003;362:2095; Ann IM 2000;132:296

Cause: The hepatitis C virus (HCV) is an RNA virus of the flavivirus family. The nucleotide sequence shows substantial variations and 6 genotypes (numbered 1 to 6), and more than 50 subtypes (designated by a letter, eg, a or b) have been identified. Genotypes 1a and 1b are the most common in the U.S., and, along with genotype 4, they are the most difficult to treat. A single individual may show variations in the sequences of the genotype that infects them (referred to as quasispecies). These may arise from mutations in response to immune surveillance.

Epidem: In developed nations the seroprevalence is 1-2%, with rates higher in Africa, Eastern Europe, and Egypt. Transfused blood was formerly a major risk, but that risk has dropped to about 1/100,000 in units completely tested (Nejm 1996;334:1685). Intravenous drug abuse is the major risk factor. Intranasal cocaine and ear piercing among males are also associated with infection (Nejm 1996;334:1691). Multiple sexual partners are also a risk factor, but the disease is not readily transmitted sexually (Hepatology 1997;26:66S). The rate of vertical transmission is less than 5% (Nejm 1994;330:744; Obstet Gynecol 1999; 94:1044). Iatrogenic spread from surgeons (Nejm 1996;334:555), needles, and organ transplantation does occur, as does spread from human bites (Lancet 1990;336:503). The risk to a health worker following needle-stick injury from an infected patient is up to 7% (MMWR Morb Mortal Wkly Rep 1998;47:1). In some studies as many as 25% have no identified risk, but 5-10% is probably closer to the truth.

Pathophys: The virus enters by deliberate injection or inadvertent breakdown of a normal barrier such as skin or mucous membranes. The virus is then taken up by hepatocytes and replication begins. There is both a humoral and cell-mediated response to infection but the immune response is usually ineffective. The development of mutant quasispecies or the effects of other HCV proteins may be important in the escape from immune clearance. The inadequate immune response not only fails to clear the virus but also causes the destruction of liver parenchyma and ultimately causes cirrhosis.

Sx: Most pts are asymptomatic or have nonspecific sx such as fatigue or joint aches (Am J Gastro 1999;94:1355). Jaundice is rare and may be seen with acute infection. In advanced disease there may be jaundice, ascites, or encephalopathy.

Si: Usually none except in advanced disease, in which signs of cirrhosis or liver failure may be present (p 42).

Crs: (Hepatology 2000;31:1014) Studies of the natural hx of hep C are hampered by short duration follow-up, retrospective design, and referral bias. About 70-85% of infected pts appear to develop a chronic hepatitis. Cirrhosis develops in perhaps 5-15% of pts per 20 yr of infection (Clin Gastroenterol Hepatol 2004; 2:183). About 6% of pts develop decompensated liver disease, 4% develop HCC, and 3.6% die as consequence of infection. Alcohol consumption of >35-50 g/day, infection after the age of 50, male gender, obesity, and HIV coinfection increase the risk of fibrosis (Lancet 2003;362:2095). Most pts die of causes other than liver disease.

Some groups have a different course. A cohort of young Irish women infected from anti-D immune globulin had only a 2% rate of cirrhosis at 17 yr (Nejm 1999;340:1228). About 50% of children infected during cardiac surgery clear the virus over 20 yr (Nejm 1999;341:866). Pts with normal transaminases have a slower rate of progression of fibrosis (Hepatology 1998;27:868). Any of the complications of end-stage liver disease may occur (p 429).

Cmplc: Cirrhosis with hepatic failure, ascites, and encephalopathy. Hepatocellular carcinoma (p 413) develops in 4% of infected pts, usually after the development of cirrhosis. Porphyria cutanea tarda (Hepatology 1992;16:1322), mixed cryoglobulinemia (Ann IM 1992;117:573), and glomerulonephritis are well established extrahepatic complications (Ann IM 1995;123:615).

Diff Dx: See p 42.

Lab: The dx is usually established by the detection of anti-HCV antibodies using an enzyme immunoassay that is highly sensitive and specific to multiple HCV antigens. With the improvement in sensitivity and specificity of the immunoassays, RIBA testing for antibodies to specific HCV proteins is rarely needed. In pts being considered for rx it is important to confirm the presence of virus itself in blood by PCR or branched DNA testing. The viral load and genotype are determined prior to beginning rx. Genotype determines the duration of rx and the fall in viral load at 12 weeks is used in the early identification of pts destined to fail rx. Those with a positive HCV ab test but negative PCR probably have cleared their infections.

Liver bx in hepatitis C shows variable degrees of portal inflammation, largely with lymphocytes, periportal interface hepatitis (formerly called "piecemeal necrosis"), inflammation, bile duct degeneration without bile duct loss, and steatosis. As with hepatitis B, biopsies are classified on a 4-point severity scale for the degree of inflammation and the degree of fibrosis. This system has replaced the old terminology that used terms such as "chronic active hepatitis" and "chronic persistent hepatitis." Bx provides information about the stage of disease and prognosis but typically does not effect initial decisions regarding rx. It may be helpful in deciding whether to treat pts with relative contraindications to rx such as depression and in those with a persistently normal ALT who are at lower risk for fibrosis. In pts who have difficulty with drug side effects, this information may help in deciding whether to continue with rx (for those with nasty looking bx) or stop rx (for milder looking bx). Liver bx has risks (p 464) and rx without bx may be more cost effective (Jama 1998;280:2088).

Rx: (Am J Med 2004;117:344)

- *General measures:* Infected pts should avoid alcohol, because no safe level of alcohol consumption has been established. Vaccines should be given for prevention of hep A, which is very morbid in pts with hep C (Nejm 1998;338:286), and for hep B.

- *Selecting candidates for antiviral rx:* The underlying but unproven assumption is that clearing viremia will result in improved outcomes. Rx is considered appropriate for adults who have persistently abnormal ALT, detectable viral RNA in serum, and evidence of inflammation or fibrosis on bx. Biopsy is not universally used in selecting rx, because pts with mild looking bx may progress to cirrhosis, and pts with mild disease respond best to rx. Pts with well compensated cirrhosis respond reasonably well to rx, but the appropriate rx for decompensated cirrhosis is unknown. Pts with persistently normal transaminases represent a group who fare better (Hepatology 1998; 27:868) and may not require rx. Some experts bx these pts and offer them rx if there is inflammation or fibrosis on bx. The elderly are more likely to die of causes other than liver disease and are treated very selectively. Pts being considered for rx should have lab studies to look for other causes of abnormal LFTs (p 43), should be offered bx for staging of disease, and should be assessed for contraindications to rx. Combination rx with interferon/ribavirin is contraindicated in severe psychiatric illness, decompensated liver disease, renal failure, pregnancy, active autoimmune illnesses, hemolytic anemia, seizures, CAD, CHF, COPD, and in unstable social situations (Jama 2003;289:2413).

- *Interferon/ribavirin for initial rx:* Ribavirin is a nucleoside analog that has antiviral effects but is ineffective as monotherapy.

Interferons (which are glycoproteins normally produced by leukocytes in response to infection) have antiviral properties but are a disappointing monotherapy. Standard rx has become the combination of ribavirin with pegylated interferon. Both pegylated interferon α-2b and α-2a are effective, and there are no convincing data that demonstrate that one is better than the other.

For **genotype 1** pts, 48 weeks of rx with weight-based dosing of ribavirin (1000 mg for pts <75 kg and 1200 mg for those >75 kg) and either 180 μg of pegylated interferon α-2a or 1.5 μg/kg of pegylated interferon α-2b are used. If viral load has not dropped by 2 logs or greater after 12 weeks then rx is stopped because chance of a sustained response is <2% (Hepatology 2002;36:S145). Viral load is rechecked at 24 weeks and rx is continued only if the virus is undetectable. Viral load is rechecked at the conclusion of rx and 24 weeks later. A sustained response (those without detectable virus 24 weeks after stopping rx) will be seen in >50% of pts.

For **genotype 2 or 3** pts, only 800 mg of ribavirin and 24 weeks of therapy are needed to achieve sustained response rates of about 80%.

• *Side effects:* Ribavirin causes predictable hemolytic anemia, with mean decrease in Hgb of 2-3 gm, that stabilizes in the first 4 weeks. In 5% of pts, the level may drop below 9.6 gm/dL. Ribavirin is teratogenic and contraception must be assured. Ribavirin may cause cough, dyspnea, rash, nausea, anorexia, and weight loss. Adverse reactions to interferon are frequent. Flulike sx after injection are common and are treated with acetaminophen and hydration. Depression, anxiety, and insomnia may require medical therapy. Depression is the most common reason for stopping rx, and it may occur in up to 50% of treated pts (Hepatology 2000;31:1207). Nausea, anorexia, and weight loss are common. Alopecia usually reverses on stopping rx. Neutropenia and thrombocytopenia are detected by routine lab monitoring. Hyperthyroidism or hypothyroidism occurs in about 3% (GE 1992;102:2155), and diabetes is a rare complication.

- *Treatment failures:* About half of pts who relapse after a response to interferon alone will have sustained virologic response to combination rx. Those who do not respond at all to interferon have a very poor response to combination rx (about 8% sustained response) (GE 2000;118:S104). Pts who failed ribavirin and nonpegylated interferon can be offered weight-based ribavirin and pegylated interferon. Pts who relapse or don't respond to combination weight-based pegylated rx can be offered rx within a clinical trial or be considered for maintenance interferon monotherapy if advanced fibrosis is seen on liver bx (see "Pts with advanced fibrosis or cirrhosis," later in this list).

- *Acute hepatitis C:* No precise definition exists for this disorder, which represent a mix of pts detected because of acute sx of liver disease or exposure to pts with hep C. Spontaneous clearance appears common in symptomatic pts (50% at 12 weeks) and the response rate to therapy is high (GE 2003;125:80). Pts without sx are more likely to develop chronic infection. A 3-6 month period of watchful waiting is probably reasonable prior to initiating rx (GE 2003;125:253).

- *HIV coinfected pts:* Response rates to combination rx using pegylated interferon α-2a and ribavirin are 40%, which is lower than that seen in pts without HIV infection (Nejm 2004;351:438).

- *Pts with advanced fibrosis or cirrhosis:* Pooled data from controlled trials suggest that the rate of fibrosis progression is lowered by rx even if viral clearance is not achieved. Several controlled trials are under way to determine if maintenance monotherapy with pegylated interferon can prevent progression of cirrhosis and hepatocellular carcinoma (Am J Med 2004;117:344).

- *Transplant:* (Semin Gastrointest Dis 2000;11:96) Hep C is now the leading reason for liver transplantation in the U.S. Infection of the graft is almost universal. Interferon and ribavirin combined and used as a prophylactic may be the best course, but studies are lacking (Am J Gastroenterol 2000; 95:2164). Despite the high reinfection rate, survival after transplant is similar to that seen in other chronic liver diseases (Nejm 1996;334:815).

- *Prevention and screening:* (MMWR Morb Mortal Wkly Rep 1998;47:1; Hepatology 1997;26:2S) Universal precautions are used in the health care setting. An NIH consensus conference suggested that changes in sexual practices are unnecessary for couples in a monogamous relationship. Razors and toothbrushes should not be shared. Pregnancy is not contraindicated and breastfeeding appears safe. The CDC recommends hep C testing in those who have used illegal injectable drugs, who have used clotting factor concentrates prior to 1987, who have received transfusions or organ transplants prior to July 1992, who are children born to hep C positive women, who are dialysis pts, who have elevated ALT, and who are workers with exposure incidents (MMWR Morb Mortal Wkly Rep 1998; 47:1). However, citing the lack of data on health outcomes of pts likely to be detected by screening, the U.S. Preventive Services Task Force found the data insufficient to recommend for or against screening of high-risk groups (Ann IM 2004; 140:465).

- *Hepatocellular carcinoma:* A sustained virologic response to interferon lowers the risk of HCC (Ann IM 1998;129:94). An RCT showed that rx with interferon reduced the risk of HCC from 38% to 4% in treated cirrhotic pts despite the fact that only 16% of pts cleared virus with rx (Lancet 1995;346:1051). Many experts screen their pts with periodic ultrasound and α-fetoprotein determinations, but there are no outcome data to support this approach in hepatitis C.

11.4 Other Causes of Viral Hepatitis

Hepatitis D (Delta Hepatitis): (Jama 1989;261:1321) The hep D virus is a defective RNA virus that requires hep B virus to replicate. Hep D infection occurs only in pts who are coinfected with hep B. In the West, the infection is seen largely in pts with risk factors such as iv drug use or hemophilia with multiple transfusions (Hepatology 1985;5:188). With effective prevention of hep B, the incidence of new delta infections in Western countries is dropping (GE 1999;117:161). Pts simultaneously infected with hep B and hep D usually recover without sequelae. More serious illness occurs when pts with chronic hep B become superinfected with hep D and severe progressive liver disease may result (Jama 1989;261:1321). Hep D infection should be considered in any pt with chronic hep B who develops unexplained jaundice, in pts with prolonged or severe apparent acute infection, and in those being considered for rx for chronic hep B. In cases of superinfection, the majority progress to clinically overt cirrhosis, but a minority have long survival with mild disease (GE 1999; 117:161). The dx is made by the detection of anti-hep D ab in pts with evidence of chronic hep B infection. In cases where the infection is rapidly cleared, the antibody response may be late and weak, but in the case of chronic infection, the antibody response is strong (Lancet 1987;1:478). Doses of interferon typically used in hep B are ineffective in hep D (Hepatology 1991; 13:1052). Higher doses (9 million U tiw) improve histology and long-term outcome (GE 2004;126:1740). Lamivudine is ineffective (Hepatology 1999;30:546).

Hepatitis E: (Epidemiol Rev 1999;21:162; Gastroenterol Clin North Am 1994;23:537) The hep E virus is an RNA virus of the calicivirus family. The disease occurs in epidemic forms and endemically in developing nations with poor sanitation. The spread is usually through water contaminated with feces. It most commonly effects pts 15 to 40 yr old. There are animal reservoirs, and zoonotic transmission has been documented (Lancet 2003;362:371). The clinical features are similar to those of hep A, and subclinical infection may occur. The dx should be considered in pts returning from endemic areas who develop jaundice without other etiology within the typical 2-9-week incubation period. Mortality rate is low (0.5-4.0%), except in pregnant women, who have fatality rates of 10-42% (mean 20%). Hep E does not lead to chronic hepatitis. Immunoassays for anti-hep E ab and PCR techniques may be used but are not commercially available. Testing may be obtained through the CDC in the U.S. Travel to endemic areas during pregnancy seems ill advised.

Hepatitis F: This virus has been described in a handful of cases in France, and its significance is unknown (J Virol 1994;68:7810).

Hepatitis G: (J Clin Gastroenterol 1997;24:62) The hep G virus was originally derived from a patient with community-acquired chronic hepatitis and was later shown to be 95% homologous with another virus called the "G.B." virus. The latter virus was derived from the plasma of a surgeon with initials G.B. and was transmitted to tamarin monkeys. In later yr 3 viruses were isolated from the tamarins, 2 of which were tamarin-derived (called the A and B viruses). The third virus isolated was named hep GB virus-C (HGBV-C). This results in confusing terminology, but the HGV and HGBV-C are the same RNA virus. The virus is found in 1-2% of U.S. blood donors and in much higher frequencies in hemophiliacs, iv drug users, and hemodialysis pts (Nejm 1996;334:1485). It can be transmitted by transfusion or vertically. It is not clear if this virus causes clinical illness. The vast majority of infected pts have no liver disease. The virus may be a causative agent in some cases of viral hepatitis or may simply be an innocent bystander to some other unknown cause of hepatitis (Nejm 1997;336:741; Nejm 1996;334:1536). The virus can only be detected by PCR. No practical serologic test exists.

Epstein-Barr Virus (EBV): Adolescents and young adults infected with EBV may present with sx and si suggestive of acute viral hepatitis, but other clues that lead to the dx of infectious mononucleosis are usually present. Older adults are less likely to have the pharyngitis and lymphadenopathy that suggest the dx. Pts over age 40 develop jaundice >25% of the time (Nejm 1999; 340:1228). Transaminases and bilirubin are elevated in 90% of patients, but levels are usually only 2-3 times normal. A heterophil ab test is usually positive, but IgM antibodies to EBV capsid antigens are more specific. A severe hepatitis (Am J Gastroenterol 1999;94:236) or fulminant hepatic failure (Liver Transpl Surg 1998;4:469) may occur.

Cytomegalovirus (CMV): This agent can cause a hepatitis similar to that of EBV though jaundice is much less common (Medicine 1986;65:124). The dx is made by the CMV-IgM test or by culture of urine and blood.

11.5 Hepatic Schistosomiasis

Am J Gastro 1991;86:1658

Five species of schistosomes cause human disease, and 200 million people are infected worldwide. Infection occurs by exposure to cercaria released by the freshwater snail host. The cercaria penetrate the skin, develop into worms, and migrate to the mesenteric vessels where eggs are laid and carried to the liver. Liver injury occurs from the inflammatory response to the eggs, and the severity depends on the worm burden and host factors. Pts may have pain, fever, diarrhea, hepatosplenomegaly, or evidence of portal HTN or variceal hemorrhage. The dx should be suspected in any patient from an endemic area (the Middle East, Saudi Arabia, Egypt, Africa, South America [especially Brazil or Venezuela], the Caribbean, the Philippines, and the Far East) who presents with these findings. The dx is made by finding eggs in feces or tissue (especially rectal bx) specimens. Liver involvement may be too patchy to make bx reliable for dx. Low attenuation branching structures (due to periportal fibrosis) may be seen on CT. Praziquantel is the usual rx.

11.6 Pyogenic Liver Abscess

Curr Opin Gastroenterol 2000;16:251

Pathophys: For discussion of amebic liver abscess see p 275. In the preantibiotic era, most liver abscess was caused by pylephlebitis (inflammation or infection of the portal vein or its tributaries) due to intraabdominal infection. Now biliary tract infection and idiopathic cases are more frequent (Surg Gynecol Obstet 1992;174:97). Endocarditis and trauma can be associated conditions. Common causative organisms include enteric gram-negative organisms (eg, *E. coli, Klebsiella*), group D *Streptococcus*, and *Staphylococcus*. More than half of isolates are polymicrobial and contain anaerobes (J Med Microbiol 1998;47:1075).

Sx/Si: The presentation is usually insidious, with malaise, anorexia, RUQ pain, and fever.

Crs: Mortality is about 10-20% and is usually seen in pts with significant comorbidities such as malignancy (Ann Surg 1990; 212:655).

Cmplc: Uncontrolled sepsis, death.

Diff Dx: The disease is usually discovered when the liver is imaged in the investigation of nonspecific abdominal sx.

Lab: Elevations in alk phos occur in >70%, but jaundice is rare in the absence of biliary obstruction. Leukocytosis is common.

X-ray: CT scanning is very sensitive (95-100%), and ultrasound is somewhat less so (South Med J 1993;86:1233).

Endoscopy: ERCP/MRCP should be considered in any patient with stones, biliary dilatation, or persistent cholestatic LFTs because of the high frequency of biliary tract disease in this group (Gastrointest Endosc 1999;50:340).

Rx: Broad-spectrum antibiotics covering the range of possible organisms in Pathophys are given pending culture results. Antibiotics are changed based on culture results and continued until CT suggests resolution or a stable appearance (in some cases CT never normalizes and a cyst remains). The mainstay of rx is percutaneous drainage (though some pts may be cured with antibiotics alone [GE 1979;77:618]). Catheter drainage is more effective than simple aspiration (by RCT [AJR Am J Roentgenol 1998; 170:1035]). Surgical rx is indicated when percutaneous methods fail or are not possible due to multiple or multiloculated abscesses.

Chapter 12

Metabolic and Inflammatory Liver Disease

12.1 Nonalcoholic Fatty Liver Disease and Nonalcoholic Steatohepatitis

Nejm 2002;346:1221; Mayo Clin Proc 2000;75:733; Ann IM 1997;126:137

Epidem: The prevalence of nonalcoholic fatty liver disease (NAFLD) is estimated between 10 and 24%. NAFLD is a spectrum of disease ranging from steatosis, to steatohepatitis, to advanced fibrosis and cirrhosis in the absence of substantial alcohol intake. Nonalcoholic steatohepatitis (NASH) is part of the spectrum of NAFLD that is found in 3% of lean pts and up to 20% of obese pts in Western countries. There is a predominance of middle-aged women with this disorder. Obesity, diabetes, and hyperlipidemia are commonly associated. However, the disease is not limited to pts with these risk factors (GE 1994;107:1103). A picture of steatosis with or without inflammation and fibrosis can be seen with starvation, TPN use, rapid weight loss, bariatric surgery, inherited metabolic defects, and a variety of drugs. These secondary causes of fatty liver disease all have unique clinical characteristics that are not further discussed here.

Pathophys: NASH is diagnosed when 3 criteria are met: (1) a liver bx shows macrovesicular fatty change and lobular or portal inflammation, with or without fibrosis; (2) there is convincing evidence

of <40 gm per week of alcohol use (about 4 drinks per week; see
p 421); and (3) there is no evidence of active infection with hep
B or C or a secondary cause of steatosis (Hepatology 1990;11:74).
Fatty liver (simple steatosis) is diagnosed when there is fatty
change without inflammation or fibrosis. The pathogenesis of
NAFLD is unknown. The accumulation of lipids in hepatocytes
in association with insulin resistance appears to be an important
first step. The progression from simple steatosis to steatosis with
inflammation and fibrosis may be the result of oxidative stress on
hepatocytes.

Sx: Most pts have no sx but some may have fatigue or RUQ
discomfort.

Si: Hepatomegaly is common. A minority present with signs of
advanced liver disease (p 42).

Cmplc: Any of the complications of end-stage liver disease may occur
(p 429).

Crs: Half of pts with NASH have stable disease over a period of yr and
the remainder have histologic worsening. About 15% of pts
progress to cirrhosis. Survival is similar to that of age-matched
controls (GE 1994;107:1103). Since there is a higher than
expected proportion of obese, diabetic females who are pts with
apparent cryptogenic cirrhosis, it has been recently postulated
that NASH is an unrecognized cause of cryptogenic cirrhosis
(Hepatology 1999;29:664). Pts with fatty liver but no inflammation or fibrosis have a low risk of progressive liver disease
(Hepatology 1995;22:1714).

Diff Dx: NASH is a consideration in pts with abnormal LFTs. The
abnormal LFTs are usually found in the process of evaluating
other medical problems. Other causes of abnormal LFTs and cirrhosis must be excluded (p 42). The most difficult differential
point is that of alcoholic liver disease. A dx of NAFLD can only
be made with liver bx. However, given the indolent nature of

NAFLD and its lack of proven rx, many physicians forgo bx (Ann IM 1997;127:410). It is assumed that pts with an unrevealing evaluation for other causes of abnormal LFTs have either fatty liver (without inflammation) or NASH. Effective rx for NASH would make the distinction between fatty liver and NASH more important.

Lab: ALT is usually >AST and are both 2-3 × the normal values. Alk phos is often mildly elevated. Bilirubin and PT are usually normal. Ferritin is elevated in more than half of pts but is generally <1000 ng/mL (GE 1994;107:1103). A variety of histopathologic changes have been described. Steatosis is seen mostly in zone 3 of the liver. Inflammation is usually mild and in the lobules without severe portal changes. Degenerating hepatocytes are present and Mallory hyalin may be seen (as in alcoholic hepatitis). Fibrosis begins in sinusoids and may progress to cirrhosis. Predictors of fibrosis include age ≥50, body mass index ≥28 kg/m^2, triglycerides ≥1.7 mmol/L, and ALT ≥2 × normal (GE 2000;118:1117). A scoring system based on these parameters can select pts unlikely to have fibrosis on bx.

X-ray: Ultrasound may show increased echogenicity consistent with fat, or CT may show evidence of fatty change. Neither study is sensitive or specific for NASH.

Rx: No effective rx for NAFLD/NASH has been identified. Gradual weight loss and exercise have been advocated and appear to result in histologic and biochemical improvement (Am J Gastro 1999;94:2467; Hepatology 2004;39:1647). However, large well-conducted studies are lacking (Am J Med 2003;115:554) and weight loss is difficult to achieve. A pilot study of ursodeoxycholic acid showed biochemical and histologic improvement at 1 yr (Hepatology 1996;23:1464), but a subsequent RCT showed no benefit (Hepatology 2004;39:770). Vitamin E has been used because of its antioxidant properties without convincing evidence of benefit (Am J Gastro 2003;98:2348). Insulin sensitizers such as pioglitazone have been effective in a pilot study (Clin Gastroenterol Hepatol 2004;2:1107), but these drugs cause weight gain and have been associated with cases of hepatotoxicity (Clin Gastroenterol Hepatol 2004;2:1059). Large RCTs are under way. Transplant has been used effectively to treat end-stage disease, though recurrence in the transplant is a risk (Transplantation 1996;62:1802).

12.2 Primary Biliary Cirrhosis

Am J Gastro 2001;96:3152; Can J Gastroenterol 2000;14:43; Lancet 1997;350:875

Epidem: There is a striking predominance in women (90%). Prevalence ranges from 5-392/1,000,000 (Semin Liver Dis 1997;17:13). Familial PBC is uncommon (1%) and seems to be related to maternally inherited factors (Gut 1995;36:615).

Pathophys: PBC is a destructive disease of small, interlobular bile ducts. It is probably due to a defect in immune regulation. Almost all pts have antimitochondrial antibodies (AMA). AMAs are directed against antigens on bile duct epithelial cells with similar antigenicity to the E2 subunit of pyruvate dehydrogenase (J Clin Invest 1993;91:2653). Immune destruction of bile ducts may be mediated in this way. A variety of infectious agents, including retroviruses, have been implicated as inciting antigenic stimuli in susceptible individuals (Am J Gastro 2004;99:2348). As bile ducts are destroyed, concentrations of hydrophobic bile acids and other hepatocellular toxins rise and cause further destruction. This causes recruitment of inflammatory cells, which produce cytokines that may promote fibrosis (Can J Gastroenterol 2000;14:43).

Sx: (Semin Liver Dis 1997;17:23) About 60% of pts are asymptomatic at dx. Fatigue occurs in more than 60% and is a frustrating problem of unknown cause. Pruritus is the second most common sx and can be severe. Some pts will have RUQ pain that usually disappears. A minority will present with a complication of end-stage liver disease such as varices or ascites. Many pts have at least one other autoimmune disease such as thyroiditis, scleroderma, rheumatoid arthritis, the CREST syndrome, or Sjögren's syndrome.

Si: (Can J Gastroenterol 2000;14:43) Findings vary with the stage of disease. In early disease, excoriations may be seen. Hepatomegaly is common (70%) and splenomegaly develops in about 35%. Jaundice, spider angiomata, and ascites are late manifestations. Xanthomas commonly occur around the eyes (xanthelasma) and less commonly occur on extremities. They disappear as disease progresses.

Crs: The rate of progression varies markedly among pts. Mean survival in asymptomatic pts is 10-16 yr compared to 7 yr in those who present with sx. Many initially asymptomatic pts develop sx within 5 yr, but a subgroup remain asymptomatic for yr. No tests are helpful in predicting who will progress (Am J Gastro 1999; 94:47). A variety of models have been employed to predict the course of advanced disease, and these can be used to determine the timing of liver transplant (Semin Liver Dis 1997;17:147). Pts with AMA-negative PBC appear to have a course similar to AMA-positive pts (Hepatology 1997;25:1090).

Cmplc: Osteoporosis is the most common bone disorder, and effective rx is lacking (Hepatology 1995;21:389). Steatorrhea and fat soluble vitamin deficiency can be seen in advanced disease. Hypothyroidism is seen in 20% of pts. Rheumatoid arthritis (10%), scleroderma (4%), CREST syndrome, and SLE have been reported (Q J Med 1996;89:5). Up to 68% of pts have xerostomia or xerophthalmia and may have dysphagia (Dysphagia 1997; 12:167). Any of the complications of end-stage liver disease may occur (p 429). Hepatobiliary malignancy is more common in

PBC (RR=46 in one referral series [Hepatology 1999;29:1396]), but malignancy is not as frequent as in other causes of cirrhosis (Am J Gastroenterol 1997;92:676). Varices are seen earlier in the course of PBC than with other liver diseases, because the portal HTN is partially presinusoidal and synthetic function may be relatively well preserved.

Diff Dx: PBC is usually considered in the evaluation of an asymptomatic pt with elevated alk phos or when a pt presents with evidence of chronic liver disease such as ascites or bleeding from varices. Some cases of PBC are detected because of autoantibody testing done for other reasons in pts with normal LFTs. This group evolves into typical PBC (Lancet 1996;348:1399). The diff dx generally includes the other causes of abnormal LFTs or cirrhosis (p 42). The chief points of confusion are sclerosing cholangitis (p 391), which produces similar LFT abnormalities, drug-induced cholestasis, and autoimmune hepatitis. When the liver bx shows bile duct lesions suggestive of PBC, but the AMA is negative and the ANA and anti-smooth muscle antibody are positive, it is difficult to confidently make a diagnosis. These pts are said by some experts to have an overlap syndrome called autoimmune cholangitis that may respond to steroids like autoimmune hepatitis (Gut 1997;40:440). To make a dx of PBC, biliary obstruction must be excluded with imaging studies, especially if the AMA is negative.

Lab: **Antimitochondrial antibody** (AMA) is 95% sensitive and 98% specific for PBC. AMAs are directed against a family of dehydrogenase enzymes, chiefly pyruvate dehydrogenase (Semin Liver Dis 1997;17:61). The major autoantigen, located on the inner mitochondrial membrane, is the E2 component of pyruvate dehydrogenase (J Hepatol 1986;2:123). Levels do not correlate with disease severity. Elevation of alk phos is the most notable laboratory abnormality in early-stage disease. The GGTP and 5'NT are elevated in a parallel fashion. ALT/AST are usually <5×

normal. Bilirubin and PT become elevated as disease progresses. Most pts have elevated cholesterol. Since the elevation is in the HDL fraction of cholesterol, the risk for heart disease is low (Hepatology 1992;15:858). Antinuclear antibody and antithyroid antibodies are common. Many other autoantibodies have been reported. Elevations of IgM and polyclonal IgG are seen.

Four pathologic stages are recognized on **liver bx.** In stage I, inflammatory cells surround a bile duct with evidence of duct epithelial degeneration. In some cases a frankly necrotic duct can be seen in a granuloma (the florid duct lesion). In stage II, fibrosis develops in the portal zones, and inflammation extends into the lobules. In stage III, fibrosis joins portal triads. Stage IV shows established cirrhosis.

X-ray: Obstruction of the bile ducts should be excluded with ultrasound or CT scan. ERCP would be reserved for cases in which PSC (p 391) was a serious consideration.

Endoscopy: Endoscopy should be performed in pts with advanced disease to identify and treat varices (p 429).

Rx:

- *Ursodeoxycholic acid:* UDCA has been evaluated in 4 RCTs (Hepatology 1995;22:759; Nejm 1994;330:1342; GE 1994;106:1284; Hepatology 1994;19:1149). A dose of 13-15 mg/kg per day is used and is usually well tolerated. There is improvement in LFTs and in pruritus for some pts. In the trial with 4-yr follow-up, the RR for death or transplant was 0.32 in the treated group (Nejm 1994;330:1342). Increasing the dose to 28-32 mg/kg/day in those with an incomplete response to standard dose rx does not appear beneficial (Am J Gastro 2001;96:3152). The drug does not improve the course of advanced disease.
- *Other medical rx:* Cyclosporine showed no convincing survival advantage compared to placebo and caused worsening of renal function in an RCT (GE 1993;104:519). Colchicine 0.6 mg po

bid improved LFTs but did not prolong survival or delay transplant in a small RCT (Hepatology 1991;14:990). Methotrexate (MTX) improves LFTs, pruritus, and histology (GE 1991; 101:1332), but the only randomized placebo controlled trial using a low dose (7.5 mg/wk) showed no benefit (GE 1999; 117:400). The combination of low-dose methotrexate and low-dose UDCA is no better than UDCA alone (J Hepatol 1997; 27:143). Uncontrolled use of MTX for colchicine failures met with partial success using a dose of 15 mg/wk (Ann IM 1997; 126:682). Based on the above, almost all pts are begun on UDCA, and some experts add colchicine or MTX in those who do not fully respond.

- *Liver transplant:* Transplant is highly effective rx (Semin Liver Dis 1997;17:137). One-yr survival is 85-90% and long-term survival is similar to that of age-matched controls. Histologic recurrence has been well documented, but recurrent disease is not rapidly progressive (Hepatology 1993;18:1392).
- *Pruritus:* Most pts have a response to cholestyramine (typically 4 gm po tid) or colestipol. Antihistamines are used in mild cases. Naloxone, ondansetron, flumecinol, tamoxifen, rifampin, phenobarbital, and plasmapheresis have all been used (Q J Med 1996;89:5).
- *Osteoporosis:* Pts should be screened for osteoporosis and treated with calcium (1500 mg/day) and vitamin D (400-800 U/day). Estrogen replacement in postmenopausal pts improves bone density (Am J Gastro 1994;89:47). UDCA does not appear to be effective (Hepatology 1995;21: 389). Transplant appears to reverse bone loss after the first few months of steroids and bed rest (Hepatology 1991;14:296).

12.3 Primary Sclerosing Cholangitis

Am J Gastro 2002;97:528; Hepatology 1999;30:325; Am J Gastro
    1998;93:515

Epidem: About 70% of pts with primary sclerosing cholangitis (PSC)
    are men. About 75% of pts have IBD. The majority of the IBD
    pts have UC (85%), but some have Crohn's. The estimated
    prevalence is 1-15/100,000 with wide geographic variation
    (Scand J Gastroenterol 1998;33:99).

Pathophys: PSC is characterized by inflammation and fibrosis of the
    intrahepatic and extrahepatic bile ducts. PSC is defined by the
    presence of bile duct strictures on cholangiography, by cholestatic
    LFT abnormalities, and by the absence of diseases that could give
    a similar picture (see Diff Dx). Immune mechanisms are thought
    to be important in the pathogenesis, especially since the disease
    is associated with IBD, autoantibodies and immunoglobulin ele-
    vations are present, and inflammation is T-cell mediated. In-
    fectious and toxic etiologies have been considered and rejected.
    Though PSC causes obliteration of larger bile ducts than PBC,
    the end result is the same: cholestasis that causes progressive
    parenchymal destruction.

Sx: Most pts come to diagnosis because of abnormal LFTs, sometimes
    detected in evaluation of their associated IBD. These pts are usu-
    ally asymptomatic. Fatigue, pruritus, jaundice, night sweats, and
    weight loss may occur as disease progresses. An important
    minority of pts (about 10%) experience attacks of fever, RUQ
    pain, and worsened LFTs in a picture that mimics bacterial
    cholangitis.

Si: In early disease, the exam is normal. As disease progresses, jaun-
    dice, excoriation from intractable pruritus, and other findings of
    end-stage liver disease may be evident (p 42).

Crs: The course of PSC is independent of the course of the associated
    IBD. A 10-yr survival of 70% was seen in a population-based

study, and median transplant-free survival appears to be about 9-12 yr (Scand J Gastroenterol 1997;32:1042). Some pts have a rapid downhill course and others go for yr without any morbidity. Prognostic models have been developed to help predict the timing of liver transplant (Mayo Clin Proc 2000;75:688; GE 1992;103:1893).

Cmplc: Cholangiocarcinoma (p 413) is seen in 10-20% of pts with PSC (Hepatology 1998;27:311). Seven percent of pts undergoing transplant have cholangiocarcinoma found in the explanted liver. It can be difficult to differentiate benign from malignant strictures. The CA 19-9 may be elevated (Mayo Clin Proc 1993;68:874), but there is no evidence that this marker allows detection at a resectable stage. Early transplant is probably the best option (Hepatology 1996;23:1105). Some data suggest that pts with PSC and UC have a greater chance of colonic dysplasia and CRC than pts with UC alone. However, the data are not adequate to justify more intense colonic surveillance for those with PSC and UC (Hepatology 1999;30:325). Osteoporosis occurs in 8% of pts with PSC compared to 30% with PBC. Osteoporosis is more likely in severe disease or with long-standing IBD (J Hepatol 1998;29:729). Any of the complications of end-stage liver disease may occur (p 429).

Diff Dx: The disease is suspected when a cholestatic pattern of LFTs is seen, especially in a pt with IBD. Cholangiography is the key to diagnosis. Several rare disorders cause a similar cholangiogram. These include HIV cholangiopathy (p 356), bile duct stricture from stones, surgery, ischemic cholangitis (Mayo Clin Proc 1998;73:380), malignancy, intraarterial chemotherapy, or congenital abnormalities. The more limited the cholangiographic abnormality, the more likely an alternative dx is present. Rarely, a pt will have LFT abnormalities suggestive of PSC, a liver bx with changes of PSC, and normal cholangiography. These pts are said to have small duct PSC (Semin Liver Dis 1991;11:11).

Lab: The alk phos is usually disproportionately elevated and rises as
disease progresses. GGTP and 5'NT are similarly elevated.
Bilirubin rises as disease advances. ALT/AST are usually less than
7× normal. With advanced disease, albumin falls and PT rises.
IgM levels are modestly elevated in half of pts. Perinuclear-
ANCA, ANA, and ASMA may be present. AMA is absent.
Liver bx can be nonspecific; the diagnosis relies on cholangiography. Bx can provide information about staging, but sampling
error is substantial (Am J Gastro 1999;94:3310). The staging is
similar to that of PBC. In stage I there is degeneration of bile
duct epithelium with an infiltrate of lymphocytes and scarring in
the portal triads. Bile ducts may proliferate, and rarely the
pathognomonic "onion skin" lesion of concentric rings of fibrous
tissue around a bile duct can be seen. In stage II, loss of bile ducts
is more prominent and inflammation and scarring expand into
the parenchyma. In stage III, fibrosis from portal zone to portal
zone is seen. In stage IV, there is frank cirrhosis.

Endoscopy: ERCP is used to obtain the quality of cholangiogram
needed for the dx, though the role of MRCP as a safer alternative
is rapidly growing. At ERCP there are multiple strictures and
dilatations of varying lengths. Outpouchings and ectatic ducts are
seen. Often this results in a beaded appearance of the bile duct.
In early disease there may be subtle changes in large ducts. In
severe disease, the intrahepatic ducts may be impossible to visualize because of strictures. Usually the intrahepatic and extrahepatic trees are involved. When only the extrahepatic ducts are
abnormal, other diagnoses (other causes of stricture) should be
strongly considered.

Rx:

- *Medical rx of underlying disease:* There is no known effective
  medical rx for PSC. Pilot studies suggest that high-dose
  ursodeoxycholic acid (UDCA at doses from 20-30 mg/kg)
  improves lab abnormalities and slows worsening of the

cholangiogram (Am J Gastro 2001;96:1558; GE 2001;121: 900). Methotrexate was ineffective in an RCT (GE 1994; 106:494). Azathioprine, colchicine, antibiotics, cyclosporine, nicotine, pentoxifylline, and prednisone are all ineffective. Higher dose and combination therapies (Am J Gastro 2000; 95:1861; Ann IM 1999;131:943) are being advocated.

- *Rx of strictures:* Some pts develop worsening LFTs or cholangitis because of a dominant stricture in the extrahepatic bile ducts. This can be treated with dilatation and short duration stenting (11 days), with improvement in LFTs and sx. There is no need for further intervention in more than 80% of pts at 1 yr and 60% at 3 yr (Am J Gastro 1999;94:2403). Bile duct perforation can occur with dilatation. For some pts, this may buy time prior to transplant, but the true effect on natural hx is unknown. A variety of other endoscopic approaches to strictures can be used (Am J Gastro 1999;94:2235). Surgical rx of strictures is now used selectively. Surgery makes later transplant more difficult, and most cirrhotics are better served with transplant (Surgery 1995; 117:146).

- *Rx of pruritus and osteoporosis:* Pruritis is treated as it is in PBC (p 390). Steatorrhea is a late finding. It may be associated with fat-soluble vitamin deficiency and replacement rx may be needed. No effective rx has yet been identified for the osteoporosis. Calcium supplements, vitamin D, and the bisphosphonates can be used.

- *Attacks of cholangitis:* There is very little published on the use of antibiotics in attacks of RUQ pain and fever. However, antibiotics are widely used at the first sign of an attack and appear to be helpful. Common choices are ciprofloxacin and Tm/S, which pts keep on hand and take at the outset of an attack. If attacks are frequent, some pts stay on prophylactic antibiotics in 3-4 week rotations (eg, rotating ciprofloxacin, Tm/S, cephalexin, ampicillin) (Hepatology 1999;30:325).

Intravenous rx is used in severe illness and occasionally in prolonged courses.

- *Liver transplant:* This is the only effective rx for pts with end-stage disease who may develop refractory episodes of cholangitis or complications of portal HTN, including variceal hemorrhage and ascites. Recent reported survivals are as high as 94% at 1 yr and 86% at 5 yr (Hepatology 1999;30:1121). The optimal timing of transplant (given the scarcity of organs and the resources needed) has not been determined. Quality of life, the presence of complications such as variceal hemorrhage, and the risk of cholangiocarcinoma if transplant is excessively delayed (Hepatology 1996;23:1105) are important factors. Transplant rejection is more common in PSC than in other diseases posttransplant, and CRC is a major cause of death (Hepatology 1995;22:451). Recurrence may occur in up to 20% of pts but does not appear to affect survival (Hepatology 1999;29:1050). CRC is an important postoperative problem, but prophylactic colectomy does not appear to be warranted (Hepatology 1998;27:685).

12.4 Autoimmune Hepatitis

Hepatology 2002;36:479; Scand J Gastroenterol Suppl 1998;225:66; Nejm 1996;334:897

Cause: Autoimmunity.

Epidem: Typically autoimmune hepatitis (AIH) is a disease of women aged 15-40, but type I disease may occur in pts of either sex at any age. Type II is almost exclusively a disease of young women.

Pathophys: There is a defect in T cell suppression of antibody producing B cells in autoimmune hepatitis. A genetic predisposition is suggested by the association with HLA loci B8, DR3, and DR4. It is thought that an environmental event, such as viral hepatitis, triggers B cell responses to hepatic surface antigens in a genetically predisposed pt. Antibody-coated cells are then cleared by natural killer cells, exposing more autoantigens. The defective T suppressor cells fail to turn down the antibody response and the process continues. This results in hepatocyte destruction, and ultimately, cirrhosis. The circulating ANA and ASMA are markers of disease and do not affect the pathogenesis.

The disease has been classified according to the autoantibodies produced (Am J Gastro 1995;90:1206). In type I (classic) autoimmune hepatitis, antinuclear antibodies (ANA), anti-smooth muscle antibodies (ASMA), perinuclear antineutrophil cytoplasmic antibodies (pANCA), asialoglycoprotein antibodies (ASGPR), and antiactin antibodies (AAA) are present. Tests for the latter 2 are not readily available. ASGPR may be of special interest since it is liver specific and may not be an epiphenomenon. In type II (representing less than 5% of the total) there are antibodies to liver-kidney microsome 1 (anti-LKM-1) and antiliver cytosol antibodies. A type III AIH had been proposed with antibodies to soluble liver antigen (SLA), but this classification was dropped by many experts when it was determined SLA pts were not clinically distinct (Lancet 2000;355:1475). SLA has now been cloned and found to be identical to cytosolic liver-pancreas antigen (Lancet 2000;355:1510). A reliable test (Gut 2002;51:259) that may be useful in cases where other markers are negative has been developed.

Sx: Many pts are asymptomatic and come to attention because of abnormal LFTs. Others have nonspecific sx of fatigue, anorexia, abdominal pain, nausea, and arthralgias. A smaller group present with jaundice or findings of advanced liver disease (p 42).

Si: The exam findings range from normal to the findings of cirrhosis and portal HTN (p 42).

Crs: Most pts respond to rx and do well. Even pts with established cirrhosis have a 10-yr survival of 90% (GE 1996;110:848). Fibrosis and cirrhosis may be reversible in some pts who respond to rx

(Ann IM 1997;127:981). Most pts require long-term or intermittent medical rx.

Cmplc: A variety of concurrent autoimmune diseases have been described, including thyroid disease, ITP, celiac disease, Sjögren's, mixed connective tissue disease, and others (Postgrad Med 1998;104:145). The risk of hepatocellular carcinoma is very low (Dig Dis Sci 2000;45:1944). Any of the complications of end-stage liver disease may occur (p 429).

Diff Dx: The dx of AIH is established by the combination of abnormal transaminases, elevated globulins ($>1.5 \times$ normal), positive titers of one of the autoantibodies listed in Pathophys (usually at $>1:80$), a compatible bx, and the absence of another cause of abnormal LFTs (p 43). Formal diagnostic criteria have been proposed (Hepatology 1993;18:998). Variants of typical AIH have been noted (Ann IM 1996;125:588). In the overlap syndrome, the serology is that of PBC but the bx looks more like autoimmune hepatitis. In autoimmune cholangitis, the bx looks more like PBC but the AMA is negative. Another troublesome group are those pts with cryptogenic chronic active hepatitis who are clinically similar to those with AIH, lack any autoantibodies, but respond to steroids (GE 1993;104:1755). Other causes of cirrhosis must be excluded (p 48).

Lab: Titers of autoantibodies are usually $>1:80$. ANA and ASMA are usually obtained and pANCA is another commercially available marker. Tests are not readily available for all of the remaining markers but can be found in specialized labs. LFTs are notable for elevated transaminases with generally mild elevations in alk phos, but a cholestatic picture may emerge in jaundiced pts. In advanced disease, PT may be abnormal. Elevations in gamma globulins are characteristic and may be a clue to AIH in pts with negative tests for available markers.

Liver Bx: Bx is used to stage the disease and to support the diagnosis but is often nonspecific. A portal infiltrate of mononuclear cells spills from the portal zones across the limiting plate of hepato-cytes and into the lobule, where it causes hepatocyte necrosis. This process had been called "piecemeal necrosis," but has been recently renamed "interface hepatitis." Fibrosis of varying degrees is present.

Endoscopy: EGD should be considered to look for varices in cirrhotic pts (p 429).

Rx: Rx with prednisone is highly effective, even in severe disease. The response rate is >80%. Depending on the severity of illness (and the preference of the treating physician) pts are treated with an initial dose of 20-60 mg po qd. Biochemical remission, marked by improvement in bilirubin, ALT, AST, and immunoglobulins, occurs within 1-3 months, and steroids are then tapered. Maintenance rx is required in most pts. To minimize the pred-nisone requirement, azathioprine in a dose of 50-150 mg is used either at the outset or as prednisone is tapered (see p 185 about azathioprine use). Azathioprine as a single maintenance agent is effective in 80% of pts when used at a dose of 2 mg/kg (Nejm 1995;333:958). Low-dose prednisone, keeping the transaminases under 5 × normal, has been advocated to minimize steroid side effects, but the approach has not been adequately studied (Hepatology 1990;11:1044). Budesonide, as an alternative to prednisone, is ineffective (GE 2000;119:1312). Tacrolimus has some efficacy (Am J Gastro 1995;90:771), but controlled studies are lacking. Cyclosporine (Am J Gastro 1999; 94:241) and mycophenolate mofetil (J Hepatol 2000;33:371) have been effec-tive in open label studies of pts who failed or did not tolerate prednisone/azathioprine. UDCA is not helpful (Hepatology 1999;30:1381). Transplant is effective but rejection (75%) and disease recurrence (25%) are frequent. The optimal immune sup-pression regimen for transplant recipients has not been deter-mined (Hepatology 2000;32:693).

12.5 Hemochromatosis

Nejm 2004;350:2383; Semin Hematol 1998;35:55

Cause: This section reviews hereditary hemochromatosis (HH), which is also called genetic or Type 1 hemochromatosis. This disorder is secondary to phenotypic expression of a mutation in the HFE gene. Juvenile hemochromatosis (a severe early onset form now called Type 2 hemochromatosis) and other rare genetic iron overload syndromes (Types 3-5) are not further discussed (reviewed in Nejm 2004;350:2383). Secondary iron overload (eg, from transfusions) is not further discussed.

Epidem: The HFE gene (see Pathophys) is found in 3-8/1000 subjects of European descent. Heterozygotes are found in 10-16% of the population. This disease does not occur in subjects without Caucasian ancestry. The Cys282Tyr mutation (see Pathophys) is most frequent in populations of Celtic or Viking origin, and the His63Asp mutation has a more global distribution. Because clinical disease does not occur in all homozygotes, the rate of clinically evident HH is 0.5-2.5/1000 in males. Phenotypic disease is 4× more frequent in men.

Pathophys: (Lancet 2002;360:1673) The gene responsible for more than 85% of the cases of HH has been identified and is called HFE (Nat Genet 1996;13:399). It encodes an HLA-like molecule. Two important mutations have been described. Cys282Tyr is the substitution of tyrosine for cysteine at amino acid 282. His63Asp is the substitution of aspartic acid for histidine at amino acid 63. In northern Europe more than 80% of affected pedigrees have one of these mutations. Most pts with HH are homozygous for Cys282Tyr, and a few (4%) are compound heterozygotes with one Cys282Tyr mutation and one His63Asp mutation. Compound heterozygotes are much less likely to develop phenotypic disease. Homozygous mutation of His63Asp rarely results in iron overload.

Dietary iron overload is not the primary defect, though clinical expression is rare in areas where there is a grain-based (not meat-based) diet. Pts with HH appear to have enhanced iron absorption. The exact mechanism of enhanced iron absorption is not well understood but may be related to defects in the regulation of hepcidin, a protein which appears to regulate the release of iron from enterocytes and macrophages into the bloodstream. Pregnancy and menses increase iron loss in women and are partially protective.

Sx: In a large cohort collected over decades, weakness/lethargy (85%), abdominal pain (60%), arthralgias (50%), and loss of libido (40%) were the most common sx (GE 1996;110:1107). As more and more pts are diagnosed at early stages, a greater proportion will be asymptomatic. A large pt survey indicated an average of 10 yr' delay between sx and dx (Am J Med 1999;106:619). Currently, the most common presenting sx is arthritis.

Clinical sx are the result of iron overload in different organ systems. Jaundice, ascites, and encephalopathy are late findings. A sudden worsening of hepatic sx should raise the question of hepatocellular carcinoma. Arthropathy is a frequent problem (40-75%) and may be a presenting complaint. It resembles DJD and progresses despite phlebotomy. A metallic or bronze hue of the skin may be present in advanced disease. Diabetes due to iron overload occurs in 30-60% of pts with advanced disease. Exocrine insufficiency is rare. Loss of libido, impotence, amenorrhea, and sparse body hair are due to iron overload effects on the pituitary. A dilated cardiomyopathy is present in 20-30% of pts with symptomatic disease, and arrhythmias may occur.

Si: Hepatomegaly is common in pts with clinical sx. Ascites is not common and may indicate heart failure. Any of the findings of advanced liver disease may be seen (p 42). Testicular atrophy and sparse body hair represent hypogonadism. Joints may show bony deformity and loss of motion, especially in the metacarpal phalangeal and proximal interphalangeal joints.

Crs: Life expectancy is normal in treated pts who do not present with cirrhosis (GE 1996;110:1107). In pts who are cirrhotic but undergo rx, survival is 80% at 10 yr. Portal HTN in HH does not result in as many complications as it does in other liver diseases (Hepatology 1995;22:1127). Pts treated with phlebotomy feel better, have decreased hepatomegaly, normalize LFTs, and require less insulin. The arthropathy and hypogonadism do not improve dramatically with phlebotomy. Analysis of death certificates suggests a vast underreporting of hemochromatosis. There is excessive occurrence of liver neoplasms (23×) and cardiomyopathy (fivefold) as causes of death in HH pts (Ann IM 1998;129:946).

Cmplc: Hepatocellular carcinoma (HCC) occurs with a RR of 200 in cirrhotic pts and ultimately occurs in 30% of these pts. *Vibrio vulnificus* infection (from warm water shellfish) is more likely to cause severe illness in hemochromatosis because of iron needed for microbial metabolism (Arch IM 1991;151:1606). Any of the complications of end-stage liver disease may occur (p 429).

Diff Dx: HH is often considered in the differential of asymptomatic abnormal LFTs and cirrhosis (p 48). Alcoholic hepatitis can mimic hemochromatosis because transferrin saturation can be very high with the release of iron from dying hepatocytes. In addition, elevations of ferritin are common in alcoholic liver disease, because ferritin is an acute phase reactant. Repeat iron studies should be done after 2-3 months of sobriety. Alcoholic cirrhosis is distinguishable from HH by bx with iron index determination (see Lab). A negative gene test does not rule out HH. Heterozygotes for HFE cause confusion because they tend to have higher than average transferrin saturations. Hepatic iron index and gene testing will clarify the dx. There are numerous other causes of iron overload, including those associated with multiple transfusions, iron loading anemias, and African iron overload, but these are generally not diagnostic pitfalls (Ann IM 1998;129:925).

Lab: (Ann IM 1998;129:925) Transferrin saturation (the ratio of Fe/TIBC multiplied by 100) is usually elevated but can be normal in young homozygous pts. Levels of >45% are investigated in a screening situation and screening detects 98% of affected individuals. If a pt has a transferrin saturation >45%, the test should be repeated after fasting, and a ferritin test should be done. If ferritin is normal, the tests should be repeated 2-3 yr later so that early HH is not missed. Ferritin reflects total body iron stores and is usually >>1000 mg/mL in symptomatic disease. In a screening situation, HH is likely if ferritin is >300 mg/mL in a man, >200 mg/mL in a woman, or if transferrin saturation is >55% on repeat testing. False-positive elevations of ferritin (which is an acute phase reactant) occur with inflammation, infection, or malignancy. LFTs can be normal in early disease, and normal LFTs do not rule out the dx of HH.

- *Liver bx:* Early findings include hemosiderin granules in periportal hepatocytes, which involves other hepatocytes as disease progresses. Fibrosis results in a micronodular (or mixed micronodular and macronodular) cirrhosis. Iron stores can be estimated from iron stains, but iron content is better measured directly on bx specimens by atomic absorption techniques. The iron content is best expressed as the hepatic iron index and is equal to micromole iron/gm dry weight/age in yr. This is useful in distinguishing alcoholic iron overload from that of HH (GE 1997;113:1270; Hepatology 1986;6:24). Most clinicians advise liver bx to confirm the diagnosis and to stage the disease, since a bx without cirrhosis means a normal life expectancy and no increased risk of HCC. Pts who are homozygous, have no hepatomegaly, have normal LFTs, and have ferritin <1000 mg/mL can be treated without bx. In this group, the chance of fibrosis is very low (GE 1999;116:193; GE 1998; 115:929).

- *Gene testing:* Gene testing is a simple means of confirming the diagnosis and allows for family screening. Most pts will be homozygous for Cys282Tyr. A few pts will be compound heterozygous, and up to 17% will be normal (GE 1999;116:193). False-negative rates in gene testing may be higher in some populations, such as Italians (GE 1998;114:996).

- *Family testing:* If probands are positive on gene tests, family members can obtain accurate information about their status (normal, heterozygous, or homozygous) through gene testing. Family members found to be homozygous are followed by periodic determinations of transferrin saturation and ferritin for evidence of phenotypic disease. Siblings have the highest yield in testing. Children should be screened since homozygote/heterozygote matings are common. One sensible strategy for probands with more than one child is to gene test the other parent (assuming parentage is well known) and to test the children only if the other parent is heterozygous (Ann IM 2000; 132:261).

- *Population screening:* Transferrin saturation is the most effective of the nongene tests for screening the population. Numerous studies suggest that screening is cost effective (GE 1994; 107:453; Arch IM 1994;154:769). There are many problems in implementation, including physician education and pt compliance (Ann IM 1998;129:962). Not all experts feel that population-based screening is justified until more is known about disease penetrance and the true disease burden in the population (Ann IM 1998;129:971). Changes can be expected when the gene test is applied to population screening.

X-ray: Chondrocalcinosis can be detected on joint x-ray in 50% of symptomatic pts.

Endoscopy: Consider EGD to look for varices in cirrhotic pts (p 429).

Rx: (Ann IM 1998;129:932)

- *Phlebotomy:* The cornerstone of rx is phlebotomy. Each unit of blood is a volume of 500 cc and contains 250 mg of iron. A typical adult male normally has 1-2 gm of iron stores, and in HH, the total burden is usually >15 gm. Pts who refuse bx and require >4 gm of phlebotomy have definite iron overload. Phlebotomy is usually well tolerated on a weekly basis. In some young, large pts, phlebotomy can be done biweekly. Some elderly pts do not tolerate phlebotomy at that rate. Phlebotomy is continued until a mild anemia occurs (Hgb just below normal). Phlebotomy is then carried out 2-6 times/yr (depending on sex and diet) for the pt's lifetime. The goal is to keep the ferritin on the low side of normal (usually <50 mg/L), but the pt should not be kept anemic.

- *Other rx:* Major dietary changes are of little benefit. Red meat can be eaten in moderation. Iron supplements should be avoided, and vitamin C (which enhances iron absorption) should be limited to 500 mg daily. Alcohol consumption should be limited (or stopped if there is cirrhosis). Shellfish from warm water should be cooked because of enhanced susceptibility to *Vibrio* infections. Testosterone is used for hypogonadism. Desferrioxamine (an iron chelator) is occasionally needed in pts who do not tolerate phlebotomy because of cardiac disease.

- *Screening for hepatocellular carcinoma:* Many experts screen their cirrhotic pts for HCC using periodic α-fetoprotein determinations and ultrasound. It is not clear that screening in these circumstances saves lives, and the optimal frequency of screening (if any) has yet to be determined (p 413).

12.6 Wilson's Disease

Mayo Clin Proc 2003;78:1126; Gastroenterol Clin North Am 1998;27:655

Cause: Autosomal recessive inheritance of mutations in the Wilson's disease gene, ATP7B, a copper-transporting protein.

Epidem: Wilson's disease (WD) is an autosomal recessive disease with a prevalence of 1/30,000 (Hepatology 1990;12:1234). It is generally diagnosed in the early teens. It can present in young children and rarely in adults in their 50s (Gut 2000;46:415).

Pathophys: WD is a multisystem disease of copper (Cu) overload. Copper is absorbed in the proximal intestine from dietary sources (shellfish, nuts, chocolate, mushrooms, and liver) and transported to hepatocytes. In hepatocytes it is incorporated into enzymes, including ceruloplasmin. Excess copper is bound in metallothionein complexes and excreted into bile. In WD, incorporation of copper into ceruloplasmin and excretion into bile are defective. The WD gene (ATP7B) appears to code for a copper-transporting ATPase. This ATPase normally serves to transport Cu intracellularly for export into serum (attached to ceruloplasmin) or into bile. More than 70 mutations of the gene have been reported, and this may account for some of the clinical heterogeneity of the disease (Am J Hum Genet 1997;61:317). After yr of defective excretion, excess Cu appears as stainable granules in hepatocytes, and eventually hepatitis and fibrosis develop. Dying hepatocytes release Cu into the circulation where it accumulates in red cells, the brain, and other organs.

Sx/Si: Several clinical presentations are possible. A hepatic presentation is seen in 40% of pts with acute hepatic failure or chronic hepatitis. Most pts have frank cirrhosis on presentation. Occasionally the liver disease is abrupt in onset. This fulminant presentation is usually accompanied by hemolytic anemia (causing very high bilirubin levels) and is more common in women. Neuropsychiatric manifestations are common and usually present at an older age. Findings include sx or si resembling Parkinson's disease, multiple sclerosis, dystonia, and choreoathetoid movements. Kayser-Fleischer rings result from copper deposition in the eye and are best detected by slit lamp exam. They are 1-3 mm in diameter, green, yellow, or brown, and they are in the periphery of the cornea. They can rarely be seen in other liver diseases (Am J Med 1992;92:643). Almost all pts have either neuropsychiatric or liver disease. Additional manifestations include renal disease (Fanconi's syndrome, stones), cardiac disease (abnormal EKG, arrhythmias), joint sx (arthritis, chondrocalcinosis on x-ray), and hematologic abnormalities.

Crs: Prior to chelating agents, WD was uniformly fatal (Arch Neurol 2000;57:276). With penicillamine, the prognosis for pts with chronic hepatitis is excellent (GE 1991;100:762). Neurologic sx improve in more than two thirds of pts. Survival for those who do not present with fulminant hepatic failure is similar to that of age- and sex-matched controls (Ann IM 1991;115:720).

Cmplc: Hepatocellular carcinoma is rare in WD (J Clin Gastro 1989;11:220). Any of the complications of end-stage liver disease may occur (p 429).

Diff Dx: The key to diagnosis is first to entertain the possibility of this rare disease. WD is most often considered in the evaluation of chronic hepatitis or abnormal LFTs (p 43) in a young pt. The diagnosis can usually be established by means of testing for ceruloplasmin and urine copper, and/or by liver bx. It is more difficult to make a dx of WD in fulminant hepatic failure because (1) ceruloplasmin may be low or urinary copper may be high in other causes of fulminant hepatic failure, (2) bx may not be obtainable because of coagulopathy, and (3) Kayser-Fleischer rings may be absent. In these cases, the hemolytic anemia or the relatively minor elevations in transaminases may be a clue.

Lab: Ceruloplasmin levels are decreased in WD because copper fails to be incorporated into ceruloplasmin and it is rapidly degraded. The ceruloplasmin level is <20 in 90% of pts (lower in some series [GE 1997;113:212]). False negatives occur with estrogens or hepatic inflammation. Normal levels are 20-40 ng/mL and decreases are seen in WD heterozygous pts, in pts with Menkes disease (an X-linked disease of poor copper absorption), in pts with protein-losing states like nephrotic syndrome, in pts suffering malnutrition, and in pts with severe liver disease. Twenty-four-hr urinary copper excretion is almost always elevated, and measurement of levels is the best noninvasive test. Linkage analysis can be used for presymptomatic testing of families if a proband is available (J Lab Clin Med 1991;118:458). Initial diagnostic testing with a gene test is not practical because there are too many possible mutations. Liver bx usually shows evidence of cirrhosis, chronic hepatitis, and excess stainable copper. The best test on bx is quantitative determination of copper levels. The results of this test may be falsely low if the sample has lots of fibrous tissue or if the specimen is mishandled. Levels may be high in other cholestatic liver diseases.

Endoscopy: Consider EGD to look for varices in cirrhotic pts (p 429).

Rx: Copper chelating drugs are highly effective. Penicillamine is the most frequently used agent and rx is lifelong. It can be used in pregnancy (Hepatology 2000;31:531). Neurologic sx largely resolve in more than two thirds of pts though deterioration (sometimes irreversible) may first occur (Q J Med 1993;86:197). Side effects, including hypersensitivity reactions, are problematic in 20% of pts. Trientene is a useful alternative (Lancet 1982; 1:643). Tetrathiomolybdate followed by zinc may be an alternative that does not cause the initial deterioration seen with penicillamine (Arch Neurol 1991;48:42). Chelators are used together with a low copper diet. Zinc has been used as an alternative to chelators and works by increasing metallothionein synthesis.

This binds copper safely in cells, but this rx has not been adequately compared to penicillamine. Liver transplant is required in fulminant hepatic failure and cures the underlying disease by providing hepatocytes without the gene defect (Hepatology 1994;19:583).

12.7 Alpha 1-Antitrypsin Deficiency

Semin Liver Dis 1998;18:217; J Inherit Metab Dis 1991;14:512

Cause: Mutation in the α_1-antitrypsin gene

Epidem: The frequency of the α_1-AT PI*ZZ phenotype (described in Pathophys) is about 0.3-0.6/1000 for whites of European descent. The PI*ZZ phenotype is almost never seen in blacks or Japanese (Respir Med 2000;94 Suppl C:S12).

Pathophys: (Nejm 2002;346:45) The α_1-AT is a protease inhibitor. Its chief function is to protect tissue against destruction by elastases produced by neutrophils. Deficiency is most often a clinical problem because of the destruction of lung tissue resulting in emphysema. The lung disease is clinically the more important adult problem (Am Rev Respir Dis 1989;140:1494) and is not reviewed here. An α_1-AT deficiency causes liver disease by a mechanism related to accumulation of high levels of the molecule in the endoplasmic reticulum of hepatocytes (Thorax 1998;53:501). Pts with complete absence of α_1-AT develop lung disease but not liver disease since there is no α_1-AT to accumulate in hepatocytes. Deficiency is classified according to the protease inhibitor (PI) system. The normal alleles are referred to as M, and a normal phenotype is called PI*MM. More than 90 allelic variants have been described, most of which are single point mutations (Am J Hum Genet 1994;55:1113). The most common variant is the Z variant. Most liver disease is associated with the PI*ZZ state. Heterozygous individuals (PI*MZ) may also have higher incidence of other liver diseases and are overrepresented in the population that ends up coming to liver transplant for any reason (Hepatology 1998;28:1058).

Sx: Only about 15% of PI*ZZ pts develop clinical liver disease. It most often occurs in infancy with presentations of neonatal hepatitis. It can present late in childhood or adolescence with portal HTN or liver failure. Asymptomatic abnormal LFTs may persist in a subgroup without clinical illness. Autopsy studies suggest that PI*ZZ is associated with cirrhosis and HCC in adults and that these pts may have no prior hx of childhood liver disease (Nejm 1986;314:736).

Si: In adults, signs of end-stage liver disease are rarely seen.

Crs: Most pts never develop liver disease. The natural hx of PI*ZZ liver disease in adulthood is not well known. The population-based studies of liver disease are all studies of children.

Cmplc: Hepatocellular carcinoma (Nejm 1986;314:736). Any of the complications of end-stage liver disease may occur (p 429).

Diff Dx: The differential dx in adulthood is usually that of abnormal LFTs or cirrhosis (p 43).

Lab: Serum levels of α_1-AT are low. If levels are low or borderline, phenotyping should be done. Liver bx, if done, shows intracytoplasmic inclusions in hepatocytes that stain strongly with PAS and resist diastase treatment. The degree of fibrosis and inflammation is quite variable.

Rx: There is no specific rx for the underlying liver disease other than to treat the complications. Transplantation cures the disorder by providing a normal phenotype (Clin Exp Immunol 1986;66:669).

12.8 Acute Intermittent Porphyria

Semin Liver Dis 1998;18:17; Lancet 1997;349:1613

Epidem: The prevalence has been estimated at 1/100,000, but the prevalence of gene mutation may be as high as 1/1700 in some regions of the world (Semin Liver Dis 1998;18:17). Attacks are rare before puberty and peak in the 30s. Most pts (80%) are women.

Pathophys: (BMJ 2000;320:1647) The porphyrias are a heterogeneous group of inherited disorders of heme synthesis. Acute intermittent porphyria (AIP) is the most clinically relevant to the gastroenterologist since it is the most common of those that present with unexplained attacks of abdominal pain. Depending on which enzyme in the heme synthetic pathway is deficient, different groups of heme precursors accumulate. These result in a variety of clinical syndromes, including the cutaneous porphyrias (reviewed in [BMJ 2000;320:1647]). In AIP deficiency of porphobilinogen, deaminase results in accumulation of the heme precursors 5-aminolevulinate (ALA) and porphobilinogen (PBG). The liver increases synthesis of these precursors in response to inadequate heme production, and massive amounts are excreted in urine. This is the presumed cause of the neurologic and psychiatric sx of the disease. Since pts have enzyme levels that are reduced but not absent, they often do well until some inciting event occurs. Only 10-15% of gene carriers develop overt disease, and many have no known family history. Attacks are often precipitated by (1) drugs (especially barbiturates and estrogens, but the list is long), (2) fasting, (3) smoking, (4) alcohol, (5) infection, (6) emotional and physical stress, and (7) estrogen peaks such as pregnancy or premenstrual phase of cycle.

Sx: (Neurology 1997;48:1678) Pts present with attacks characterized by abdominal pain (80%), nausea and vomiting (50%), constipation (50%), tachycardia (40%), dark urine (25%), and fever (16%). Neuropsychiatric manifestations include limb weakness (40%) and delirium (22%). Less frequently, cranial nerve abnormalities, seizures, depression, and psychosis may occur. Muscle weakness may progress to frank paresis of the extremities. Cranial nerve involvement may cause bulbar paralysis, respiratory failure, and death.

Si: (Neurology 1997;48:1678) There may be physical exam evidence of proximal muscle weakness, a mild sensory neuropathy, hyporeflexia, or hypertension during acute attacks.

Crs: Attacks may be fatal in a small percentage of pts, especially when the diagnosis is delayed or management is inappropriate. The risk of future attacks correlates with remission levels of PBG in the urine (Medicine 1992;71:1). However, the course is not readily predictable and some unfortunate pts have continued attacks without inciting factors.

Diff Dx: Clinically identical attacks may be seen with AIP, variegate porphyria, hereditary coproporphyria, and plumboporphyria, which can be distinguished by their patterns of urine and fecal porphyrins (BMJ 2000;320:1647). Acute attacks may mistakenly be thought of primarily as psychiatric illness, and misdiagnosis is common. Muscle weakness with respiratory involvement can mimic Guillain-Barré syndrome.

Lab: The diagnosis is made by detecting elevated urinary levels of ALA and PBG during an attack. This can be done on spot urine but is best performed by an experienced reference lab on a 24-hr sample. Levels may normalize between attacks. Additional tests of urine and feces can be used to distinguish AIP from other, rarer porphyrias with similar sx (coproporphyria and variegate porphyria). Urine may turn dark on exposure to light because of precipitation of PBG. Hyponatremia, leukocytosis, or abnormal LFTs are seen in about 20% of pts (Neurology 1997; 48:1678).

Rx: The precipitating cause should be identified and treated. A comprehensive list of forbidden medicines should be consulted (Medicine 1992;71:1). Morphine or meperidine may be used for pain. Fluids with 10% glucose are given. Heme arginate (hematin) (3 mg/kg/day qd $\times$ 4 days) is the drug of choice and should be given early in an attack (Arch IM 1993;153:2004). It reduces synthesis of ALA and is highly effective in aborting attacks. It does not reverse established neuropathy. The duration of remission induced by heme arginate can be prolonged by tin protoporphyrin (GE 1993;105:500). Seizures should be treated with an agent that does not induce porphyrins, such as gabapentin (Neurology 1995;45:1216). Family members should be screened for asymptomatic disease so that preventative measures can be undertaken. Prevention is done by avoiding known precipitants.

Chapter 13

Neoplastic Liver Disease

13.1 Hepatocellular Carcinoma

Lancet 2003;362:1907; Postgrad Med J 2000;76:4

Cause: (Nejm 1999;340:798) The vast majority of cases of hepatocellular carcinoma (HCC) are due to chronic hep B or chronic hep C infection (RR = 100-200). In the U.S., where infection rates are lower, viral hepatitis still accounts for 71% of HCC (Hepatology 1993;18:1326). Cirrhosis of any cause is a risk. The cirrhosis of hep B, hep C, or hemochromatosis is associated with a relative risk of >100. Other causes of cirrhosis (eg, alcohol, PBC, Wilson's, α_1-AT deficiency, autoimmune disorders) are associated with a much lower RR of 2-5. Glycogen storage disease, tyrosinemia, and porphyria cutanea tarda are causative. Aflatoxin (a toxin from *Aspergillus* found in a variety of stored foods like peanuts, corn, and rice), anabolic steroids, and thorium dioxide (an obsolete radiographic contrast medium) are apparent toxic causes.

Epidem: The incidence of HCC varies widely by region and correlates with chronic hep B infection. The highest rates are in Asia and sub-Saharan Africa, where 10-25% of the population is infected by hep B and the HCC incidence is 30-120/100,000 per yr in men. In Japan, HCC is the third leading cause of cancer death, largely due to hep C (Nejm 1993;328:1797). Incidence in southern Europe is 5-10/100,000 per yr (Brit J Surg

1998;85:1319). The incidence in the U.S. has risen over the past 3 decades from 1.4/100,000 to 2.4/100,000 per yr, and the disease is occurring at a younger age. This is probably a result of the increasing incidence of hep C infection. Blacks are affected twice as often as whites and men 3 times as often as women (Nejm 1999;340:745).

Pathophys: The mechanisms by which viral hepatitis causes HCC are unknown. Chronic inflammation and increased hepatocyte turnover are probably important. There may be direct oncogenic effects of the viruses as well. Aflatoxin induces p53 mutations, allowing unrestrained cell proliferation (Lancet 1991;338:1356).

Sx: Weight loss, RUQ pain, malaise, and jaundice are the typical sx of advanced disease. Sudden clinical decompensation in a pt with established cirrhosis is a second common presentation. With the advent of detection by screening, many pts are asymptomatic.

Si: RUQ mass, hepatomegaly, irregular liver edge, bruit over the liver, stigmata of chronic liver disease (p 42), tumor-induced fever.

Crs: The tumor grows locally, compromises hepatic function, invades blood vessels, and spreads to lungs and then to distant sites. Median survival without rx is 3-6 months after the onset of sx. Five-year survival of pts treated with transplant for small lesions is similar to the survival of pts undergoing transplant for any reason. Five-year survival for those undergoing successful resection is 20-40% (see Rx). Five-year survival in the fibrolamellar variant is better (66%).

Cmplc: Paraneoplastic syndromes are frequent. These include hypercholesterolemia (11%), hypoglycemia (2.8%), hypercalcemia (1.8%), and erythrocytosis (2.5%) (Cancer 1999;86:799).

Diff Dx: The differential is that of a hepatic mass (p 418). Pts with masses with α-fetoprotein (AFP) levels >10,000 ng/mL and no evidence of a germ cell tumor can be diagnosed without bx. If a pt is cirrhotic and has two imaging studies showing a nodule

>2 cm with hypervascularization or one such imaging study and an AFP level >400 ng/mL, then HCC is very likely (J Hepatol 2001;35:421). The remainder require imaging-directed bx. Some authors advise against bx because of the risk of seeding the bx tract (N Z Med J 1996;109:469). A cavernous hemangioma should be ruled out prior to bx by MRI or by tagged rbc scan if the initial imaging study suggests that possibility. The dx should always be considered when a pt with cirrhosis has a clinical deterioration.

Lab: Serum α-fetoprotein (AFP) is elevated in 80% of pts with HCC. Elevations occur in hep B, hep C, germ cell tumors, pregnancy, and other causes of cirrhosis. The gross appearance of HCC ranges from a discrete nodule to a diffuse lesion. The fibro-lamellar variant of HCC is a large, hard tumor with bands of fibrous tissue that arises in a noncirrhotic liver. The fibrolamellar variant carries a better prognosis with aggressive surgery (Hepatology 1997;26:877).

X-ray: Ultrasound is the most commonly used initial test for detection. Either helical CT or MRI can then be used to assess the extent of growth and vascular involvement. There is no clear evidence to suggest that either modality is consistently superior (Postgrad Med J 2000;76:4). Lesions are frequently missed on imaging studies. A sensitivity of 63% was seen in pts whose CT was compared to their explanted liver after transplant (Radiology 1994;193:645).

Rx:

- *Resection and transplant:* (Ann IM 1998;129:643) Only a small proportion (10% in Western countries) of pts with HCC are candidates for cure by resection or transplantation. Resection is widely used in pts who do not have cirrhosis (since they tolerate wide resections) or in selected Child-Pugh grade A (p 51) cirrhotic pts with small lesions. The finding of a wedged hepatic vein pressure gradient of >10 mm Hg (a measure of the degree of portal HTN) identifies pts fit for resection (GE 1996;111:1018). Survival after curative resection is only 20-40% at 5 yr and recurrence is 70%. Many of the recurrences are probably new primary lesions. If the resected specimen shows histologic findings suggestive of recurrence (Ann Surg 1993;218:145), transplant is a consideration. Transplantation has the advantage that it can be performed in pts with advanced cirrhosis who do not tolerate wide resections. Transplant rids the pt of a diseased liver that is very likely to generate new lesions even if the first lesion is cured in the resection. Initial transplant experience in unselected pts who received no adjuvant rx was poor, with only 9% of pts free of disease at 2 yr, perhaps because HCC implanted in the donor liver (Surgery 1991;110:726). However, if transplantation is reserved for pts with a single lesion <5 cm in diameter or no more than 3 lesions each <3 cm, then recurrence-free survival climbs to 83% at 4 yr (Nejm 1996;334:693). About 25% of pts preoperatively thought to meet these criteria are found to have more advanced disease in the explanted liver.

- *Ablation for local control:* In pts with unresectable disease, chemoembolization reduces tumor growth at the risk of acute liver failure. There is no survival benefit (Nejm 1995; 332:1256). Chemoembolization is done with cisplatin mixed in the oily solvent lipiodol that remains selectively in the tumor. Many centers use different variations of chemoembolization as a temporizing measure while pts await liver transplant (Ann IM 1988;108:390). Percutaneous ethanol injection of small lesions (Cancer 1992;69:925) and cryotherapy (Brit J Surg 1998;85:1171) have been tried, but controlled data are lacking.

- *Chemotherapy:* Chemotherapy after transplantation for small tumors is unlikely to be of benefit since those pts do well with surgery alone. For more advanced lesions, chemotherapy is disappointing with overall response rates of 20% and survival of 2-6 months with a variety of regimens (Postgrad Med J 2000; 76:4). Intraarterial chemotherapy has been used, but has not been adequately studied.

- *Screening:* (GE 2004;127:S108) The routine screening of cirrhotic pts for HCC is controversial. A large randomized trial of Chinese pts with hep B showed a 37% reduction in mortality with screening with AFP and US every 6 months (J Cancer Res Clin Oncol 2004;130:417). A similar trial in Western pts is unlikely to be done. Screening is not strongly supported by the data (Am J Gastro 2000;95:1535) but is widely practiced (Am J Gastro 1999;94:2988). Some studies suggest that screening detects lesions before they become unresectable (Hepatology 2000;32:842; Ann Surg 1995;222:375). Screening can be done by AFP determinations, US, or CT scan. These modalities can be used alone or in combination. Studies are often repeated on a q 6 month basis. Screening might be helpful to pts with Child's grade A cirrhosis (who can be treated with resection) and to Child's grade B pts if transplant is readily available. Screening is unlikely to be cost effective in pts with Child's grade C cirrhosis (these pts should have transplants in any event) and in the elderly with comorbidities. Consensus conferences have advocated screening, but no widely endorsed practice guidelines are available (J Clin Gastro 2002;35:S86).

- *Prevention:* Universal vaccination of Taiwanese children against hep B has resulted in a dramatic drop in chronic infection and in the incidence of HCC (Nejm 1997;336:1855). A reduction in incidence of HCC was seen in one trial of interferon for hep C (Lancet 1995;346:1051) but not in a prospective cohort study (Hepatology 1998;28:1687). Elimination of aflatoxin from stored food may be of benefit.

13.2 Hepatic Masses

Semin Liver Dis 1993;13:423

There are many lesions that can present as hepatic masses, and the diagnostic approach and diff dx are fully reviewed elsewhere (see Semin Liver Dis 1993;13:423). Common considerations include:

- *Hepatic adenoma:* These lesions are most often associated with oral contraceptive use. They typically present as palpable or radiographic masses in women. Because of the risk of rupture or malignant transformation, surgical resection is indicated, and preoperative bx is avoided because the lesions are vascular.

- *Focal nodular hyperplasia:* These lesions are masses with a thick central stellate scar. They can cause pain, but rupture is rare and malignant transformation is not seen. CT, MRI, or ultrasound may detect the characteristic scar that distinguishes these lesions from more serious tumors. Bx should be avoided because of the risk of bleeding.

- *Cavernous hemangioma:* These lesions are very common (found at up to 20% of autopsies) and are usually asymptomatic. They can grow and cause pain, but rupture is rare. They may be detected by several imaging studies, but MRI is the most sensitive for distinguishing them from malignant tumors. Only symptomatic lesions should be treated with surgery and bx should be avoided.

- *Cysts:* (J Am Coll Surg 2000;191:311) Simple cysts are commonly seen on imaging studies. They are generally asymptomatic but can enlarge and cause sx. Neoplastic cysts are usually detected because of papillary projections and multiloculations on imaging studies. They are treated surgically. Cysts may be seen after trauma. Hydatid cysts (from *Echinococcus*) need to be considered in endemic areas (Gastroenterol Clin North Am 1996;25:655).

- *Other lesions:* Hepatobiliary cystadenomas are detected by their septations and should be resected. Focal fatty infiltration, HCC (see section 13.1), metastatic disease, and abscess can present as masses.

Chapter 14

Drug- and Toxin-Induced Liver Disease

14.1 Alcoholic Liver Disease

Mayo Clin Proc 2001;76:1021; Postgrad Med J 2000;76:280

Cause: Excessive intake of ethanol. For practical purposes, alcohol has been defined in units. A unit is 1 oz of spirits, 12 oz of beer, or 4 oz of wine, and it contains about 10-12 gm of alcohol. Most individuals developing alcoholic liver disease (ALD) consume more than 35 units/week. A safe level of 21 units/week for men and 14 units/week for women has been proposed.

Epidem: Alcohol is the major cause of cirrhosis in Western countries. The risk of alcoholic liver disease is higher in those who consume >30 gm daily (Gut 1997;41:845), though only 5% of pts with this level of consumption have overt disease. Risk climbs markedly with increasing consumption. Female sex, drinking without food, binge drinking, and drinking concentrated beverages or multiple types of beverages increase risk.

Pathophys: Three forms of ALD are recognized. Steatosis **(alcoholic fatty liver)** occurs in 90-100% of heavy drinkers and is reversible with abstinence. However, **cirrhosis** develops in 30% of pts who drink more than 40 units/week, and fibrosis in 37% (Lancet 1995;346:987). In **acute alcoholic hepatitis,** there is hepatocyte ballooning and necrosis with cholestasis, but no evidence of cirrhosis. This occurs in about 10-35% of heavy drinkers. **Alcoholic cirrhosis** is the most severe form of injury and is seen in 8-20% of heavy drinkers. Histologically, there are bridges of fibrosis that develop between central veins and portal tracts. This creates a micronodular pattern of regenerating nodules.

Multiple factors are thought to mediate alcoholic liver injury (Postgrad Med 1998;103:261). Ethanol is oxidized to acetaldehyde by alcohol dehydrogenase, and then to acetate. Changes that occur in the redox potential of the cell from this oxidation have harmful effects on lipids and carbohydrate metabolism. Acetaldehyde binds to proteins, creating antigenic targets and starting an inflammatory cascade. Iron deposition may play a role.

Sx: Many pts are asymptomatic and come to evaluation because of abnormal LFTs detected at a checkup or as part of an alcohol detoxification evaluation. Pts may have nonspecific complaints of anorexia, malaise, or abdominal pain, which are often related to their alcoholism. The most crucial point is eliciting the alcohol hx. A variety of screening questionnaires have been developed. The CAGE questionnaire is widely used. It consists of 4 questions:

C: Have you ever felt the need to **cut** down your drinking?
A: Have you ever felt **annoyed** by criticism of your drinking?
G: Have you ever felt **guilty** about your drinking?
E: Have you ever taken a drink first thing in the morning **(eye opener)**?

Two or more positive responses suggest problem drinking. Pts often lie about their alcohol use, and hx from family members may be critical.

Si: In steatosis there is often hepatomegaly. In alcoholic hepatitis the pt looks ill, and there may be fever, jaundice, spiders, tender hepatomegaly, ascites, or encephalopathy. Alcoholic cirrhosis causes signs of end-stage liver disease (p 42) that cannot be distinguished from signs caused by other liver diseases.

Crs: Five-year survival in cirrhosis is 35-50%. Survival is much better in abstinent pts than in those who continue to drink. The prognosis in acute alcoholic hepatitis can be determined from laboratory parameters (see Lab).

Cmplc: HCC is a risk in cirrhotic pts (p 413). Any of the complications of end-stage liver disease may occur (p 429).

Diff Dx: The diff dx may be that of abnormal LFTs, cirrhosis, or jaundice (p 42).

Lab: LFTs, CBC with diff, and PT should be obtained. Transaminases are elevated in alcoholic hepatitis, usually in a pattern of AST>ALT with neither more than 7 × the upper limit of normal. GGTP is frequently elevated. In advanced disease, albumin drops and the PT is elevated. An elevated MCV can be a clue to alcoholism, and a random alcohol level can be informative. In alcoholic hepatitis a severity score, called the discriminant function, is calculated as 4.6 × (pt's PT − control PT) + bilirubin (mg/dL) (GE 1978;75:193). A score of >32 or spontaneous encephalopathy is associated with high mortality (>30%). Leukocytosis is common in alcoholic hepatitis. Thrombocytopenia can be seen with portal hypertension or as a result of toxic effects of alcohol on bone marrow. Pts should have appropriate tests to exclude other causes of abnormal LFTs (p 43), and all should be tested for hep C. Liver bx is prognostic and can confirm the diagnosis. It is usually not necessary to perform bx.

X-ray: Ultrasound should be performed to rule out obstruction or tumor. Pts with alcoholic cirrhosis may not dilate their bile ducts in response to obstruction (because of severe fibrosis), so caution in interpretation is warranted.

Endoscopy: Consider EGD to look for varices in cirrhotic pts (p 429).

Rx: ACG guidelines for management (Am J Gastro 1998; 93:2022) include:

- *Abstinence:* This is the most important factor in successful rx but the most difficult to achieve. Individual counseling, support groups such as Alcoholics Anonymous, and other structured rx programs have variable efficacy. Drug rx such as naltrexone or acamprosate may have a role in reducing consumption (Jama 1999;281:1318).

- *Nutritional support and supplements:* In hospitalized pts with severe disease, enteral feedings improve outcome (GE 1992;102:200). Pts with cirrhosis rapidly recruit alternative fuels such as skeletal muscle, and prolonged starvation should be avoided. A nighttime snack and early morning feeding are important. Expensive formulations of branched chain amino acids (which may reduce encephalopathy) are usually not needed. Thiamine, folate, and multivitamins should be routinely given.

- *Corticosteroids for alcoholic hepatitis:* Two RCTs demonstrate that a course of prednisolone 40 mg po qd (for 4 weeks followed by a taper) reduces mortality in pts with severe alcoholic hepatitis (Nejm 1992;326:507; Ann IM 1989;110:685). In these trials, pts with encephalopathy or a high discriminant function (described above) were treated. Pts with active bleeding, active infection, renal failure, pancreatitis, or poorly controlled diabetes should be excluded. The long-term benefits are unknown.

- *Other drug rx:* Propylthiouracil 300 mg po qd for up to 2 yr reduced mortality from 25 to 13% in an RCT of pts with ALD, but the data have not been replicated and the drug is not widely used (Nejm 1987;317:1421). Colchicine was effective in prolonging median survival in an RCT, but methodologic flaws and the lack of a confirmatory study have stopped its widespread use (Nejm 1988;318:1709). A variety of therapies are investigational (Postgrad Med J 2000;76:280).

Pentoxifylline 400 mg po tid improved short-term survival in a single RCT of severe alcoholic hepatitis (GE 2000;119:1637).

- *Liver transplant:* Liver transplant is effective in ALD and has survival comparable to transplant for other liver diseases (Surgery 1992;112:694).

14.2 Drug-Induced Liver Injury

There are more than 600 described drug, chemical, and herbal causes of liver injury. Several patterns of liver injury may be seen, including acute hepatocellular injury, cholestasis, granulomatous hepatitis, chronic hepatitis, vascular injury, fulminant hepatic failure, and neoplasia. Drugs should be suspected in all cases of asymptomatic LFTs or clinically overt liver injury. A methodical listing of all the pt's current and recent medicines is the cornerstone of diagnosis. Herbal remedies should not be overlooked (Jama 1995;273:502). A current reference (such as the American Hospital Formulary) should be used to research each drug, and a list of suspected agents should be made. A literature search for case reports can be helpful when the reference source provides scanty information. Given the long list of offending agents, it is not possible to provide a meaningful review of the individual agents in a text of this size. Excellent reviews are available (Nejm 2003;349:474).

14.3 Acetaminophen Overdose

Postgrad Med 1999;105:81; Lancet 1995;346:547

Cause: Intentional overdose with suicidal intent, excessive doses without suicidal intent, and therapeutic doses in a pt predisposed to toxicity (usually because of alcohol) (Hepatology 1995; 22:767).

Epidem: Fifty percent of exposures to toxic doses are seen in children, and 63% of poisonings are accidental (Am Fam Phys 1996;

53:185). Accidental misuse has higher morbidity and mortality and is common in alcoholics (Nejm 1997;337:1112).

Pathophys: About 5-10% of ingested acetaminophen is converted via the P450 enzyme system to a toxic metabolite N-acetyl-p-benzoquinoneimine (NAPQI). Normally the sulfhydryl groups of glutathione rapidly bind this metabolite and inactivate it. However, when high levels of NAPQI overwhelm the available glutathione, binding occurs with sulfhydryl groups of hepatic proteins, causing hepatocyte necrosis (Postgrad Med 1999;105:81). Intentional overdose is the most common presentation. However, those with enhanced activation of P450 systems (due to alcohol and a variety of drugs) or those with reduced glutathione stores (cirrhosis, starvation, alcoholism, or eating disorders) can develop toxicity without intentional overdose.

Sx/Si: Following intentional overdose, there is anorexia, nausea, and vomiting for the first 24 hr. From 24 hr to 48 hr the pt improves. Thereafter some pts develop sx and si of liver failure with RUQ pain, hepatomegaly, jaundice, somnolence, confusion, coma, and oliguria. By day 6-7 those destined to recover will begin to improve.

Crs: Of untreated pts with levels in the toxic range, 1-2% die of liver failure.

Cmplc: Fulminant hepatic failure, renal failure, acidosis.

Diff Dx: The diff dx may be that of fulminant hepatic failure (p 49) or abnormal LFTs (p 43).

Lab: In a single-dose ingestion, acetaminophen levels are obtained serially and are plotted on a nomogram to determine if they cross the toxic threshold that requires rx (Ann EM 1991;20:1058). PT/INR and LFTs are followed serially to look for evidence of hepatic damage. Cr is obtained daily to look for evidence of renal failure. Acid-base status is assessed at 24 hrs, because acidosis is common in severe toxicity. A toxic screen to look for other ingestions is indicated (Dig Dis Sci 2000;45:1553).

Rx: Charcoal is given if less than 1 hr has elapsed since substantial overdose. Depending on the acetaminophen level, the time since ingestion, host factors, and stage of illness, rx with N-acetylcysteine is given. The drug is uniformly effective in preventing fatality if given within 16 hr of ingestion (Nejm 1988; 319:1557). The iv formulation may be more consistently effective (because of nausea and vomiting) and is now FDA approved in the U.S. The oral formulation is widely used as first-line treatment. The duration varies depending on the clinical course. Prolonged courses are indicated in fulminant hepatic failure. Those caring for such pts must consult a comprehensive source (eg, Lancet 1995;346:547) for details. In the U.S., consultation with the Rocky Mountain Poison and Drug Center (303-739-1123) may be valuable for current protocols. A transplant center should be contacted for advice if there is evidence of developing severe liver damage (ALT/AST > 1000 U/L). The rx of fulminant hepatic failure is complex and belongs in specialty centers (Lancet 1997;349:1081).

Chapter 15

Complications of End-Stage Liver Disease

15.1 Portal Hypertension and Variceal Hemorrhage

Gastroenterol Clin North Am 2003;32:1079; Nejm 2001;345:669

Cause: Rupture of varices secondary to portal hypertension, defined as portal venous pressure >5 mm Hg.

Epidem: Most varices are associated with cirrhosis, and the epidemiology of varices is that of the underlying cause of cirrhosis.

Pathophys:
- *Portal HTN:* The portal vein forms from the confluence of the superior mesenteric and splenic veins. Portal pressure can rise because of increased outflow resistance or increased portal inflow. Increased resistance can be due to (1) prehepatic causes (portal vein thrombosis); (2) hepatic causes (cirrhosis, inflammation with hepatocyte swelling, mass, regenerating nodules); or (3) posthepatic causes (hepatic vein obstruction; see Budd-Chiari syndrome p 451). Increased portal inflow results from peripheral vasodilatation and the hyperdynamic circulation of cirrhosis due to an imbalance of vasodilators and vasoconstrictors.
- *Varices and bleeding risk:* In portal HTN, the increase in pressure causes the opening of collateral vessels. Most of these vessels are in the retroperitoneum. The most troublesome collaterals are veins intrinsic to the distal esophagus and

proximal stomach that become dilated and tortuous (Lancet 1997;350:1235). As variceal pressure rises, wall tension and the risk of bleeding also rise (Hepatology 2000;32:842). Direct pressure measurements are not readily available to most clinicians, and risk must be estimated by other criteria. Three clinical criteria are used to predict risk: (1) variceal size, (2) Child-Pugh grade (p 51), and (3) the presence of red wales (endoscopically identified longitudinal, dilated venules on varices that look like whip marks) (Nejm 1988;319:983). Varices are called size **F1** if they are small and straight, **F2** if enlarged, tortuous, and occupying less than one third of the lumen circumference, and **F3** if coiled and occupying more than one third of the circumference of the lumen (Nejm 1988;319:983).

- *Unusual varices:* Isolated gastric varices can occur with splenic vein thrombosis (Am J Gastro 1984;79:304). Ectopic varices can form in the duodenum, in adhesions to the abdominal wall, in surgical anastomoses, and at ostomies (Hepatology 1998;28:1154).
- *Portal hypertensive gastropathy (PHG)* (Am J Gastro 2002; 97:2973): PHG is a lesion seen in the stomach of pts with portal HTN. Microscopically, it represents an area of microvascular ectasia and perivascular fibrosis. Endoscopically, it is recognized as multiple small erythematous areas outlined by subtle lines giving a cracked sand or snakeskin appearance to the mucosa. In more severe disease there is oozing and more prominent red spots, and lesions may be seen in body, fundus, and antrum. In the largest series followed endoscopically over 3 yr, acute bleeding was rare (2.5% over 3 yr) and chronic bleeding was seen in 11% (GE 2000;119:181). Disease parallels the severity of portal HTN and may worsen or improve spontaneously.

Sx: Pts present with sx of UGI bleeding (p 33). Hematemesis and melena are common.

Si: Melena or hematochezia are typical. Pts may become encephalo-pathic. Other stigmata of portal HTN may be present (ascites, splenomegaly), and other findings of chronic liver disease may be present (p 42).

Crs: About 50% of cirrhotics have varices. Cirrhotics without varices develop them at 5-15%/yr. Varices become large (and therefore at risk to bleed) at a rate of 4-10%/yr. Only about one third of pts with varices bleed, but each bleeding episode carries a 20-30% risk of death. Rebleeding often occurs within 48 hr of the initial bleed, but risk remains high for 6 weeks. Rebleeding is most fre-quent in pts with severe liver failure, massive initial bleed, ongoing alcoholism, HCC, large varices, or renal failure (Gastroenterol Clin North Am 2000;29:337). Untreated pts rebleed or die within a yr about 70% of the time. Isolated gastric varices are at very high risk for bleeding (Hepatology 1992;16:1343). Pts with small varices have a low risk of bleeding (8% at 4 yr), but a worsening Child-Pugh grade (p 51) may sug-gest variceal enlargement and a higher risk of bleeding (Am J Gastro 2000;95:503).

Cmplc: Variceal hemorrhage can lead to death, SBP (p 441), renal failure, and aspiration pneumonia.

Diff Dx: The differential of variceal hemorrhage is that of upper gi bleeding. The differential for portal HTN is that of causes of cir-rhosis (p 48, Evaluation of Cirrhosis), causes of thrombosis of the portal vein or its tributaries (p 455), and Budd-Chiari (p 451).

Lab: See "Approach to Acute Bleeding," p 34. An elevated PT in a pt with evidence of UGI bleeding may be a clue to varices as the cause.

X-ray: Radiographs are not indicated in the evaluation of bleeding. Imaging may be needed to evaluate the underlying cause of portal HTN, especially to rule out malignancy and to evaluate portal vein patency. MR angiography is better than Doppler ultrasound for this purpose (AJR Am J Roentgenol 1993;161:989).

Endoscopy: (Semin Liver Dis 1999;19:439) Varices are easily diagnosed at endoscopy as bluish veins, and size is best estimated after air insufflation. **Endoscopic sclerotherapy** (EST) is performed by the injection of a sclerosant (eg, sodium tetradecyl sulfate, polidocanol, or ethanolamine) into or around variceal channels. Sessions are continued every week or 2 until varices in the distal 5 cm are eliminated. Follow-up EGD is done q 3 months × 6 months, then q 6-12 months to look for recurrence. Complications include fever, retrosternal pain, pleural effusions, esophageal ulcers (which may bleed in up to 20%), esophageal stricture, perforation from full-thickness necrosis, and mediastinitis (Endoscopy 1992;24:284). **Endoscopic variceal ligation** (EVL) is replacing sclerotherapy. In this technique, a 1-cm barrel wrapped with rubber bands on its outside is attached to the end of the endoscope. The varix is sucked into the hollow portion of the barrel. A band is deployed off the barrel and wraps itself around the base of the varix. The band and the clotted varix fall off a few days later, leaving a small ulceration. This technique has fewer associated complications than sclerotherapy (see Rx).

Rx: Because of the frequency and high mortality associated with variceal bleeding, a bewildering number of clinical studies and meta-analyses have been published. These are very well reviewed in Brit J Surg 1995;82:1023, and the bottom lines are as follows:

- *Prevention of a first variceal bleed:* The nonselective beta-blockers (propranolol and nadolol) reduce the incidence of a first bleed by about 45% (for one meta-analysis, see Ann IM 1992;117:59). Ideally, pts would have the dosage adjusted on the basis of portal pressure gradients, but in practice, the dosage is adjusted until resting heart rate is reduced 25% or until pulse is 50-60. Sclerotherapy as primary prophylaxis is not recommended. A large RCT showed that sclerotherapy was effective at decreasing bleeding but was associated with increased mortality for unclear reasons (Nejm 1991;324:1779). In an RCT, EVL appeared more effective than propranolol in preventing a first bleed from large varices (Nejm 1999; 340:988). This study was unusual for its finding of a high rate of bleeding on propranolol, and further studies are warranted before considering this as the first-line approach (Nejm 1999; 340:1033).

- *Rx of acute bleeding:* Endoscopic control of bleeding is the rx of choice for acute hemorrhage (Hepatology 1995;22:332). EVL is preferred over sclerotherapy because eradication occurs more quickly, with lower mortality and fewer complications (major RCT, Nejm 1992;326:1527; meta-analysis, Ann IM 1995; 123:280). Octreotide, a somatostatin analogue with a longer half-life, has become the drug of choice for acute bleeding episodes. This agent appears to be as effective as sclerotherapy (Gut 1997;41:526). The addition of octreotide (50 μg iv bolus and 50 μg/hr as a continuous infusion for 5 days) to EVL lowers early rebleeding compared to ligation alone (Lancet 1995;346:1666) or sclerotherapy alone (Nejm 1995;333:555). Vasopressin is effective but is no longer used because of cardiac vasoconstriction. Prophylaxis against SBP (p 441) should be given. Gastric varices are difficult to treat and injection with cyanoacrylate glue has become a widely used initial rx (Gastroenterol Clin North Am 2003;32:1079).
- *Prevention of recurrent bleeding:* Sclerotherapy has been well shown (in 8 trials) to be superior to placebo in the prevention of further bleeding. Ligation has been shown to be superior to sclerotherapy regarding rebleeding rate, mortality, and complications (meta-analysis, Ann IM 1995;123:280). Beta-blockers

are effective in preventing recurrent bleeding compared to placebo (meta-analysis, Lancet 1990;336:153), but in practice most pts have endoscopic obliteration with EVL. The addition of beta-blockers to a course of endoscopic obliteration improves outcome (Hepatology 2000;32:461). The addition of isosorbide mononitrate may be beneficial but is often poorly tolerated (Lancet 2003;361:952). Pts with an episode of variceal bleeding should be evaluated for liver transplantation.

- *TIPS:* (Gastroenterol Clin North Am 2000;29:387) A transjugular intrahepatic portosystemic shunt (TIPS) is a stent placed between a hepatic vein and an intrahepatic portion of the portal vein. It can be placed in 90% of pts, with a 10% complication rate and a 2% procedure-related death rate (Radiographics 1993;13:1185). Complications include mechanical events during placement (such as bleeding, rupture of the capsule), complications of shunting (encephalopathy in 15% [Gut 1996;39:479] and worsened liver function), and stent-related complications (hemolysis, infection, stenosis). The established indications for TIPS are active variceal bleeding despite endoscopic rx (including a second attempt) and prevention of recurrent variceal hemorrhage in pts awaiting liver transplantation (Jama 1995;273:1824). TIPS may also be useful in refractory ascites and Budd-Chiari (GE 1996;111:1700). Initially, a TIPS behaves like a surgical shunt with decompression of the portal system. A TIPS is much more prone to occlusion than a surgical shunt. Occlusion due to clot or stent kinking can occur within weeks in about 3-10% of cases. Recurrent portal HTN from stenosis due to pseudointimal hyperplasia occurs frequently (about 60%). This problem can be treated with repeated dilatations (GE 1997;112:889). Right-sided heart failure is a catastrophe if it develops in a TIPS pt, because the elevated right atrial pressure is transmitted directly to the portal system, causing recurrent varices. As long as the stent is patent, esophageal varices resolve, but fundic varices often do not because of splenorenal collaterals or massive splenomegaly excessively feeding the short gastric vessels (GE 1997;112:889). Monitoring with Doppler is commonly done but can miss significant stenosis. Some centers do periodic angiography and/or endoscopy.

- *Surgical shunts and decompression:* (Gastroenterol Clin North Am 2000;29:387) A variety of surgical shunts to decompress the portal system have been described. All shunts reduce bleeding but are accompanied to varying degrees by encephalopathy and worsened liver failure. A side-to-side anastomosis of IVC to portal vein reduces bleeding and ascites, but is prone to clot and makes transplant surgery more difficult. Distal splenorenal shunt (joining a transected splenic vein to the left renal vein) lowers pressure in varices but does not reduce portal inflow, and so ascites is a problem with this technically demanding operation. Esophageal transection with an automated suturing device and other devascularization procedures are not widely used. These procedures may be alternative salvage strategies (Hepatology 1992;15:403) for those who fail endoscopic rx and TIPS.

- *Balloon tamponade:* Balloon tamponade is effective in controlling hemorrhage in 80-90% of pts, but complications and early rebleeding are common (Scand J Gastroenterol Suppl 1994; 207:11). Aspiration pneumonia occurs in 10% of pts and orotracheal intubation is routinely used. The 4-lumen Sengstaken-Blakemore tube has esophageal and gastric balloons and an aspiration port and is most often used. The Linton-Nachlas tube has a bigger gastric balloon and is used for gastric varices. It is important to make sure that the position of the gastric balloon within the stomach is confirmed radiographically to prevent accidental inflation in the esophagus. The tube must be deflated for 30 minutes q 4-6 hr and duration of use must be minimized. Generally, tubes are a temporizing measure used in desperate circumstances when endoscopic and pharmacologic methods fail while awaiting TIPS.

- *Portal hypertensive gastropathy (PHG):* Rx is that of the underlying portal HTN with medical rx, TIPS, or shunt (Dig Dis 1996;14:258). In a small trial, propranolol was effective in reducing bleeding (Lancet 1991;337:1431).

15.2 Ascites

Nejm 2004;350:1646; Hepatology 1998;27:264

Cause: (Nejm 1994;330:337) Ascites can be secondary to portal HTN or due to a variety of conditions in which portal pressures are normal. Causes of ascites associated with portal HTN are cirrhosis (the vast majority), alcoholic hepatitis, heart failure, hepatic metastases, fulminant hepatic failure, Budd-Chiari, venoocclusive disease, myxedema, and fatty liver of pregnancy. Causes of ascites without portal HTN include peritoneal carcinomatosis, TB, pancreatic ascites (from a disrupted pancreatic duct), biliary ascites (bile in the belly usually from a biliary surgery mishap), chylous ascites (milky ascites from disrupted lymphatics often associated with malignancy [Am J Gastro 2002;97:1896]), nephrotic syndrome, bowel obstruction/infarction, and serositis from connective tissue disease. The serum-ascites albumin gradient is used to separate these 2 groups (see Lab).

Epidem: Varies with underlying cause.

Pathophys: (Lancet 1997;350:1309) The pathogenesis of ascites due to cirrhosis is complex and incompletely understood. Cirrhotics develop increased cardiac output, decreased peripheral vascular resistance, and splanchnic vasodilatation. This is probably a result of an imbalance between vasodilating and vasoconstricting substances. This leads the neurohumoral system to detect a decreased effective circulating volume. This causes: (1) increased activity of the renin-angiotensin-aldosterone system; (2) increased levels of ADH; (3) increased sympathetic nervous system activity; and (4) alterations in intrarenal factors such as kallikrein and endothelin. These 4 factors result in reduced renal blood flow and retention of sodium and water.

Sx: Pts may present with bloating or pain if ascites develops rapidly.

Si: Ascites can be detected by bulging flanks, shifting dullness, or a fluid wave (p 43). The physical exam can be misleading. Findings of associated malignancy or other underlying diseases (such as end-stage liver disease) may be present.

Crs: About 50% of cirrhotics will develop ascites over 10 yr. Cirrhotic ascites is a poor prognostic sign with a 2-yr survival of 50%. A striking 40% of pts with ascites will develop hepatorenal syndrome (HRS) within 4 yr (GE 1993;105:229). The course of noncirrhotic ascites is dependent on the underlying disease.

Cmplc: SBP (p 441), and HRS (p 446).

Diff Dx: Analysis of ascitic fluid and imaging the abdomen are usually sufficient to determine the cause of ascites.

Lab: Ascitic fluid is obtained by paracentesis to determine the underlying cause and to look for evidence of SBP in pts with a clinical deterioration. Paracentesis is safe even with mild to moderate defects in coagulation (PT $<2 \times$ the normal value, platelets counts 50-100,000). Fresh frozen plasma or platelets are not needed prior to the procedure with these moderate hemostatic defects (Transfusion 1991;31:164). Risks are hematoma, infection, or, rarely, massive bleeding. Cell counts, albumin, total protein, culture (in blood culture bottles to improve sensitivity [Arch IM 1987;147:73]), and Gram stain are useful in most instances. The **serum-ascites albumin gradient** is calculated by subtracting the ascites albumin (in mg/dL) on an initial paracentesis from the serum albumin obtained the same day. A gradient of ≥1.1 gm/dL is indicative of portal HTN as the cause of ascites (Ann IM 1992;117:215). Total protein of <1.0 gm/dL predicts a high future risk of SBP. Cytology is obtained if the pt is not a known cirrhotic, has other findings to suggest malignancy, or has an ascites cell count of >500 lymphocytes. TB culture and AFB smear is considered if the cell counts show a large number of lymphocytes and the albumin gradient is <1.1. Triglycerides are obtained if the specimen looks milky to prove the presence of chylous ascites. Neutrophil counts >250 cell/mm^3 indicate infection (see SBP p 441). Most pts with infected ascites have SBP but some have peritonitis secondary to an intraabdominal infection, such as a perforated viscus. In many of these cases, ascites total protein is >1.0 gm/dL, ascites LDH > serum LDH, and ascites glucose is <50 mg/dL (GE 1990;98:127). Pancreatic ascites (from a disrupted pancreatic duct) is identified by high amylase in ascitic fluid.

X-ray: Ultrasound is very sensitive for the detection of ascites, and all pts with suspected ascites should undergo an imaging study to confirm the ascites and to look for evidence of malignancy. Cardiac echo may be needed to evaluate a cardiac cause of ascites.

Rx: (Hepatology 1998;27:264)
- *Diet:* Ascites disappears to the extent that sodium excretion exceeds sodium intake. The first step in rx is to limit intake. A 2-gm Na diet (=88 mEq of Na) is about all that can be realistically expected. Extensive teaching is needed for the pt and his or her personal chef. Fluid restriction is needed only if there is significant hyponatremia. Restricting fluids to 1500 mL if Na falls below 130 seems prudent. Bed rest is not needed.
- *Diuretics:* (Nejm 1994;330:337) The combination of furosemide 40 mg po qd and spironolactone 100 mg po qd is a starting point for rx that often results in speedy diuresis without hypokalemia. Spironolactone can be given in one dose

in the AM since the drug half-life is very long in cirrhosis (GE 1992;102:1680). If weight or urine Na excretion has not responded, then the dose should be doubled. The unusual pt who fails to respond can be treated with up to 160 mg furosemide and 400 mg spironolactone. Amiloride can be used in place of spironolactone (starting at 10 mg and increasing to 40 mg). This avoids gynecomastia, which can be seen with spironolactone and amiloride has a faster onset of action (Adv Intern Med 1990;35:365).

- *Monitoring rx:* The pt monitors weight, aiming to lose 1 lb per day (or more if peripheral edema is present). If there is inadequate weight loss, urine volume and urine Na are measured to estimate Na balance. If a pt has a good response to diuretics, a high urinary excretion of Na is expected. The net Na balance can be calculated if urine Na and volume are measured. For example, if a pt on diuretics makes 2 L of urine with a urine Na concentration of 80 mEq Na/L, the pt's urinary Na excretion is 160 mEq/day. If the pt is compliant with a 2-gm Na diet, the intake is 88 mEq (there is 44 mEq Na in one gram NaCl). Therefore, the pt's net loss of Na is calculated as: **88 mEq** (what was eaten in a 2-gm Na diet) − **160 mEq** (sodium excreted in 2 L of urine at 80 mEq/L) = **72 mEq** net loss of Na per day. Since the average L of ascites has 128 mEq of Na in it (Adv Intern Med 1990;35:365), the pt would lose 72/128=0.56 L of ascites per day. If the pt has urine with a high volume and sodium content but fails to lose ascites, then diet noncompliance is likely. If urine Na and volume are low, then the response to diuretics has not been adequate and doses should be increased if possible. Rx is monitored with periodic lytes, BUN, and Cr to assess for excessive azotemia or electrolyte disturbances. Diuretic doses often need to be reduced in pts who respond well.
- *Tense ascites:* A total paracentesis should be performed at the outset in tense ascites for more rapid sx relief.

- *Refractory ascites:* About 10% of pts are resistant to diuretics. Repeated therapeutic paracentesis is effective for this group. The use of volume expanders to protect against azotemia is controversial. An RCT compared the use of 40 gm of albumin after each paracentesis vs placebo and showed that albumin prevented azotemia and hyponatremia (GE 1988;94:1493). However, mortality was not affected. Several small series indicate that clinically important azotemia is uncommon, and many experts question the importance of albumin given its great expense (GE 1991;101:1455). Use of the plasma expander dextran 70 is a cheaper alternative to albumin (Dig Dis Sci 1992;37:79), but its use does not have the support of an RCT as does albumin. Given the safety of albumin, the use of 8 gm of albumin for every L of ascites removed has been recommended (Lancet 1997;350:1309). TIPS (p 434) is an alternative in refractory ascites. It is effective in preventing recurrent ascites but does not appear to improve survival compared to large volume paracentesis (GE 2003;124:634; GE 2002;123:1839). The chief disadvantages of TIPS are shunt stenosis, hepatic encephalopathy, and cost. It may be best for pts without severe liver failure in whom repeated paracentesis is not practical or desired by the pt. Liver transplantation is the ideal rx for pts with refractory ascites since it is the only intervention that will improve the otherwise dismal prognosis.
- *Shunts:* Peritonovenous shunts (eg, the LeVeen or Denver shunts) were developed in the 1970s as physiologic rx of ascites. Their value is severely limited by poor long-term patency and complications, including adhesion formation, that can make transplant difficult. Their use should be restricted to pts who have refractory ascites, are not transplant candidates, and are unable to have repeated paracentesis (Hepatology 1998;27:264).

- *Malignant ascites:* Repeated paracentesis is the usual rx. Some pts with ascites from massive intrahepatic metastases may respond to diuretics (GE 1992;103:1302).
- *Hepatic hydrothorax:* This is defined as a pleural effusion in a pt with cirrhosis and no evidence of cardiopulmonary disease. It is due to movement of ascites across defects in the diaphragm and is seen in 4-10% of pts with ascites. It can be debilitating and is managed with thoracentesis, diuretics, TIPS, or transplant (Am J Med 1999;107:262).

15.3 Spontaneous Bacterial Peritonitis

Nejm 2004;350:1646; J Hepatol 2000;32:142; Semin Liver Dis 1997;17:203

Cause: Bacterial infection. Gram-negative aerobic bacteria and nonenterococcal *Streptococcus* are the most common organisms.

Epidem: The prevalence of spontaneous bacterial peritonitis (SBP) in cirrhotics on hospital admission is 10-30%.

Pathophys: Most episodes of SBP are thought to occur by translocation of bacteria from gut to mesenteric lymph nodes (J Hepatol 1994;21:792). Translocation implies movement of bacteria across an intact gut. Some cases may occur from seeding from another source (eg, lung, urinary tract).

Sx/Si: Some pts present with obvious peritonitis with severe pain, fever, abdominal tenderness, hypotension, and leukocytosis. Others present with milder sx of pain or with nonspecific sx such as worsened encephalopathy and azotemia. About one third of pts may be initially asymptomatic (Hosp Pract 2000;35:87).

Crs: Survival after SBP is only 30-50% at 1 yr.

Cmplc: Encephalopathy, renal failure, and death.

Diff Dx: SBP is considered in pts with ascites who develop sx of pain, infection, or clinical deterioration. The major differential point is that of peritonitis secondary to an intraabdominal process. Pts with secondary peritonitis often are infected with more than one organism and do not respond to antibiotics. They may have ascites with glucose <50 mg/dL, ascites LDH > serum LDH, or protein >1.0 gm/dL (GE 1990;98:127).

Lab: A diagnostic paracentesis should be done on admission to hospital or if during hospitalization pts develop abdominal pain, fever, leukocytosis, renal failure, or unexplained encephalopathy. SBP is diagnosed when PMN count is >250/mm³, though counts are usually greater than 500/mm³. If the tap is bloody, subtract 1 PMN for each 250 RBC present. Culture is obtained directly into blood culture bottles at the bedside. Culture will be negative in half of pts with suggestive sx and elevated PMN counts. Pts with PMN count >250/mm³ and negative cultures are labeled "neutrocytic ascites" and have a clinical course and prognosis indistinguishable from culture-positive SBP (Dig Dis Sci 1992;37: 1499). Those with counts <250/mm³ and positive ascites cultures have bacterascites (Dig Dis Sci 1995;40:561). Repeat tap is done to determine which pts had early SBP and which had transient seeding of ascites, perhaps from another source such as pneumonia or UTI.

Rx:

- *Acute infection:* Antibiotics are begun when paracentesis shows PMN counts >250/mm³. Cefotaxime 2 gm iv q 8 is the most studied choice. Aminoglycosides must be avoided. A variety of other agents including ceftriaxone, ceftazidime, amoxicillin-clavulanic acid, ciprofloxacin, norfloxacin, and ofloxacin are effective. If the pt develops SBP while on quinolone prophylaxis, cefotaxime should be used though quinolone resistance is uncommon (J Hepatol 1997;26:88). A follow-up tap may be done 2 days later, and a 25% decrease in PMN count is expected. If rx appears to be failing, antibiotics are changed and the possibility of secondary peritonitis is reconsidered. The addition of iv albumin (1.5 gm/kg on dx and 1 gm/kg on day 3) to cefotaxime improves renal function and survival (mortality 10% in albumin/antibiotic group and 29% in antibiotic alone group by RCT) (Nejm 1999;341:403). Albumin should be considered, especially in pts with impaired renal function, but is very expensive (U.S. $5-25/gm). Pts with SBP should be evaluated for transplant because of the poor prognosis.

- *Prophylaxis:* The International Ascites Club expert panel has developed the following guidelines (J Hepatol 2000;32:142). Antibiotic prophylaxis should be given to cirrhotics with UGI bleeding (meta-analysis [Hepatology 1999;29:1655]). Oral norfloxacin 400 mg q 12 for 7 days is an effective regimen (GE 1992;103:1267), but combinations of other agents (amoxicillin-clavulanic acid with quinolones) have been used. In pts who have had a previous episode SBP, norfloxacin 400 mg/day is suggested because of a 40-70% risk of recurrence (GE 1992;103:1267). If ascites protein is >1.0 gm/dL, antibiotic prophylaxis is only needed during acute bleeds. If protein is <1.0 gm/dL, risk of SBP is higher but it is not clear that pro- phylaxis is appropriate, and experts cannot reach consensus. A regimen of ciprofloxacin 750 mg po q week is low cost and reduces the risk of SBP from 22% to 4% over 6 months in pts with low-protein ascites (Hepatology 1995;22:1171).

15.4 Hepatic Encephalopathy

Nejm 1997;337:473; Am J Gastro 1997;92:1429; Aliment Pharmacol Ther 1996;10:681

Pathophys: The pathogenesis of hepatic encephalopathy (HE) is not well understood. Elevations in blood ammonia are important, and most effective therapies are directed at lowering levels. Ammonia worsens brain function by inhibiting neurotransmis- sion and synaptic regulation. Increased levels of serotonin (synthesized from high levels of tryptophan found in HE) and its metabolites may contribute to the sleep disturbance and depression seen in HE (The Neurologist 1995;1:95). It has been hypothesized that endogenous benzodiazepines, acting at GABA-benzodiazepine binding sites, contribute to HE. Alterations in the blood-brain barrier, zinc deficiency, manganese deposition, and disturbed ATPase function may play roles (Mayo Clin Proc 2000;75:501).

Precipitants: There are several common clinical events that may precipitate HE by a variety of mechanisms. Increased ammonia production may result from excessive dietary protein, digested blood in UGI bleeding, constipation, or infection. Ammonia may more easily cross the blood-brain barrier in hypokalemia, azotemia, and alkalosis. Decreased clearance of hepatic toxins may result from worsening liver function, HCC, TIPS, surgical shunting, or hypotension. Benzodiazepines or other psychoactive drugs may potentiate the abnormalities of HE. Fulminant hepatic failure (p 49) causes an encephalopathy associated with severe cerebral edema, and is not discussed here.

Sx: Early-stage HE (called subclinical HE) is subtle. It causes impairment of complex activities such as driving a car or balancing a checkbook. As disease worsens there may be increasing levels of confusion, disorientation, and personality change, progressing to somnolence, stupor, and finally coma.

Si: Early-stage HE may only be evident on psychometric tests (such as connecting dots). Pts initially may have a mild tremor that may progress to asterixis. Asterixis is a momentary loss of tone that results in a flapping motion. It is best demonstrated by having the pt extend the wrists while holding arms outstretched. Asterixis can be seen in the tongue. As disease progresses, reflexes become hyperactive, and rigidity may develop. When coma develops, asterixis may not be detectable.

Crs: Generally the course is that of the underlying liver disease. Some pts have acute encephalopathy due to a reversible precipitant, and others have chronic sx in the absence of precipitants.

Diff Dx: The differential is broad. Important considerations are subdural hematoma (especially in alcoholics with coagulopathy), intracranial trauma, meningitis, stroke, tumor, abscess, and Wernicke's encephalopathy. Metabolic abnormalities such as hypoglycemia, hypoxia, uremia, electrolyte abnormalities, and encephalopathy induced by drugs should be considered.

Lab: In the evaluation of other causes of mental status change and possible precipitants of HE, a CMP, CBC, oxygen saturation, toxicology screen, urinalysis, and a paracentesis are usually indicated. EEG abnormalities are well described but are not pathognomonic. EEG is not usually helpful or necessary. A lumbar puncture may be selectively indicated.

X-ray: MRI or CT of the brain may be needed to exclude structural diseases.

Rx: Any precipitants should be identified and treated. In the early stages of rx, dietary protein can be restricted if necessary (to as low as 20 gm/day, increasing as the pt improves). In the long term, protein intake must be increased to the needed 1.0-1.5 gm/kg/day (BMJ 1999;318:1364). **Lactulose** is the cornerstone of rx, though high-quality trials supporting its use are lacking (BMJ 2004;328:1046). It works by reducing ammonia levels (and potentially levels of other toxins), by its cathartic effect, and by lowering colonic pH. The reduction in colonic pH decreases urease production by bacteria and traps ammonia in the lumen by converting it into hydronium ion. Lactulose is given in divided doses totaling 30-100 gm (or 45-150 mL) daily. The dose is adjusted to produce 3-4 soft stools daily. If sx are severe, 30 gm are given every 2 hr until the pt stools vigorously. Lactulose enemas can be given if oral rx is not possible. Pts with subclinical encephalopathy benefit from lactulose, and there should be a low threshold to empirically treat any pts with any suggestive sx in the setting of cirrhosis (Hepatology 1997;26:1410). Lactitol is a more palatable alternative not available in the U.S.

Neomycin (4-6 gm daily in divided doses) can be used to kill urease-producing bacteria. It is effective as a single agent or it can be added to lactulose in refractory cases. Ototoxicity and nephrotoxicity can result from prolonged use of neomycin because some is absorbed systemically. **Metronidazole** (Gut 1982;23:1) and **rifaximin** (J Hepatol 2003;38:51) are antibiotic alternatives to neomycin. Metabolism of ammonia to urea is zinc dependent, and zinc repletion may be important in deficient pts. **Sodium benzoate** reduces ammonia production and is an inexpensive alternative (Hepatology 1992;16:138).

Aromatic amino acids may produce false neurotransmitters that worsen encephalopathy. A diet rich in **branched chain amino acids** may be useful in malnourished cirrhotics who do not tolerate oral protein (Hepatology 1984;4:279). The use of branched chain preparations in parenteral formulations is usually unnecessary (Hepatology 1994;19:518).

15.5 Hepatorenal Syndrome

Lancet 2003;362:1819

Pathophys: The dx of hepatorenal syndrome (HRS) requires: (1) chronic or acute liver disease with liver portal HTN; (2) Cr >1.5 or Cr clearance <40 cc/min; (3) no evidence of shock, bacterial infection, excessive fluid loss, or recent use of nephrotoxic drugs; (4) no sustained response to 1.5 L of saline as a challenge; (5) proteinuria <500 mg/day; and (6) no evidence of obstruction on ultrasound. Variable features include a urine volume <500 mL/day, urine Na <10 mEq/L, urine osmolality < plasma osmolality, serum Na <130, and no hematuria (Liver

Transpl 2000;6:287). When renal failure progresses rapidly (50% worsening in under 2 weeks), the disorder is called type 1 HRS. In type 2 HRS there is steady deterioration over weeks to months.

HRS is functional in that kidneys from pts who die of HRS can be successfully transplanted with normalization of renal function. The imbalance of vasoconstrictors and vasodilators as a result of the cirrhosis seems crucial. It has been hypothesized that some other direct message is sent from liver to kidney resulting in the intense vasoconstriction, but the nature of that message has not been determined. Precipitating events are volume depletion, paracentesis, overdiuresis, bleeding, infection, x-ray dye, NSAID use, and worsening liver function.

Sx: Those with type 1 HRS usually have Child-Pugh grade C cirrhosis (p 51) and have the clinical findings of advanced liver disease with jaundice. Those with type 2 HRS are likely to have less severe liver disease and usually have diuretic resistant ascites.

Si: Those of end-stage liver disease (p 42).

Crs: Most pts with type 1 HRS die within 2 weeks. Those with type 2 survive a few months.

Diff Dx: HRS is a dx of exclusion made when renal failure occurs in the setting of advanced liver disease. Almost all pts have ascites. Other causes of renal failure need to be excluded, including volume depletion, nephrotoxic drugs, intrinsic renal disease, sepsis, and obstruction.

Lab: See definition of HRS in Pathophys.

X-ray: Ultrasound is indicated to rule out obstruction.

Rx: Inadequate central volume is excluded by monitoring central volume, often with a Swan-Ganz catheter. Diuretics are stopped, nephrotoxic agents are held, and infection is treated. If the pt gets better with these measures, he or she does not have HRS. A variety of medical therapies have been tried without success. Preliminary evidence supports the combination of terlipressin (an ADH analogue that is a splanchnic vasoconstrictor) and albumin (Hepatology 2002;36:941). Terlipressin is not available in the U.S. N-acetylcysteine has been of benefit in a small, uncontrolled trial (Lancet 1999;353:294). The use of midodrine (a vasoconstrictor) with octreotide (which inhibits endogenous vasodilator release) was effective in a small number of pts with type 1 HRS (Hepatology 1999;29:1690). Noradrenaline and albumin were effective in a pilot study (Hepatology 2002; 36:374). TIPS has been effective in improving renal function in a small number of pts (Hepatology 1998;28:416). Dialysis and peritoneovenous shunting do not improve outcome, unless as a bridge to transplant. Liver transplant is effective, but survival is diminished compared to transplantation in pts without HRS (Transplantation 1995;59:361).

15.6 Hepatopulmonary Syndrome

Lancet 2004;363:1461; Ann IM 1995;122:521

This syndrome is the combination of pulmonary vascular abnormalities with hypoxemia in the setting of advanced liver disease. Pts have intrapulmonary vascular dilatations and direct arteriovenous shunts. Hypoxia often worsens in the upright position. Diagnosis is confirmed by echocardiography and lung scanning. Liver transplant is especially beneficial in pts whose hypoxemia responds to 100% oxygen (and presumably have fewer shunts) (Mayo Clin Proc 1997; 72:44).

15.7 Portopulmonary Hypertension

Lancet 2004;363:1461; Clin Chest Med 1996;17:17

A small number of pts with advanced liver disease develop pulmonary hypertension due to a vasoconstrictive/obliterative process of pulmonary vessels. Pts present with dyspnea and near syncope. The dx is confirmed by right heart catheterization. Prostacyclin (a pulmonary vasodilator) improves hemodynamics and may be a bridge to liver transplant (Hepatology 1999; 30:641). Transplant mortality is high if pulmonary hypertension is moderate to severe.

Chapter 16

Vascular Liver Disease

16.1 Budd-Chiari Syndrome

Nejm 2004;350:578; J Clin Gastro 2000;30:155; Brit J Surg
1995;82:1023

Cause: Budd-Chiari syndrome is caused by obstruction of the normal
hepatic venous outflow. This can occur at the level of the hepatic
veins or in the vena cava. Many diseases can result in venous
obstruction. **Mechanical** causes include congenital membranous
obstruction of the IVC (common in Asia) or posttraumatic, postsurgical, or invading malignancy such as HCC. **Hypercoagulable**
causes include paroxysmal nocturnal hemoglobinuria; poly-
cythemia vera; other myeloproliferative disorders; deficiencies of
protein C, S, or antithrombin III; estrogens; or other hypercoagulable states. About 30% of cases are idiopathic.

Epidem: In a large U.S. series, 83% of pts were women, and the mean
age was 37 yr (range 14-68) (Ann Surg 1990;212:144).

Pathophys: There are 3 hepatic veins that drain the liver. The course
of the Budd-Chiari syndrome is determined by the degree of
obstruction of these veins and the acuity of onset. When obstruction occurs there can be increase in the direct flow from the caudate lobe to the IVC. This results in caudate hypertrophy that
may be seen on imaging studies. Venous obstruction causes
hypoxia and increased sinusoidal pressure, with resultant
hepatomegaly and varying degrees of liver failure. When onset is

sudden and massive, fulminant hepatic failure may occur (p 49). When the obstruction is gradual or limited, portal hypertension (ascites and varices) is a greater problem than hepatocellular failure.

Sx: The sx can vary widely, as indicated. There may be evidence of RUQ pain from Glisson's capsule distention, distention from ascites, and a complaint of generalized weakness (Lancet 1993;342:718).

Si: Ascites is almost universal. Tender hepatomegaly is common with acute presentations. Prominent veins may be seen over the abdominal wall or back. Those with acute presentations may also have evidence of hepatic encephalopathy or hepatorenal syndrome. Those with chronic presentations predominantly have findings of portal HTN and cirrhosis. Leg edema is common with IVC obstruction.

Crs: Mortality is almost universal if the disease is not treated. The course varies widely depending on the extent and acuity of obstruction and the underlying predisposing condition. If hepatic venous drainage can be restored, the majority of pts survive long-term (Gut 1999;44:568).

Cmplc: Liver failure, variceal hemorrhage, encephalopathy.

Diff Dx: The disease needs to be considered in any pt presenting with ascites and a tender liver. Some pts present with evidence of portal hypertension or cirrhosis. The usual pitfall in dx is to fail to consider this unusual disease. Once this disease is considered, the dx can usually be made by imaging studies. The broad diff dx is that of jaundice or cirrhosis (p 48).

Lab: Liver bx, which is characteristic, shows centrilobular congestion and necrosis with dilated sinusoids. LFTs vary widely depending on the severity of illness. Transaminases are typically 8 × normal and alk phos 3 × normal. Hypoalbuminemia and elevated PT are common.

X-ray: Doppler ultrasound of the hepatic veins is the initial study. Positive exams are confirmed by angiography. CT or MRI may show evidence of clot. Hypertrophy of the caudate lobe may be seen on any imaging study.

Rx: Pts whose obstruction is due to malignancy should receive palliative care. Thrombolysis can be used in acute thrombosis. Those with a reversible degree of liver failure and focal obstruction (eg, IVC web, short lengths of hepatic vein occlusion) can be treated with angioplasty (Lancet 1993;342:718) with or without stent placement. Anticoagulation is used after angioplasty (Gut 1999;44:568). If the clot is too extensive but liver dysfunction is not too severe, a surgical shunt is used. Shunts can work well even if cirrhosis is present (Am J Surg 1996;171:176). With severe liver dysfunction, liver transplantation is the best option, with a TIPS as a temporizing measure (Am J Gastro 1999; 94:603). An underlying hematologic disorder should be sought and treated if found.

16.2 Venoocclusive Disease

Venoocclusive disease (VOD) is a nonthrombotic obliteration of the intrahepatic veins by loose connective tissue (Am J Med 1986; 81:297). It causes jaundice, RUQ pain, ascites, weight gain, and hepatomegaly. It is almost exclusively seen in stem cell transplant pts. No single rx is highly effective, and morbidity and mortality are substantial (Br J Haematol 1999;107:485; Mayo Clin Proc 2003;78:589).

16.3 Ischemic Hepatitis (Shock Liver)

Am J Med 2000;109:109; J Clin Gastro 1996;22:126

Epidem: The epidemiology is that of the underlying cardiac disease that predisposes to the illness.

Pathophys: The precise mechanism of hepatic injury in ischemic hepatitis is unknown. Hypotension is the typical inciting insult. However, hypotension alone does not explain the syndrome. Trauma pts are hypotensive but rarely develop ischemic hepatitis. The major difference between pts with trauma and ischemic hepatitis is that the latter group almost always have heart failure (Am J Med 2000;109:109). CHF causes passive congestion of the liver with resultant necrosis, and in severe cases can cause cardiac cirrhosis (Sherlock S and Dooley J. Diseases of the liver and biliary system. 10th ed. Boston: Blackwell Science, 1997:196-199). A sudden ischemic insult presumably causes abrupt hepatocellular damage in a pt predisposed to injury by underlying passive congestion from CHF.

Sx/Si: Usually pts are critically ill, and they may have many sx and signs associated with CHF.

Crs: The course is determined by the underlying illness.

Cmplc: There are no convincing data to suggest liver sequelae.

Diff Dx: The major differential points are viral hepatitis and toxic hepatitis from drugs. However, those illnesses are usually not associated with such a sudden and massive rise and rapid fall of transaminases.

Lab: Pts with underlying CHF commonly have elevated bilirubin (>2 mg/dL in one-third of pts, and at times much higher) with normal alkaline phosphatase and mild transaminase abnormalities. With an acute bout of ischemic hepatitis, the laboratory picture is so distinctive that the dx is easy to make. Following a clinical insult, typically hypotension in a CHF pt, there is a rapid rise of transaminases to >20-200 × normal (Am J Gastro 1992; 87:831). The values then fall steadily over the next week to normal or near normal. The PT/INR is often elevated (J Clin Gastroenterol 1998;26:183). Hypoglycemia occurred in one-third of pts in one adult series (J Clin Gastro 1998;26:183). Bx is not needed, but if done (at autopsy), shows midzonal (GE 1984; 86:627) or centrilobular necrosis (Dig Dis Sci 1979;24:129).

Rx: The rx is that of the underlying hypotension and cardiac illness.

16.4 Portal Vein Thrombosis

Am J Gastro 2002;97:535; Am J Med 1992;92:173

Portal vein thrombosis is a rare cause of portal HTN. It occurs in young children (usually due to intraabdominal infection) and in middle-aged adults. Causes include cirrhosis, neoplasia (pancreatic cancer and HCC), infection, pancreatitis, myeloproliferative disorders, and hypercoagulable states. Many other uncommon causes have been described. The dx is made by Doppler ultrasound of the portal vein. If that is a limited quality study, MR angiography is done. In acute cases there may be a role for thrombolysis or anticoagulation. In chronic cases, rx is usually directed at associated variceal hemorrhage.

Chapter 17

Liver Disease in Pregnancy

Am J Gastro 2004;99:2479; Nejm 1996;335:569

Liver disease in pregnancy may represent a disease present at conception, a disease acquired unique to pregnancy, or a disease acquired coincident with but not unique to pregnancy. Pregnancy results in several changes in LFTs that might be interpreted as pathologic. Albumin falls 10-60% in the second trimester, and alk phos rises to 2-4 × normal in the third trimester. Transaminases remain normal. There are several hepatic disorders unique to pregnancy, including:

Hyperemesis gravidarum, intractable vomiting seen in the first trimester, can be associated with mild transaminase abnormalities (usually <2 × normal).

Intrahepatic cholestasis of pregnancy presents as pruritus, generally in the third trimester of pregnancy. Jaundice follows pruritus in 20-60% of women. Bilirubin is usually <6 mg/dL, alk phos is 4 × normal, and transaminases are 2-10 × normal. Serum bile acids are markedly elevated. There is an increased risk of premature delivery or stillbirth. Vitamin K is given prophylactically to prevent deficiency due to malabsorption. Cholestyramine or ursodeoxycholic acid can be used to treat the pruritus (Hepatology 1992;15:1043).

Preeclampsia/eclampsia is a disorder in which the liver is one of several target organs. Abnormal transaminases are frequent in moderate to severe disease but are usually less than 500 U/L. **Hepatic rupture** is a rare, catastrophic event typically associated with preeclampsia/eclampsia.

HELLP syndrome and acute fatty liver of pregnancy are discussed in the following sections.

17.1 HELLP Syndrome

Obstet Gynecol 2004;103:981; J Perinatol 1999;19:138; Am Fam Phys 1999;60:829

Cause: Unknown.

Epidem: HELLP is a catchy acronym for hemolysis, elevated liver enzymes and low platelets. Pts with HELLP are a subset of the pts with hypertensive disorders of pregnancy who are at risk for a more severe course. HELLP has an incidence of about 2-6/1000 pregnancies and is seen in about 4-12% of pts with preeclampsia or eclampsia (Am Fam Phys 1999;60:829). The onset is usually in the third trimester.

Pathophys: (Jama 1998;280:559) The pathophysiology of this disorder, like that of preeclampsia, is not understood. Endothelial injury from a placental toxin and an enhanced thrombotic tendency may be important. Platelets become activated, resulting in vasospasm, platelet aggregation, and further damage. In the liver, damage to endothelium results in fibrin deposition in hepatic sinusoids with hemorrhage and hepatocyte necrosis. The disorder usually occurs with preeclampsia but may occur on its own.

Sx: RUQ pain is an important clue. Malaise, nausea, vomiting, and headache are typical. Seizures may occur.

Si: Hypertension (>30/15 over baseline or >140/90) is present in 85%. RUQ tenderness and edema are common. Hyperreflexia may be detected.

Crs: Maternal mortality is 1-4% from a variety of causes, including hepatic rupture, pulmonary embolus, and hypoxic encephalopathy. Perinatal mortality is 5-20% and is largely dependent on gestational age and birth weight.

Cmplc: Hepatic rupture is a dreaded complication that occurs in 1% of pts. Ascites, pleural effusions, pulmonary edema, or multisystem organ failure may occur.

Diff Dx: The findings may suggest viral illness, musculoskeletal pain, cholecystitis, hepatitis, PUD, pyelonephritis, nephrolithiasis, ITP, other microangiopathic anemias, and acute fatty liver of pregnancy (Jama 1998;280:559).

Lab: Hemolysis is proven by a low haptoglobin and sometimes occurs with evidence of a microangiopathic process (schistocytes, burr cells). ALT and AST are elevated and platelets are <100,000/mL. Proteinuria is typical.

Rx: Most authors (but not all [Br J Obstet Gynaecol 1995;102:111]) recommend delivery as soon as there is a reasonable chance of fetal survival. Bed rest, magnesium sulfate to prevent seizures, and blood pressure control are adjunctive therapies. Steroids are given for fetal lung maturity and may also have a beneficial effect on platelets and LFTs (Am J Obstet Gynecol 1999;181:304).

17.2 Acute Fatty Liver of Pregnancy

Semin Perinatol 1998;22:134; Nejm 1996;335:569

Cause: Unknown.

Epidem: This is a rare disorder occurring in 1/13,000 deliveries. It is more common in a first pregnancy or when the mother is carrying multiple fetuses.

Pathophys: The pathogenesis is unknown. The hallmark of the disorder is microvesicular fatty infiltration of hepatocytes. The disorder may represent an abnormality of mitochondrial function.

Sx/Si: Pts present in the third trimester. The most common initial sx are nausea and vomiting (76%), abdominal pain (43%), anorexia (21%), and jaundice (16%). Pruritus is uncommon. Late findings can include asterixis or coma, and deterioration can occur rapidly. Half of pts have preeclampsia. The liver is usually normal or small.

Diff Dx: Considerations include HELLP, viral or drug hepatitis, and biliary tract disease. In HELLP the bilirubin is usually <5 mg/dL, and hypoglycemia is rare. In practice it is not essential to distinguish the HELLP syndrome from acute fatty liver of pregnancy by liver bx since the rx is the same for both.

Crs: Maternal mortality is less than 10% with disease recognition and rx (Semin Perinatol 1998;22:134). Fetal mortality is <20% (Nejm 1996;335:569). Recurrence is uncommon with a subsequent pregnancy, but it does occur. The illness resolves rapidly with delivery.

Lab: ALT is elevated but is typically <1000 U/L. Bilirubin is usually elevated, except in mild cases. Hypoglycemia and elevated PT are common in severe disease. Thrombocytopenia is common but DIC is seen only in more severe cases.

X-ray: US may show fat and excludes biliary obstruction as the cause of jaundice.

Rx: Rx is prompt delivery and supportive care for hypoglycemia, coagulopathy, and encephalopathy. Liver transplant has been used in rare instances (Hepatology 1990;11:59).

Chapter 18

Procedures

Comment: It is important that a clinician be able to describe to the pt the experience and the more common complications of endoscopy prior to referral for the procedure. This is especially common in open-access systems where the endoscopist may not meet the pt until minutes before the procedure. The list of complications listed here is not comprehensive but is a reasonable list to use in discussions with pts.

18.1 Upper Endoscopy (EGD)

Description: The pt is kept npo, brought to the unit, and an iv is placed. The pt lies left lateral decubitus and is sedated. A mouthpiece is placed to protect the teeth. The endoscope is passed and the upper tract examined. Gagging and belching may occur but are usually minor. Breathing is not significantly affected by the instrument. It is not generally painful and takes 10-15 minutes after sedation. Amnesia is common but not universal. If abnormalities are seen, biopsies (which are painless) may be taken and strictures may be dilated (see p 72). Pts cannot drive or work for 24 hr after the exam because of the sedation.

Complications: (Gastrointest Endosc Clin N Am 1996;6:287) Perforation (<1/5000 if no dilatation, <1/500 if esophageal dilatation is needed), bleeding, infection, adverse reaction to sedation, failure to detect important abnormalities. Minor problems include sore throat (not commonly) and iv site phlebitis.

18.2 Colonoscopy

Description: The pt undergoes a bowel prep, generally with polyethylene glycol solution or sodium phosphate. The pt is kept npo, brought to the unit, and an iv is placed. The pt lies left lateral decubitus and is sedated. The colonoscope is advanced to the cecum in >19/20 cases. Cramps are common during the advance, but the sedation makes it very tolerable for most pts. Sometimes the pt changes positions or the assistant palpates the abdomen to aid the advance of the scope. Polyps are removed and biopsies are taken, both of which are generally painless. The exam lasts 15-40 minutes depending on the quality of the prep, the ease of the exam, and the need for rx. The pt may feel gassy, bloated, or crampy because of insufflated air for up to several hr after the procedure. Pts cannot drive or work for 24 hr after the exam because of the sedation.

Complications: (Gastrointest Endosc Clin N Am 1996;6:343) Risks include perforation (<1/1000 if no polypectomy; higher with polypectomy) that may require urgent surgery, possibly with a temporary colostomy. Bleeding is uncommon and occurs in 0.07% of diagnostic studies and in 1.2% of procedures with polypectomy. Bleeding is more common after the removal of large polyps. Bleeding might require transfusion, a second procedure (for endoscopic control of bleeding), or surgery. Infection, adverse reaction to sedation, and failure to detect important abnormalities may occur. Minor problems include iv site phlebitis and perianal irritation from the prep and scope.

18.3 Sigmoidoscopy

Description: Same as colonoscopy, though the exam generally is done without sedation and usually takes less than 10 minutes.

Complications: (Gastrointest Endosc Clin N Am 1996;6:343) Same as with colonoscopy, though the perforation rate is much lower (1-2/10,000).

18.4 Endoscopic Retrograde Cholangiopancreatography

Description: The pt experience for endoscopic retrograde cholangiopancreatography (ERCP) is the same as for EGD, but the position on the table is semiprone. The exam takes 10-60 minutes depending on complexity. Stones may be removed or stents placed, depending on the findings. The exam is generally done in situations where therapy is likely to be needed.

Complications: (Gastrointest Endosc Clin N Am 1996;6:379) Pancreatitis is the most frequent complication of ERCP and occurs in 3-7% of pts. It can be severe but is usually not. Perforation or bleeding may occur in 1-2% after sphincterotomy. These are usually managed without surgery. Cholangitis may occur if the biliary tree is obstructed, and antibiotics are usually given prophylactically. The other complications are those of EGD.

18.5 Percutaneous Endoscopic Gastrostomy

Description: A diagnostic EGD is done, and the pt is placed supine with the scope in the stomach. An area about two thirds the distance from umbilicus to left costal margin is prepped, draped, and injected with lidocaine. A catheter with a stylet is passed into the stomach, and through the catheter a long suture is passed and brought out through the mouth when the endoscope is withdrawn. The feeding tube is attached to the suture (several techniques exist) and the tube is pulled into place in the stomach.

Mild discomfort at the site is common for 2-3 days. When the tube is no longer needed, it is usually pulled out by traction through the abdomen and the hole rapidly seals over. Oral intake is possible with the tube in place.

Complications: (Gastrointest Endosc Clin N Am 1996;6:409) Because most pts undergoing PEG are ill, complications are frequent. Major complications occur in 2.7% of pts and include aspiration, peritonitis, perforation, gastrocolic fistula, necrotizing fasciitis, tumor implant at stoma, tube migration, or accidental removal. Minor complications include wound infection and leakage and occur in 6-7% of pts. Procedure-related death occurs in 0.7% of pts.

18.6 Liver Biopsy

Description: The pt lies supine, and an area in the midaxillary line overlying the liver is identified for bx, usually using ultrasound. The area is prepped and draped, and lidocaine is injected. The pt is asked to inhale, exhale, and stop breathing, at which time the bx is obtained. The bx is an odd sensation that many people liken to being punched, but the immediate pain is usually minimal. Over the minutes following the bx, pain often increases and is sometimes felt in the shoulder. Pain is managed in some pts with analgesics. In only a tiny percentage of pts is the pain severe. The pt is observed for 2-6 hr and discharged. About 3% of pts having bx require admission.

Complications: (Ann IM 1993;118:96) Complications occur in up to 3% of patients and include severe pain, bleeding, bile peritonitis, hemothorax (rare), and perforation of a viscus (rare). Most complications resolve without intervention. Transfusion can be required. Death occurs in 0.01% of pts.

18.7 Liver Transplantation

Postgrad Med 2004;115:73; Dis Mo 1999;45:150; Int Surg 1999;84:297

Description: Liver transplantation is the most useful rx for end-stage liver disease. Practice guidelines have been developed (Liver Transpl 2000;6:122). The most common indications are end-stage chronic viral hepatitis, alcoholic liver disease, cryptogenic cirrhosis, PBC, PSC, and fulminant hepatic failure. Pts should be evaluated for transplant when their survival without a transplant becomes less than it would be with a transplant. This includes pts with Child-Pugh grade B or C cirrhosis (p 51), diuretic resistant ascites, HRS, SBP, severe encephalopathy, and variceal hemorrhage. Quality of life, rather than life expectancy, may be the issue for pts with pruritus, recurrent bouts of cholangitis, or sx of the portopulmonary syndrome. The major contraindications are HIV positivity, active alcohol or illicit drug use, extrahepatic malignancy, cholangiocarcinoma, systemic infection, lack of portal venous inflow, and advanced cardiopulmonary disease. Pts need adequate social and family supports to deal effectively with the complexities of posttransplant rx. Pts undergo a comprehensive evaluation of cardiopulmonary status, renal function, portal vein patency, psychosocial, psychiatric, and financial circumstances.

   The major limitation is the scarcity of organs. In the U.S., the United Network for Organ Sharing (UNOS), has developed a system for organ allocation based on disease severity. Since 2002, allocation is based on the Model for End-Stage Liver Disease (**MELD**) score (Hepatology 2001;33:464). This score is based on objective criteria including bilirubin, creatinine and INR; time on the transplant list is no longer a factor. Because of the scarcity of organs, the wait is long and varies by geographic location. Split liver transplantation allows living donor transplantation and doubles the organs available for cadaveric transplantation. Its role is evolving (Ann Surg 1999;229:313).

The liver is harvested from the donor and can last up to 12 hr in preservative solution. Through a large bilateral subcostal incision with xiphoid extension, the native liver is removed after the pt is put on venous bypass. The anastomoses are made beginning with the vena cava followed by the portal vein to allow reperfusion. The bile duct is done with an end-to-end anastomosis, except in PSC when a Roux-en-Y choledochojejunostomy is done.

Complications: Within the first 3 days, hemorrhage, graft nonfunction, and hepatic artery thrombosis may occur. Acute cellular rejection, neurologic complications, and biliary complications occur in the first few weeks. Late complications include opportunistic infections and ductopenic rejection. Lymphoproliferative disorders are the major malignancy seen in transplant pts. Many diseases can recur in transplant pts, especially hepatitis B and hepatitis C.

Long-Term Rx: Immunosuppression is usually achieved with cyclosporine or tacrolimus along with azathioprine and prednisone. This multidrug rx results in a number of problems, including HTN, azotemia, obesity, diabetes, infection, and bone disease. The complications of immunosuppression will be addressed with new regimens (Q J Med 1999;92:547).

18.8 Enteral Nutrition

Dis Mo 1997;43:349; GE 1995;108:1280

Description: Enteral nutrition via feeding tubes is widely used in hospitalized pts. Tube feeding is considered for all pts who go 1-2 weeks without nutrition, who cannot take adequate oral calories, and in whom a feeding tube can be placed. Nasoenteric tubes are used for short-term feeding. If a tube can be placed

beyond the third portion of the duodenum, there is a reduced risk
of aspiration, so this should be attempted. Most pts can be fed
with bolus infusions, but continuous infusions are used for jejunal
feeding or in pts with reflux. PEGs are indicated when prolonged
tube feeding is expected. Isotonic polymeric formulations are
almost always sufficient to meet nutritional needs. Additional
free water is usually required. Elemental formulas are reserved for
pts with short bowel syndrome.

Complications: Aspiration can occur after gastric feeding. The risk
can be minimized by elevation of the head of the bed with
feeding, continuous rather than bolus feeding for those at risk,
checking for gastric residuals, and monitoring symptoms.
Diarrhea is common and may have many causes that should be
evaluated and treated. Many uncommon nasoenteric tube complications may occur and care must be taken to avoid feeding the
lungs!

18.9 Parenteral Nutrition

Dis Mo 1997;43:349

Description: Parenteral nutrition (PN) can be lifesaving in severely
malnourished pts who cannot be fed enterally. Its efficacy has
been established in a limited number of conditions. However,
there is no clear benefit of PN in many of the conditions in
which it is used (Jama 1998;280:2013). It should only be used
where the enteral route is not available. Specific indications are
beyond the scope of this summary. PN can be given through a
peripheral vein in large volume solutions or through a central
vein in more concentrated solutions. The formulation of PN is
based on an assessment of nutritional status and the underlying
disease. Elements of the PN formula include (1) protein given as
amino acids (0.8-1.5 gm/kg per day depending on clinical state);
(2) glucose to provide about 50-60% of calorie requirements;

(3) lipid emulsion to provide 25-30% of calorie requirements; (4) electrolytes (including Na, K, phosphate, Cl, and acetate if a source of bicarbonate is needed); (5) vitamins; and (6) trace elements (zinc, copper, chromium, and manganese). H2RAs and heparin may be added. Some other trace elements (iodine, selenium, molybdenum) may be needed in prolonged PN. Vitamin K is not included in multivitamin preparations and is given separately.

Complications: Numerous complications occur from the central venous catheter. These include pneumothorax, air embolus, hemothorax, catheter sepsis, and venous thrombosis. Metabolic abnormalities that result from parenteral feeding include hyperglycemia and electrolyte abnormalities. Elevated transaminases are common at the beginning of rx and usually resolve. Cholestasis, steatosis, and steatohepatitis may develop (GE 1993;104:286), and hepatic failure has been seen with long-term feeding. Refeeding syndrome may occur in severely malnourished pts.

Chapter 19

Pearls in Gastroenterology

- Today's pearls are tomorrow's fecaliths.
- The National Institute of Diabetes and Digestive and Kidney Diseases (NIDDK) is a valuable resource for pt education materials. Information is distributed through the National Digestive Diseases Information Clearinghouse (NDDIC). Publications are available online, and copies suitable for distribution to pts can be ordered at their Web site: http://catalog.niddk.nih.gov/materials.cfm?CH=NDDIC.
- GERD is a frequently mismanaged illness. Physicians often underestimate the impact GERD has on quality of life and dismiss it as a minor problem not worthy of aggressive therapy (p 53).
- H. pylori is not an important contributor to the pathophysiology of GERD. There is a strong inverse relationship between H. pylori infection and severe forms of GERD, such as Barrett's esophagus (p 55).
- PPIs must be given 30 min to 1 hr prior to breakfast for optimal effect, because they require meal-stimulated parietal cell pH drop for effective binding. H2RAs should not be given prior to PPI doses because they block PPI binding (see p 61).
- Many pts with dysphagia and recurrent episodes of food impaction will not volunteer this important hx unless asked. Since most dysphagia is readily treatable, this sx must not be overlooked (p 9).

- Pts with reflux-related strictures should be maintained on PPIs (not H2RAs) to reduce the risk of recurrence (see p 74).
- Though surveillance for Barrett's esophagus is widely performed in the United States, its benefits are far from proven, its costs are high, the yield is modest, and the optimum surveillance strategy has not yet been determined (p 67).
- Gastritis is best considered a histologic term. There are no consistent sx or endoscopic findings that correlate with the microscopic appearance of gastritis (see p 105).
- There is little point to obtaining an upper gi series in the evaluation of dyspepsia. The sensitivity of UGI series for ulcers and esophagitis is limited. If the UGI series shows a gastric ulcer, EGD is done to rule out malignancy, and if the UGI is negative EGD is still needed for diagnosis (p 4).
- In pts with refractory peptic ulcers, ongoing NSAID use must be excluded by random salicylate levels, NSAID levels, and questioning of relatives. Pts who continue to use NSAIDs in the face of ulcer disease have a high incidence of stenosis and multiple operations (p 119).
- Consider the possibility of past or present physical or sexual abuse in pts with complaints that sound functional and do not respond readily to routine measures and in pts who have seen multiple providers for the same complaint (p 162).
- Colorectal cancer is the second leading cause of cancer death in the United States, with a lifetime incidence of 6% (p 219).
- Most cases of colon cancer associated with the hereditary nonpolyposis colon cancer syndrome (HNPCC) go unrecognized because clinicians are unaware of its existence (p 242).
- Diverticular bleeding is arterial. Thus, it tends to be fairly large volume and abrupt in onset (p 165).
- Fecal incontinence is frequent, but pts are reluctant to discuss it. They will often complain of excessive flatus, diarrhea, and urgency rather than recognize incontinence as the cause of sx (p 294).

- Acute mesenteric ischemia (p 303), chronic mesenteric ischemia (p 305), and ischemic colitis (p 306) are 3 distinct syndromes with differing symptoms and signs. They are frequently misdiagnosed.
- All too often, pts suffer with undiagnosed fecal impactions or are not aggressively and promptly treated after the diagnosis is made (p 297).
- Contrary to traditional teaching, there is no evidence that fatty food intolerance, belching, or bloating are sx of gallbladder disease (p 335).
- HIDA scan with ejection fraction is widely used to select pts for cholecystectomy with suspected acalculous gallbladder disease, but there is no high-quality evidence to support the value of this approach (p 6).
- The painful rib syndrome is a commonly overlooked cause of RUQ pain, for which there is a characteristic history and exam (p 356).
- Genetic hemochromatosis pts will be found in almost all primary care practices, but the onset of sx is typically 10 yr prior to the time of diagnosis (p 399).
- The incidence of hepatocellular carcinoma is rising in the West and will continue to do so because of hepatitis C (p 413).
- Pts with cirrhosis should undergo endoscopy to look for varices, because prophylactic medical therapy reduces the bleeding rate (p 429).
- Ischemic hepatitis (shock liver) has a spiking pattern of transaminases that is diagnostic in the appropriate clinical setting (p 453).
- An elevated PT in a patient with evidence of UGI bleeding may be a clue to varices as the cause (p 429).
- A comprehensive list of gi Web site, including links to clinical guidelines and pt information, can be found at http://www.medmark.org/gastro/.

- The best names for authors of gi literature include: **Butt** (Medicine 1987;66:472), **Terdimann** (Am J Gastro 1999;94:2344), and **Neugut** (Am J Gastro 1993;88:1179).

Index

elevated, approach to, 50
Proton pump inhibitors
    in GERD, 61
    in ulcer disease, 118
Pruritus ani, 296
Pseudocyst
    pancreatic, 321
Pseudodiverticulosis
    esophageal, 104
Pseudo-obstruction
    acute colonic, 210
    chronic, 212
Pyogenic liver abscess, 380

R

Radiation enteritis, 213
Radiation proctitis, 213
Ranitidine bismuth citrate
    in H. pylori, 113
Red blood cell scan, 36
Red wales, 430
Reflux
    gastroesophageal, 53
Regional enteritis. See Crohn's disease
Reiter's syndrome, 269
Ribavirin, 373
Ring
    esophageal, 72
Ringed esophagus, 75
Rotor syndrome, 49
Rowasa, 195
Rumination syndrome, 97

S

Salmonella, 266
Schatzki's rings, 10
Schistosomiasis

hepatic, 379
Scleroderma, 54
Sclerosing cholangitis, 391
Screening
    for colorectal cancer, 231
    for FAP, 249
    for hemachromatosis, 403
Serum-ascites albumin gradient, 437
Sexual abuse, 162
Shigella, 268
Shock liver, 453
Short bowel syndrome, 204
Short segment Barrett's esophagus,
    68
Sigmoidoscopy, 462
Sister Mary Joseph's node, 138
Sitzmarks, 20
Sliding hiatal hernia, 132
Sludge, 321
Smooth muscle relaxants, 160
Sodium benzoate, 446
Solitary rectal ulcer syndrome, 298
Somatostatinoma, 333
Sorbitol, 16, 26
Spastic disorders of esophagus, 93
Sphinter of oddi dysfunction, 352
Splanchnicectomy, 330
Spontaneous bacterial peritonitis, 441
Sprue
    celiac, 200
Steatorrhea, 32
Stercoral ulcer, 297
Stool
    72 hour collection, 29
    electrolytes and osmoles, 29
    lactoferrin, 24
    laxative screen, 30
    wbc, 24
Stress ulcer, 124
Stricture